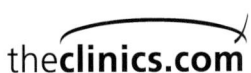

A. Simon Turner, BVSc, MS
CONSULTING EDITOR

VETERINARY CLINICS OF NORTH AMERICA

Equine Practice

Advances in Reproduction

GUEST EDITOR
Elaine M. Carnevale, DVM, PhD

December 2006 • Volume 22 • Number 3

SAUNDERS

An Imprint of Elsevier, Inc.
PHILADELPHIA   LONDON   TORONTO   MONTREAL   SYDNEY   TOKYO

W.B. SAUNDERS COMPANY
A Division of Elsevier Inc.

Elsevier, Inc., 1600 John F. Kennedy Blvd., Suite 1800, Philadelphia, PA 19103-2899

http://www.vetequine.theclinics.com

VETERINARY CLINICS OF NORTH AMERICA: Volume 22, Number 3
EQUINE PRACTICE   ISSN 0749-0739
December 2006   ISBN 1-4160-3823-X
Editor: John Vassallo; j.vassallo@elsevier.com

Copyright © 2006 by Elsevier Inc. All rights reserved. No part of this publication may be reproduced or transmitted in any form or by any means, electronic or mechanical, including photocopy, recording, or any information retrieval system, without written permission from the Publisher.

Single photocopies of single articles may be made for personal use as allowed by national copyright laws. Permission of the publisher and payment of a fee is required for all other photocopying, including multiple or systematic copying, copying for advertising or promotional purposes, resale, and all forms of document delivery. Special rates are available for educational institutions that wish to make photocopies for non-profit educational classroom use. Permissions may be sought directly from Elsevier's Rights Department in Philadelphia, PA, USA: phone: (+1) 215 239 3804, fax: (+1) 215 239 3805, e-mail: healthpermissions @elsevier.com. Requests may also be completed on-line via the Elsevier homepage (http://www.elsevier. com/locate/permissions). In the USA, users may clear permissions and make payments through the Copyright Clearance Center, Inc., 222 Rosewood Drive, Danvers, MA 01923, USA; phone: (978) 750-8400, fax: (978) 750-4744, and in the UK through the Copyright Licensing Agency Rapid Clearance Service (CLARCS), 90 Tottenham Court Road, London WIP 0LP, UK; phone: (+44) 171 436 5931; fax: (+44) 171 436 3986. Other countries may have a local reprographic rights agency for payments.

The ideas and opinions expressed in *Veterinary Clinics of North America: Equine Practice* do not necessarily reflect those of the Publisher. The Publisher does not assume any responsibility for any injury and/or damage to persons or property arising out of or related to any use of the material contained in this periodical. The reader is advised to check the appropriate medical literature and the product information currently provided by the manufacturer of each drug to be administered to verify the dosage, the method and duration of administration, or contraindications. It is the responsibility of the treating physician or other health care professional, relying on independent experience and knowledge of the patient, to determine drug dosages and the best treatment for the patient. Mention of any product in this issue should not be construed as endorsement by the contributors, editors, or the Publisher of the product or manufacturers' claims.

Veterinary Clinics of North America: Equine Practice (ISSN 0749-0739) is published in April, August, and December by Elsevier Inc., 360 Park Avenue South, New York, NY 10010-1710. Business and Editorial Offices: 1600 John F. Kennedy Blvd., Suite 1800, Philadelphia, PA 19103-2899. Customer Service office: 6277 Sea Harbor Drive, Orlando, FL 32887-4800. Subscription prices are $165.00 per year for US individuals, $265.00 per year for US institutions, $83.00 per year for US students and residents, $193.00 per year for Canadian individuals, $324.00 per year for Canadian institutions, $209.00 per year for international individuals, $324.00 per year for international institutions and $105.00 per year for Canadian and foreign students/residents. To receive student/resident rate, orders must be accompanied by name of affiliated institution, date of term, and the *signature* of program/residency coordinator on institution letterhead. Orders will be billed at individual rate until proof of status is received. Foreign air speed delivery is included in all *Clinics* subscription prices. All prices are subject to change without notice. **POSTMASTER:** Send address changes to *Veterinary Clinics of North America: Equine Practice*, Elsevier Periodicals Customer Service, 6277 Sea Harbor Drive, Orlando, FL 32887-4800, USA; phone: 1-800-654-2452 [toll free number for US customers], or 1-407-345-4000 [customers outside US]; fax: 1-407-363-1354; e-mail: usjcs@elsevier.com

Reprints. For copies of 100 or more, of articles in this publication, please contact the Commercial Reprints Department, Elsevier Inc., 360 Park Avenue South, New York, New York 10010-1710. Tel. (212) 633-3813, Fax: (212) 462-1935 email: reprints@elsevier.com.

Veterinary Clinics of North America: Equine Practice is covered in *Index Medicus, Excerpta Medica, Current Contents/Agriculture, Biology and Environmental Sciences,* and *ISI.*

Printed in the United States of America.

ADVANCES IN REPRODUCTION

CONSULTING EDITOR

A. SIMON TURNER, BVSc, MS, Diplomate, American College of Veterinary Surgeons; Professor, Department of Clinical Sciences, College of Veterinary Medicine and Biomedical Sciences, Colorado State University, Fort Collins, Colorado

GUEST EDITOR

ELAINE M. CARNEVALE, DVM, PhD, Assistant Professor, Department of Biomedical Sciences; Animal Reproduction and Biotechnology Laboratory, College of Veterinary Medicine and Biomedical Sciences, Colorado State University, Fort Collins, Colorado

CONTRIBUTORS

JASON E. BRUEMMER, MS, PhD, Associate Professor, Department of Animal Sciences, Equine Reproduction Laboratory, Animal Reproduction and Biotechnology Laboratory, Colorado State University, Fort Collins, Colorado

STEFANIA BUCCA, DVM, The Irish Equine Centre, Johnstown, Naas, County Kildare, Ireland

ELAINE M. CARNEVALE, DVM, PhD, Assistant Professor, Department of Biomedical Sciences; Animal Reproduction and Biotechnology Laboratory, College of Veterinary Medicine and Biomedical Sciences, Colorado State University, Fort Collins, Colorado

DEAN HENDRICKSON, DVM, MS, Diplomate, American College of Veterinary Surgeons; Professor of Surgery; Department of Clinical Sciences, James L. Voss Veterinary Teaching Hospital, Colorado State University, Fort Collins, Colorado

KATRIN HINRICHS, DVM, PhD, Diplomate, American College of Theriogenologists; Department of Veterinary Physiology and Pharmacology and Department of Large Animal Clinical Sciences, College of Veterinary Medicine and Biomedical Sciences, Texas A&M University, College Station, Texas

BILL L. LASLEY, PhD, Department of Population Health and Reproduction, University of California-Davis, Davis, California

IRWIN K.M. LIU, DVM, PhD, Department of Population Health and Reproduction, University of California-Davis, Davis, California

PAUL R. LOOMIS, MS, President, Chief Executive Officer, Select Breeders Service, Colora, Maryland

LISA J. MACLELLAN, PhD, Seven Creeks Equine, Euroa, Victoria, Australia

MARGO L. MACPHERSON, DVM, MS, Diplomate, American College of Theriogenologists; Associate Professor, Reproduction, Department of Large Animal Clinical Sciences, College of Veterinary Medicine, University of Florida, Gainesville, Florida

PATRICK M. MCCUE, DVM, PhD, Department of Clinical Sciences, College of Veterinary Medicine and Biomedical Sciences, Colorado State University, Fort Collins, Colorado

CAROL L. MOELLER, MS, Senior Research Associate, Animal Reproduction and Biotechnology Laboratory, Department of Biomedical Sciences, College of Veterinary Medicine and Biomedical Sciences, Colorado State University, Fort Collins, Colorado

LEE MORRIS, BVSc, DVSc, Diplomate, American College of Theriogenologists; Registered Specialist-Veterinary Reproduction, EquiBreed Ltd, Cambridge, New Zealand

CORALIE J. MUNRO, BS, Department of Population Health and Reproduction, University of California-Davis, Davis, California

J.C. OUSEY, MSc, PhD, Senior Research Scientist, Equine Fertility Unit, Department of Veterinary Medicine, University of Cambridge, Newmarket, Suffolk, United Kingdom

JANET F. ROSER, PhD, Department of Animal Science, University of California-Davis, Davis, California

HEYWOOD R. SAWYER, PhD, Research Professor, Department of Medical Education and Public Health, College of Health Sciences, University of Wyoming, Laramie, Wyoming

EDWARD L. SQUIRES, PhD, Diplomate, American College of Theriogenologists (Hons); Animal Reproduction and Biotechnology Laboratory, Colorado State University, Fort Collins, Colorado

MATS H.T. TROEDSSON, DVM, PhD, Diplomate, American College of Theriogenologists; Diplomate, European College of Animal Reproduction; Professor of Theriogenology and Director of Equine Research Programs, Department of Large Animal Clinical Sciences, College of Veterinary Medicine, University of Florida, Gainesville, Florida

D.N. RAO VEERAMACHANENI, BVSc, MScVet, PhD, Professor, Animal Reproduction and Biotechnology Laboratory, Department of Biomedical Sciences, College of Veterinary Medicine and Biomedical Sciences, Colorado State University, Fort Collins, Colorado

KAREN E. WOLFSDORF, DVM, Diplomate, American College of Theriogenologists; Hagyard Equine Medical Institute, Lexington, Kentucky

ADVANCES IN REPRODUCTION

CONTENTS

Preface   xi
Elaine M. Carnevale

Advanced Methods for Handling and Preparation
of Stallion Semen   663
Paul R. Loomis

> Clinical reproduction in the horse more closely parallels human clinical reproduction than in other domestic farm animals. Horse breeders rarely include fertility as a selection criterion when making mating decisions; in most breeds, there is no licensing or approval of stallions. This has led to a significant number of stallions in the breeding pool that possess desirable performance traits but are subfertile for a variety of reasons, some of them genetically transmitted between generations. Therefore, semen characteristics can vary greatly among stallions within the breeding population. A champion stallion is not gelded or culled for poor semen quality or the inability of his spermatozoa to withstand semen preservation techniques. Rather, equine theriogenologists go to great lengths to maximize reproductive performance using any and all means available. Therefore, advanced methods for processing and selecting stallion semen provide the clinician with valuable tools for handling poor-quality semen or for obtaining spermatozoa for assisted reproduction procedures.

Collection and Freezing of Epididymal Stallion Sperm   677
Jason E. Bruemmer

> The ability to harvest and preserve epididymal sperm from a stallion after simple elective castration, a catastrophic injury, or severe acute illness and subsequent death has been realized, allowing for the preservation of genetics that would have been lost otherwise. Currently, the care taken to collect the testes and epididymides properly, coupled with proper packaging and shipping, could

make the greatest contribution to salvaging viable sperm. As advances in assisted reproductive techniques continue, more offspring may be obtained from stored epididymal sperm from valuable stallions.

Sperm Morphology in Stallions: Ultrastructure as a Functional and Diagnostic Tool 683
D.N. Rao Veeramachaneni, Carol L. Moeller, and Heywood R. Sawyer

Conventional light microscopic evaluation of a seminal ejaculate does not fully avail potential indicators of functional impairment in spermatozoal organelles. The technique of critical quantitative evaluation of morphologic features of individual structural components of spermatozoa at a light microscopic level in conjunction with critical qualitative evaluation of spermatozoal organelles at an ultrastructural level, as described in this article, is a valuable clinical tool. Compared with a battery of sperm function assays used in human andrology clinics, this relatively less expensive and simple technique is an efficient functional and diagnostic tool.

Advanced Insemination Techniques in Mares 693
Lee Morris

Advanced artificial insemination techniques, such as deep uterine, hysteroscopic, oviductal, and intrafollicular insemination, are described in the context of the different types of spermatozoa that are now available for insemination, including fresh, chilled, frozen, sex-sorted, and epididymal spermatozoa. The implementation of these new technologies answers and poses questions about the interactions of sperm and oocytes in vivo.

Breeding-Induced Endometritis in Mares 705
Mats H.T. Troedsson

Endometritis is a common cause of infertility in broodmares. In the past, the condition was believed to be exclusively the result of bacterial contamination of the uterus. Treatment strategies were focused on preventing bacteria from entering the uterus and on treating mares with signs of endometritis with antibiotics. More recent research on uterine defense mechanisms has increased our understanding of the pathophysiology of equine endometritis. Additional causative agents have been identified, and we have learned to separate uterine infections and a physiologic breeding-induced endometritis resulting from uterine exposure to semen.

Management of Postfixation Twins in Mares 713
Karen E. Wolfsdorf

Methods to manage twins after fixation include natural reduction, dietary reduction, transvaginal ultrasound-guided aspiration, surgical removal, craniocervical dislocation, and transabdominal ultrasound-guided injection. Of these, results have been inconsistent with regard to producing a single healthy foal, except for craniocervical dislocation. This new technique enables the twin to be reduced before complete placenta formation has occurred, allowing the remaining fetus to use the entire endometrial surface and grow to its full potential.

Hormone Profiles and Treatments in the Late Pregnant Mare 727
J.C. Ousey

Evaluation of hormone profiles in late pregnancy is one of the major determinants of fetoplacental compromise in equine clinical practice. Use of hormone therapies is subjective and reflects, to a large extent, our lack of understanding about the endocrine relations between the mare, placenta, and fetus. This article describes the normal endocrine events in late gestation, the abnormal hormone patterns associated with fetoplacental dysfunction, and the hormone interventions that are currently used or could be used to improve pregnancy outcome.

Diagnosis of the Compromised Equine Pregnancy 749
Stefania Bucca

Identification of a compromised pregnancy in the mare requires the exhaustive collection of a database that includes past and recent reproductive and medical histories and a variety of parameters indicating fetal distress and possibly suggesting neonatal compromise. Judicious interpretation of findings and serial recording of data throughout gestation may help in the early detection of abnormal fetomaternal exchange pathways. Some sources of compromise may be identified, and the impact on fetomaternal well-being may be calculated. Appropriate preventive or corrective measures may then be implemented to minimize the risks of an unfavorable outcome.

Diagnosis and Treatment of Equine Placentitis 763
Margo L. Macpherson

Equine placentitis is a complex disease that has devastating consequences for horse owners. Placentitis is a significant cause of foal loss annually. Prompt diagnosis and treatment of the disease are paramount for survival of the affected neonate. This article discusses current information on pathogenesis of the disease as well as diagnostic and therapeutic options.

Laparoscopic Cryptorchidectomy and Ovariectomy in Horses 777
Dean Hendrickson

> Laparoscopic surgery has become commonplace in the field of equine urogenital surgery. As with most surgical procedures, the limiting factors in developing new surgical techniques are limited to the patient size and demeanor, the skills of the surgeon, and the available equipment. Some of the greatest benefits of laparoscopic surgery in the horse include better visualization of the important structures; tension-free amputation of the testes or ovaries, which generally leads to less postoperative pain; and the ability to evaluate the transected stump carefully to make sure there is no hemorrhage. This article is limited to the use of laparoscopy for cryptorchidectomy and ovariectomy.

Granulosa Cell Tumors of the Equine Ovary 799
Patrick M. McCue, Janet F. Roser, Coralie J. Munro, Irwin K.M. Liu, and Bill L. Lasley

> The granulosa cell tumor is the most common ovarian tumor in mares. A clinical diagnosis can be made based on the presence of a unilaterally enlarged ovary and a small inactive contralateral ovary. Endocrine testing may be beneficial to confirm a diagnosis. Surgical removal of the tumor eliminates the adverse effect on pituitary function and results in resumption of follicular development and ovulation in the opposite ovary over time.

Superovulation in Mares 819
Edward L. Squires

> Recently, a commercial product has been made available (equine follicle-stimulating hormone [eFSH]) for superovulating mares. This has provided the practitioner with a hormonal product that is readily available for enhancing multiple ovulations. Additional benefits of stimulating multiple follicles include an increased number of follicles available for oocyte collection, availability of extra embryos for embryo freezing, enhancement of fertility in subfertile mares, and advancement of the first ovulation of the year. This article provides a short historical background, but most of it centers on the use of eFSH for stimulation of follicular development and ovulation in mares.

Vitrification of Equine Embryos 831
Elaine M. Carnevale

> Vitrification can be used successfully to cryopreserve equine embryos. Embryos for vitrification should be collected from donor mares' uteri when they are 300 μm or less in diameter, however, and at the morula or early blastocyst stage of development. No special equipment is required for vitrification; the straw containing

the embryo is exposed to vapor for 1 minute before plunging it into liquid nitrogen. Warming of the straw requires no special equipment, and the embryo can be transferred directly from the straw into a recipient's uterus. Vitrification has been repeatedly successful when the procedure is used with small embryos and provides a method for the rapid cryopreservation of equine embryos.

Collection, Evaluation, and Use of Oocytes in Equine Assisted Reproduction 843
Elaine M. Carnevale and Lisa J. Maclellan

Assisted reproductive techniques have been developed to obtain pregnancies from subfertile mares and stallions and to salvage gametes after death. In recent years, these procedures have been used for clinical cases with repeated success. Although new developments occur, the basis for the success and future development of assisted reproductive techniques is our ability to collect and handle the equine oocyte successfully. This article focuses on important clinical aspects of oocyte collection and evaluation and briefly discusses the clinical use of assisted reproductive procedures in the horse.

Equine Cloning 857
Katrin Hinrichs

Equine cloning is now in use as a clinical technique. It is available commercially, and its efficiency seems to be increasing. The foals produced by cloning may differ in some phenotypic and behavioral traits from the original animal but should produce offspring that reflect those that the original donor animal would have produced. This is especially true in the case of male animals, where the mitochondrial DNA is not passed to the progeny. Results of pregnancies due in 2006 should add significantly to our understanding of the factors affecting production of viable cloned foals and of the similarities and differences among cloned foals and between these foals and the donor animals.

Index 867

FORTHCOMING ISSUES

April 2007
    Trauma and Emergency Care
    Eileen K. Sullivan, DVM, *Guest Editor*

August 2007
    Evidence-Based Veterinary Medicine
    David Ramey, DVM, *Guest Editor*

December 2007
    Urinary Tract Disorders
    Harold C. Schott II, DVM, PhD, *Guest Editor*

RECENT ISSUES

August 2006
    Advances in Diagnosis and Management of Infection
    Louise L. Southwood, BVSc, PhD
    Guest Editor

April 2006
    Medical Case Management
    Jennifer M. Macleay, DVM, PhD, *Guest Editor*

December 2005
    Therapies for Joint Disease
    Troy N. Trumble, DVM, PhD, *Guest Editor*

The Clinics are now available online!

Access your subscription at:
www.theclinics.com

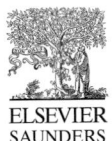

Preface

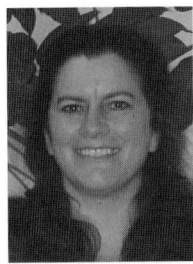

Elaine M. Carnevale, DVM, PhD
Guest Editor

Advances in equine reproduction have been numerous in recent years. Research and clinical efforts have resulted in a better understanding of basic reproductive physiology, and the incorporation of molecular biology has provided new avenues of research. Considering the limited funding available for reproductive research, one has to be impressed by the extent of recent advances in reproduction. The authors that have contributed to this issue include academic researchers and clinical innovators, each with new or accumulated information to benefit and update the equine practitioner.

Articles within this issue do not follow a specific theme. They are designed to present a relatively concise update to the equine practitioner in the field of reproduction. Comprehensive reviews and developments in clinical aspects of reproduction are included. However, a significant portion of this issue describes advances in breeding technologies. As these technologies have advanced, many breed registries have changed their rules to allow for the use of new procedures for handling and preserving equine gametes and embryos. Many of the new procedures, including advanced methods of handling sperm and artificial insemination, can assist the clinician and breeder in obtaining pregnancies with limited or compromised sperm. Superovulation is only now being developed as a repeatable procedure for clinical use, and we are beginning to understand its benefits and limitations in the mare. The development of methods to vitrify embryos will provide the practitioner with a more flexible and clinically relevant procedure, compared with more conventional methods of cryopreservation. In recent years, we have explored methods to salvage equine genetics. Gametes can be collected from ovaries or testes after the death of a valuable horse and used to produce additional offspring. Our ability to collect and handle the equine oocyte has resulted in methods to reliably produce offspring from subfertile horses and has increased our understanding of equine reproduction. The final article deals with equine cloning, an ultimate method of salvaging valuable genetics and a topic of interest and debate within the equine industry.

I would like to thank the authors for their contributions and efforts in advancing the science and art of equine reproduction. I would like to thank John Vassallo and Dr. Simon Turner for their help in the publication of this issue. Finally, I would like to recognize the clinicians, researchers, breeders, and breed associations who have supported and advanced our understanding of equine reproduction.

Elaine M. Carnevale, DVM, PhD
Department of Biomedical Sciences
College of Veterinary Medicine and Biomedical Sciences
Colorado State University
Fort Collins, CO 80523, USA

E-mail address: emc@colostate.edu

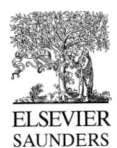

Advanced Methods for Handling and Preparation of Stallion Semen

Paul R. Loomis, MS

Select Breeders Service, 1088 Nesbitt Road, Colora, MD 21917, USA

Since the advent of artificial insemination, practitioners and researchers have been concerned with semen handling techniques. Practices that minimize damage and maximize viability, survival, and fertility of spermatozoa are required for assisted reproductive technologies (ARTs). Many procedures for processing semen and ARTs require the separation of spermatozoa from seminal components. Semen is composed of a heterogeneous population of viable and nonviable spermatozoa suspended in secretions from various accessory sex glands. Semen may also contain other cells (eg, leukocytes, epithelial cells, erythrocytes, immature germ cells) and contaminants (eg, bacteria, viruses, urine). Sperm separation techniques are used by practitioners and researchers for several reasons. One reason is to concentrate spermatozoa and remove seminal plasma before cooling or freezing semen. Another reason is to separate spermatozoa from seminal plasma and to select an enriched population of viable spermatozoa from the ejaculate. The purpose of this article is to outline reasons and procedures for separation and selection of equine spermatozoa.

Semen collection

Natural mating provides a "closed-loop system." Spermatozoa are exposed to an appropriate environment from ejaculation, directly into the female reproductive tract, until fertilization in the oviduct. Because semen is ejaculated through the open cervix and into the uterus of an estrous mare, prolonged exposure of spermatozoa to seminal fluids is minimized. The stallion ejaculates in a series of five to eight jets or fractions. The composition of each fraction varies. The first secretions (presperm) contain no spermatozoa and are primarily from the bulbourethral glands. The next

E-mail address: paulloomis@selectbreeders.com

two or three jets contain most spermatozoa (sperm-rich fractions), and the final fractions contain few spermatozoa and are composed primarily of secretions from the seminal vesicles [1–5]. Semen processing requires interruption of nature's closed-loop system. Therefore, a primary concern is to do no harm when handling ejaculated spermatozoa. Spermatozoa collected using an artificial vagina (AV) and manipulated in the laboratory can be damaged by deviations in temperature, osmotic pressure, and exposure to contaminants. Damage can also be caused by prolonged exposure to components of seminal plasma and to byproducts of metabolism during incubation. The practitioner's goal should be to obtain a complete ejaculate with a single mount and minimal sexual stimulation of the stallion before collection of semen, optimizing the potential to obtain an ejaculate with relatively low volume and high sperm concentration. As is discussed later, this type of ejaculate is preferable when semen preservation protocols are used. Ejaculate volume but not total sperm output is affected by the amount of sexual stimulation before ejaculation [6,7]. In a retrospective study of 6897 ejaculates collected from 71 stallions, Sieme and coworkers [7] demonstrated the relation between the number of mounts required for ejaculation and quantitative (volume and concentration) and qualitative (progressive motility after 24 hours of storage at 5°C) semen parameters. An increase in the number of mounts resulted in increased seminal volume, decreased sperm concentration, and decreased progressive motility after 24 hours at 5°C. One simple and practical technique to decrease the collected seminal volume and, conversely, increase sperm concentration is to void the presperm (bulbourethral gland secretions). This is done by diverting the stallion's penis away from the AV for a few seconds after the stallion has mounted and while the presperm is emitted.

Multiple mounts in the same AV, without changing the collection vessel or liner, increase the amount of presperm and contaminants (detritus and water-soluble lubricant) in collected semen. Contamination of semen with small amounts of water-soluble lubricant significantly increased the osmolarity [8,9] and decreased the pH [10] of semen, leading to a reduction in sperm quality. Excessive amounts of water-soluble lubricant should be avoided, and if multiple mounts are required for ejaculation, the collection vessel should be changed or emptied between mounts.

Processing semen for cooling

Cooled semen technology has had a major impact on the equine breeding industry, especially over the past 15 years, with the acceptance of cooled semen by most of the major breed registries. Optimum retention of sperm motility at 5°C is dependent on several factors, including adequate dilution of seminal plasma ($\geq 3:1$ ratio) with an appropriate extender and cooling at a controlled rate [11]. Sperm motility, viability, membrane integrity, and fertility are best maintained when seminal plasma is diluted to 25% or less of its original volume and the total sperm concentration is 25 to 50 × 10^6/mL [12–14]. The standard insemination dose in the industry for cooled shipped semen is 1 billion progressively motile spermatozoa before cooling. Ejaculates with low sperm concentrations require centrifugation or collection of sperm-rich fractions using an open-ended AV [12,15] to concentrate spermatozoa and allow for adequate removal of seminal plasma and extension of semen. It is standard practice in our laboratory to centrifuge semen that has an initial total sperm concentration of less than 100 × 10^6/mL or a progressively motile sperm concentration of less than 67 × 10^6/mL. Briefly, semen is extended at a 1:1 ratio with a nonfat, skim milk, glucose extender at 37°C. The extended semen (in 40-mL aliquots) is loaded into 50-mL centrifuge tubes with conical bottoms and centrifuged at approximately 400g for 12 minutes. After centrifugation, supernatant (30 mL) is aspirated from each tube using a sterile syringe, and the remaining 10 mL of spermatozoa, extender, and seminal plasma is mixed and further diluted with fresh extender to a volume of 40 mL. Based on sperm recovery after centrifugation, a 75% recovery of the initial number of spermatozoa is assumed. The volume of extended semen per dose can then be adjusted to include 1 × 10^9 progressively motile spermatozoa for packaging. We have used this technique on numerous stallions over many years to improve retention of sperm motility significantly during cooled storage, as has been reported by others [16]. The loss of 25% of spermatozoa from stallions that produce low sperm numbers or are booked to a large number of mares is not ideal, however. New techniques for centrifuging semen over dense cushions are discussed later and could prove to be more efficient for such stallions.

Role of seminal plasma

Seminal plasma has been shown to be detrimental to stallion spermatozoa during storage [12,17,18], and most protocols involve dilution or partial removal of seminal plasma before cooling. Recently, the role of seminal plasma in protecting spermatozoa in the mare's reproductive tract and mediating the postbreeding inflammatory response has been elucidated [19,20]. After the introduction of spermatozoa into the mare's reproductive tract, spermatozoa trigger an inflammatory response. In most mares, this is a normal physiologic response; however, in susceptible mares, the duration of this inflammatory response is prolonged and results in postbreeding endometritis. Seminal plasma modulates the duration of postbreeding endometritis and plays an important role in sperm transport and elimination of dead spermatozoa. Proteins in seminal plasma selectively protect live spermatozoa from binding and phagocytosis by polymorphonuclear neutrophils while promoting elimination of dead spermatozoa. In addition to the vital role of seminal plasma in the mare's reproductive tract, the absence of seminal plasma during storage results in poor maintenance of sperm motility [13]. Therefore, protocols that involve removal of all seminal plasma should be avoided; generally, 5% to 20% of seminal plasma should be retained after centrifugation. Love and coworkers [21] cooled spermatozoa in the presence of seminal plasma, however, and reported a reduction in DNA integrity, as measured by the sperm chromatin structure assay, although sperm motility was maintained. They concluded that sperm motility and DNA integrity are protected when semen is centrifuged to remove the seminal plasma and spermatozoa are resuspended in Kenney-type extender supplemented with high-potassium Tyrode's medium [22]. In the study, the reduction in DNA integrity was observed after prolonged exposure (24 and 48 hours) of spermatozoa to seminal plasma. The authors noted that previous studies demonstrated a beneficial effect of seminal plasma through antioxidant properties that protect DNA from oxidative degradation. Moore and colleagues [23] reported that the exposure of spermatozoa to 20% seminal plasma for 2 to 6 hours before cryopreservation was detrimental to postthaw motility, whereas when spermatozoa were exposed to 80% or less seminal plasma for 15 minutes at 22°C before packaging and freezing, postthaw motility and viability were not affected.

Frozen semen processing

Most protocols for cryopreservation of stallion spermatozoa involve the removal of all or most ($\geq 95\%$) seminal plasma by centrifugation and resuspension of sperm pellets in an extender. Spermatozoa are concentrated, allowing sufficient cells to be packaged in a small volume for freezing. Spermatozoa are often packaged in one to eight 0.5-mL straws or in a single 4- to 5-mL maxistraw. Removal of most of the seminal plasma helps to eliminate its detrimental effects on sperm survival during freezing [24]. Recently, seminal plasma has been added back to sperm pellets for up to 80% of the original semen volume without significantly reducing the percentages of motile or viable spermatozoa after cryopreservation [23]. The results of similar preliminary experiments in our laboratory (P.R. Loomis, MS, unpublished data, 2003) are in agreement with these findings. We saw no reduction in postthaw motility when up to 40% seminal plasma was added back to sperm pellets before cryopreservation as long as the final glycerol concentration of the extended semen was adjusted to accommodate the reduced volume of freezing extender. Some investigators [5,25] have reported that seminal plasma is beneficial to stallion spermatozoa cryosurvival and that inclusion of up to 20% of the original semen volume had no detrimental effect on postthaw motility. Other researchers [26] reported that spermatozoa frozen with 5% seminal plasma exhibited better postthaw quality (motility and glass wool/Sephadex [GWS] filtration yield) when compared with spermatozoa frozen with 0% and 25% seminal plasma, however. Although the ideal amount of seminal plasma to add back to sperm pellets after centrifugation is controversial, 5% to 20% seminal plasma is generally considered appropriate.

Centrifugation "cushions"

Centrifugation of stallion semen can be harmful, especially when spermatozoa are packed tightly at the bottom of the tubes after vigorous centrifugation. Stallion semen is usually diluted and centrifuged for 10 to 15 minutes at between 400g and 600g to achieve a soft pellet. Total sperm recovery of approximately 75% is generally accomplished with this technique. Attempts to increase recovery rates by increasing centrifugation time or force usually result in a decrease in semen quality. Weiss and coworkers [27] reported that sperm quality was better when semen was centrifuged at 600g for 10 minutes compared with 1000g for 2 minutes or 2000g for 2 minutes. The concept of layering a dense solution (0.25 mL) below the extended semen to provide a "cushion" for spermatozoa during centrifugation was introduced by Cochran and colleagues in 1984 [28]; initially, a glucose-ethylenediaminetetraacetic acid (EDTA) buffer and, later, freezing extender containing egg yolk and 4% glycerol were used. A higher percentage of motile spermatozoa were obtained after centrifugation using this cushion technique. No benefit was reported to using a glucose-EDTA cushion when evaluating the motility and acrosomal integrity of spermatozoa after freezing and thawing, however [29]. Revell and coworkers [30] used a cushion technique that involved layering a dense solution (60% wt/vol) of iodixanol in water (OptiPrep; Axis-Shield PoC AS, Oslo, Norway) below diluted stallion semen before centrifugation. The density of the solution (1.32 g/mL at 20°C) prevented spermatozoa from compacting at the bottom of the tube; therefore, more rigorous centrifugation could be used to increase sperm recovery. One investigator (D.D. Varner, DVM, MS, DACT, personal communication, 2006) used OptiPrep (30 μL) layered in the bottom of a specially designed glass centrifuge tube ("nipple tube"; Pesce Laboratory Sales, Kennett Square, Pennsylvania) before centrifugation at 400g for 20 minutes to achieve good sperm recovery from centrifuged semen. When using this technique, they simply resuspended the sperm pellet and OptiPrep in extender, and the spermatozoa has been used to obtain excellent pregnancy rates. When using such a dense cushion, even after vigorous centrifugation, spermatozoa are suspended in a band below the supernatant and above the cushion material. When larger volumes of OptiPrep are used in 50-mL centrifuge tubes with conical bottoms, the supernatant and the cushion material should be carefully aspirated from above and below the spermatozoa before resuspension of the spermatozoa in extender.

Recently, two proprietary products (Eqcellsire, IMV, L'Aigle, France; Cushion Fluid, Minitube, Landshut, Germany) were introduced to aid in obtaining higher sperm recovery after centrifugation of stallion semen. Both products are described as dense, inert, isotonic solutions that have similar functions. The Eqcellsire method and a conventional technique were compared for percent recovery, postthaw motility (% rapid motility), and fertility [31]. The Eqcellsire method involved (1) dilution of semen (1:1 ratio) with an optically clear diluent (Eqcellsire A) to which 2% egg yolk and antibiotics (penicillin, 50,000 IU/L, and gentamicin, 50 mg/L) are added, (2) loading of diluted spermatozoa (40–45 mL) into 50-mL conical-bottomed centrifuge tubes, (3) gentle layering of Eqcellsire B (3.5 mL) on the bottom of the centrifuge tube below the diluted semen, (4) centrifugation at 1000g for 20 minutes, (5) aspiration of the supernatant above and the cushion material below the concentrated band of spermatozoa found at the interface of the two solutions, and (6) resuspension of spermatozoa in freezing extender. For the conventional technique, semen was diluted in INRA 82 plus 2% egg yolk and centrifuged for 10 minutes at 600g [32]. Total sperm recovery using the Eqcellsire method was significantly ($P<.02$) higher than conventional centrifugation (99% versus 77%, respectively), resulting in a 28% increase in the number of straws produced. Postthaw semen quality and fertility were not different for semen processed with the two techniques.

Sperm recovery, postthaw motility, membrane integrity, acrosomal status, and mitochondrial membrane potential were compared for ejaculates of "good" and "bad" freezers centrifuged by three different techniques before freezing [33]. Treatments included (1) conventional centrifugation with semen diluted to a final sperm concentration of 50×10^6/mL with INRA 82, loaded into 50-mL plastic tubes, and centrifuged for 10 minutes at 600g; (2) a layer of Cushion-Fluid (5 mL) as a cushion below semen diluted as in the conventional method and centrifuged for 20 min at 1000g; and (3) semen diluted as in the conventional method, loaded into a siliconized conical glass tube, and centrifuged for 20 minutes at 1000g without a cushion. Sperm recovery was improved by using a cushion technique versus conventional centrifugation (83% versus 75% recovery, respectively), and no significant difference in postthaw semen quality was observed. The recovery rate using the cushion technique (83%) in this study was not as high as previously reported [31], potentially because a milk-based extender was used instead of an optically clear extender. Therefore, visualizing the interface between the sperm pellet and supernatant was more difficult with the milk-based extender and possibly resulted in the aspiration of more spermatozoa. The two diluents may also have different viscosities, which would lead to different sperm sedimentation rates during centrifugation. A lower recovery rate (81%) was reported [31] when an opaque milk-based diluent (INRA 82 plus egg yolk) was used with the cushion technique. Interesting findings in the study by Knop and colleagues [33] were that the highest sperm recovery was obtained using the siliconized glass tubes without a cushion (92%) and that no detrimental effect on postthaw semen quality was observed despite the high centrifugation speed.

Sperm separation techniques

The techniques discussed thus far have focused on separating spermatozoa, other cells, and debris from seminal plasma. These centrifugation techniques do little to improve the percentage of viable spermatozoa in the sample or to remove contaminants or other cells. Several techniques for sperm separation have been developed and for more than 20 years have been widely used in human [34] and bovine [35] ARTs. Semen separation techniques have been used for low-dose insemination of sexed and unsexed semen, intracytoplasmic sperm injection (ICSI), and gamete intrafallopian transfer (GIFT) in the horse. Of practical interest to the equine practitioner is the use of sperm separation techniques to enrich a semen sample with a higher percentage of viable spermatozoa before insemination of mares. This could pertain to poor-quality fresh ejaculates or to damaged spermatozoa after cooling or freezing.

The first successful separation of motile from nonmotile spermatozoa was done by filtering diluted semen through a column of small glass beads [36]. Numerous techniques have since been used to separate spermatozoa. There are three basic approaches to differential sperm separation: (1) motile sperm migration (swim-up [SU], swim-down techniques); (2) sperm adherence techniques (eg, glass wool [GW], glass beads, Sephadex [FS] filtration); and (3) density gradient centrifugation (eg, bovine serum albumin [BSA]; Percoll [Sigma Chemical Company, St. Louis, Missouri]; PureSperm, Nidacon International AB, Goteborg, Sweden).

Sperm migration

The most simple method to separate motile spermatozoa from the other components of semen is a SU technique. Semen is carefully overlaid with culture medium. The sample is incubated, allowing the motile spermatozoa to swim from the semen layer into the culture medium. In the mare, only highly motile spermatozoa complete the migration through the uterotubal junction to populate the oviduct, and in theory, the SU technique mimics the selection of motile spermatozoa that occurs in the female reproductive tract [35]. The standard SU technique has been modified for bovine and human spermatozoa by adding hyaluronic acid, a glycosaminoglycan found in the female reproductive tract, to the SU medium. The addition of hyaluronic acid resulted in a significantly higher recovery of motile and membrane-intact spermatozoa [37,38]. Although this technique does provide a purified population of motile spermatozoa, the yield is extremely low (10%–20%); therefore, the SU procedure is most appropriate for harvesting small numbers of motile spermatozoa for techniques like in vitro fertilization (IVF) or ICSI and, possibly, low-dose hysteroscopic insemination. The SU technique has been used with semen from fertile stallions, with a significant increase in progressive motility and significant decreases in sperm head and tail abnormalities: 8.1% and 10.5% of total and progressively motile spermatozoa, respectively, were recovered [39]. The SU technique has also been used with poor-quality frozen-thawed semen from a subfertile stallion to obtain acceptable spermatozoa for ICSI [40].

Because low yield and small processing volumes are associated with the SU technique, it is not appropriate for separating spermatozoa from whole ejaculates for cooling or freezing. The presence of dead or dying spermatozoa in an ejaculate has been reported to be detrimental to motility and fertility of the remaining spermatozoa [41,42]. Therefore, removing dead or dying spermatozoa from the ejaculate could help to maximize the postprocessing quality of frozen and cooled semen. Techniques that could be used for processing poor-quality ejaculates before artificial insemination or cryopreservation include filtration (sperm adherence) and density gradient centrifugation.

Sperm adherence techniques

There is a tendency for dead and damaged spermatozoa to stick to glass surfaces [43,44] and to be bound or trapped by hydrated FS (polysaccharide beads) filters. Acrosome- and plasma membrane–intact spermatozoa pass through columns of FS and GW. This technique has been used to remove dead spermatozoa from ejaculates of semen before cryopreservation, significantly increasing the motility and fertility of frozen-thawed spermatozoa from low-fertility bulls [45]. Based on the different surface charges for dead and live spermatozoa, this technique was modified to include gels of positively and negatively charged celluloses and FS, referred to as Sephadex ion-exchange (FS + IE) filtration [46]. GWS trapping of stallion spermatozoa with damaged acrosomes or plasma membranes was reported to be highly correlated with the fertility of frozen-thawed stallion semen [47]. Columns of GWS are prepared by first packing a small amount of GW at the bottom of a plastic syringe with the plunger removed. Tubing is attached to the tip of the syringe and clamped before layering FS gel over the GW. The 20% FS gels are prepared by adding FS particles (20 g, G-10 or G-15; Sigma Chemical Company) to an appropriate buffer or semen extender, allowing the FS to swell during incubation for 0.5 to 1 hour. Extended semen is then layered over the FS gel and filtered through the GWS column. An enriched population of spermatozoa is recovered in the filtrate for further processing. FS + IE filter columns are prepared in a similar fashion, but the two (positive and negative charged) cellulose gels are layered above the FS gel before the addition of extended semen.

Density gradient centrifugation

This technique is based on the separation of spermatozoa into subpopulations with different specific gravities. A suspension of colloidal silica particles coated with polyvinylpyrrolidone (PVP; Percoll) or covalently bound hydrophilic silane (PureSperm) is placed in a centrifuge tube as a continuous or multilayered discontinuous gradient. Often, a two-layer discontinuous gradient is prepared by layering a 40% to 45% solution over an 80% to 90% solution of Percoll or PureSperm. Semen is layered over the gradient, and the tubes are centrifuged. Density gradient centrifugation separates spermatozoa based on motility and morphology, because most of the normal spermatozoa pass through the gradients and are located in the pellet at the bottom of the tube. Most of the nonmotile or morphologically abnormal spermatozoa, premature germ cells, other cells, and extender components are found trapped at the interface between the gradients or suspended in one of the two gradients [48,49]. Although Percoll has been the most widely used material for density gradient separation of spermatozoa, concerns over the potential toxicity of unbound PVP from Percoll and the possibility that it may contain endotoxins resulted in its removal from human clinical use. Subsequently, silanized silica products, such as PureSperm, were developed; these products were presumably safer [34,50].

Specific application of sperm separation techniques

Limited studies have been published on the application of sperm selection techniques in the horse. With the increased use of semen preservation and ARTs, however, it is useful to develop sperm separation and selection techniques for stallion semen. Separation of spermatozoa from seminal plasma is required for semen preservation. Also, selection of viable from nonviable spermatozoa, before or after preservation, can yield commercially acceptable insemination doses from poor-quality ejaculates. The removal of dead and dying spermatozoa from poor-quality semen of subfertile stallions may improve fertility; however, this remains to be demonstrated.

Selection of spermatozoa is important for some ARTs, such as GIFT. For GIFT, spermatozoa are transferred with oocytes into recipients' oviducts. Centrifugation through a discontinuous Percoll gradient was used to select spermatozoa and achieve pregnancies using GIFT in which 1×10^5 progressively motile spermatozoa were transferred with oocytes [51]. In a subsequent study [52], a pregnancy rate of 82% was obtained when fresh unextended spermatozoa were selected through a Percoll gradient, and 2×10^5 spermatozoa were transferred along with oocytes for GIFT.

Percoll density gradient has been used to select and concentrate motile spermatozoa for low-dose hysteroscopic inseminations [53]; in the study, a conception rate of 64% was achieved using only 1×10^6 motile spermatozoa deposited at the uterotubal junction. Pregnancy rates were not different after deep uterine horn inseminations of 25×10^6 spermatozoa selected by Percoll gradient centrifugation versus the same number of unselected spermatozoa, however [54].

Nie and colleagues [54] evaluated methods of spermatozoa selection for use with deep horn insemination of low numbers of equine spermatozoa. Pregnancy rates were compared after insemination of 25×10^6 total spermatozoa without selection or selected by GWS filtration or a discontinuous (90%:50% ratio) Percoll density gradient. Contrary to findings with bovine spermatozoa [45], no significant increase in fertility was observed after insemination with selected spermatozoa, although pregnancy rates tended to be higher after inseminations with spermatozoa selected by GWS filtration than with unselected spermatozoa.

A discontinuous Percoll gradient was used to improve the motility, longevity, and viability of thawed stallion spermatozoa [55]. Frozen-thawed semen was centrifuged through a Percoll gradient before dilution and incubation or diluted in extender and incubated after thawing without Percoll processing. Immediately after thawing and at 60 minutes of incubation at 38°C, the Percoll-processed spermatozoa had significantly higher postthaw motility and viability than unselected spermatozoa.

The new generation of gradients using silane-coated colloidal silica particles (PureSperm, labeled as Equipure and BoviPure for species-specific applications) was evaluated for enhancing the quality of stallion spermatozoa [49]. Extended stallion semen was centrifuged through a two-layer (40% and 80%) discontinuous gradient of EquiPure, resulting in an increased percentage of total and progressively motile spermatozoa. In addition, the mean percentage of morphologically normal spermatozoa tended to be higher in the processed versus the unprocessed semen. The 40% and 80% Percoll gradients contained significantly more morphologically abnormal spermatozoa (proximal droplets, detached heads, abnormally shaped midpieces, bent or coiled tails, and premature germ cells) than the pelleted spermatozoa that had completely passed through the gradients. Mendes and coworkers [50] reported that PureSperm was as effective as Percoll for separating frozen-thawed bovine spermatozoa for in vitro fertilization, in agreement with similar studies with human spermatozoa [56,57].

Because stallions are not selected based on fertility or semen quality, an application of particular interest to equine theriogenologists is the use of sperm selection techniques to improve the quality and potential for cryopreservation of asthenospermatozoaic (low-quality) ejaculates from stallions that would otherwise be unsuitable for cooled or frozen semen preservation. The aim of these techniques would be to concentrate while removing dead, dying, and abnormal sperm that may negatively affect fertility. FS and FS + IE filtrations have been used to improve semen quality from low-grade buffalo ejaculates before cryopreservation [58]. The filtration system containing FS + IE columns removed immotile, dead, and abnormal spermatozoa from low-quality ejaculates; spermatozoa from the filtered semen survived the stresses of cryopreservation better than the unfiltered ejaculates. Motility and percentages of normal acrosomes, morphology, and intact plasma membranes were significantly improved by FS and FS + IE filtration at all stages of semen processing. Postthaw motility in FS + IE versus unfiltered semen was approximately 40% versus 20%, respectively.

Researchers in Germany recently reported results of an extensive study aimed at examining techniques for sperm selection, with the goal of improving cooled and frozen stallion semen quality [39]. In an initial experiment, the effectiveness of various sperm separation techniques was compared for the separation of the higher quality spermatozoa from normal stallion ejaculates. SU, GW, and GWS techniques all produced significant improvement in progressive motility and sperm-head morphology. Continuous Percoll gradient resulted in a significant decrease in semen quality when compared with controls in this study, however. The percentages of total and progressively motile spermatozoa recovered after the various treatments were 8.1% and 10.5% for SU, 52.5% and 40.4% for Percoll, 33.4% and 47.4% for GW, and 37.2% and 54.5% for GWS. In a second experiment, techniques for sperm selection were applied to whole ejaculates to improve the quality of spermatozoa after cooling and freezing. Standard centrifugation was compared with GWS filtration and filtration using Leucosorb filters (Pall Corporation, East Hills, New York). In a previous experiment by this group, stallion semen filtered through L4 filters (precursor of the Leucosorb filters from the same manufacturer) had a significant increase in semen quality as well as fertility compared with semen processed by standard centrifugation techniques. Spermatozoa filtered by GWS or Leucosorb filters had a higher percentage of progressively motile spermatozoa immediately after processing. Leucosorb-filtered semen maintained significantly higher progressive motility at 24 and 48 hours after cooling than semen that had been processed by standard centrifugation techniques. A significantly higher percentage of membrane-intact spermatozoa was also recovered from both filtration treatments versus centrifugation. Total sperm recovery was significantly lower with both filtration techniques compared with centrifugation; however, because of the selective nature of the filtration, the percentage of progressively motile spermatozoa recovered was not different. Recovery of progressively motile spermatozoa for centrifugation, GWS, and Leucosorb filtration was 67.6%, 68.8%, and 63.3%, respectively. GWS and Leucosorb filtration processing of semen before cryopreservation resulted in significantly higher progressive motility of spermatozoa after thawing (49.6% and 47.1%, respectively) than was achieved with standard centrifugation before freezing (32.1%). No differences were detected in the percentage of membrane-intact or acrosome-intact spermatozoa after thawing for any of the procedures. A third experiment was conducted to compare per cycle pregnancy rates for mares inseminated with GWS- or Leucosorb-processed fresh-cooled semen with semen processed by standard centrifugation before extension and cooling. Unlike the results of the previous Leucosorb fertility trial, no significant difference was detected in per cycle pregnancy rates, and the authors concluded that although GWS and Leucosorb filtration significantly improved semen quality, the effects on fertility are still unknown.

Summary

Clinical reproduction in the horse more closely parallels human clinical reproduction than in other domestic farm animals. Horse breeders rarely include fertility as a selection criterion when making mating decisions; in most breeds, there is no licensing or approval of stallions. This has led to a significant number of stallions in the breeding pool that possess desirable performance traits but are subfertile for a variety of reasons, some of them genetically transmitted between generations. Therefore, semen characteristics can vary greatly among stallions within the breeding population. A champion stallion is not gelded or culled for poor semen quality or the inability of his spermatozoa to withstand semen preservation techniques. Rather, equine theriogenologists go to great lengths to maximize reproductive performance using any and all means available. Therefore, advanced methods for processing and selecting stallion semen provide the clinician with valuable tools for handling poor-quality semen or for obtaining spermatozoa for assisted reproduction procedures.

References

[1] Mann T, Minotakis CS, Polge C. Semen composition and metabolism in the stallion and jackass. J Reprod Fertil 1963;5:109–22.
[2] Mann T. Biochemistry of stallion semen. J Reprod Fertil Suppl 1975;23:47–52.
[3] Kosniak K. Characteristics of the successive jets of ejaculated semen of stallions. J Reprod Fertil Suppl 1975;23:59–61.
[4] Magistrini M, Lindeberg H, Koskinen E, et al. Biophysical and ^{1}H magnetic resonance spectroscopy characteristics of fractionated stallion ejaculates. J Reprod Fertil Suppl 2000;56:101–10.
[5] Katila T, Anderson M, Reilas T, et al. Post-thaw motility and viability of fractionated and frozen stallion ejaculates. Theriogenology 2002;58:241–4.
[6] Ionata LM, Anderson TM, Pickett BW, et al. Effect of supplementary sexual preparation on semen characteristics of stallions. Theriogenology 1991;36:923–37.
[7] Sieme H, Echte A, Klug E. Effect of frequency and interval of semen collection on seminal parameters and fertility of stallions. Theriogenology 2002;58:313–6.
[8] Devireddy RV, Swanlund DJ, Alghamdi AS, et al. The effect of collection and cooling conditions on water transport characteristics of equine spermatozoa. Theriogenology 2002;58:233–6.
[9] Duoos L, Troedsson MHT, Alghamdi AS, et al. The importance of osmotic pressure for the quality of fresh, cooled and cryopreserved equine spermatozoa. Theriogenology 2002;58:261–4.
[10] Limone LE, Shaughnessy DW, Gomez-Ibanez S, et al. The effect of artificial vagina lubricants on stallion sperm motion measures and semen pH during cooled storage. Theriogenology 2002;58:333–6.
[11] Varner DD, Blanchard TL, Love CC, et al. Effects of cooling rate and storage temperature on equine spermatozoa, motility parameters. Theriogenology 1988;29:1043–51.
[12] Varner DD, Blanchard TL, Love CC, et al. Effect of semen fractionation and dilution ratio on equine spermatozoal motility parameters. Theriogenology 1987;28:709–18.
[13] Jasko DJ, Moran DM, Farlin ME, et al. Effect of seminal plasma dilution or removal on spermatozoal motion characteristics of cooled stallion semen. Theriogenology 1991;35:1059–67.
[14] Jasko DJ, Martin JM, Squires EL. Effect of insemination volume and concentration of spermatozoa on embryo recovery in mares. Theriogenology 1992;37:1233–9.
[15] Tischner M, Kosniak K, Bielanski W. Analysis of the pattern of ejaculation in stallions. J Reprod Fertil 1974;41:329–35.
[16] Brinsko SP, Crockett EC, Squires EL. Effect of centrifugation and partial removal of seminal plasma on equine spermatozoal motility after cooling and storage. Theriogenology 2000;54:29–36.

[17] Pickett BW, Sullivan JJ, Byers WW, et al. Effect of centrifugation and seminal plasma on motility and fertility of stallion and bull spermatozoa. Fertil Steril 1975;26:167–74.
[18] Jasko DJ, Hathaway JA, Schaltenbrand VL, et al. Effect of seminal plasma and egg yolk on motion characteristics of cooled stallion spermatozoa. Theriogenology 1992;37:1241–52.
[19] Troedsson MHT, Lee C-S, Franklin RD, et al. The role of seminal plasma in post-breeding uterine inflammation. J Reprod Fertil Suppl 2000;56:341–9.
[20] Troedsson MHT, Desvousges A, Alghamdi AS, et al. Components in seminal plasma regulating sperm transport and elimination. Anim Reprod Sci 2005;89:171–86.
[21] Love CC, Brinsko SP, Rigby SL, et al. Relationship of seminal plasma level and extender type to sperm motility and DNA integrity. Theriogenology 2005;63:1584–91.
[22] Padilla AW, Foote RH. Extender and centrifugation effects on the motility patterns of slow-cooled stallion spermatozoa. J Anim Sci 1991;69:3308–13.
[23] Moore AI, Squires EL, Graham JK. Effect of seminal plasma on the cryopreservation of equine spermatozoa. Theriogenology 2005;63:2372–81.
[24] Amann RP, Pickett BW. Principles of cryopreservation and a review of cryopreservation of stallion spermatozoa. Equine Vet Sci 1987;7:145–73.
[25] Aurich JE, Kuhne A, Hoppe H, et al. Seminal plasma affects membrane integrity and motility of equine spermatozoa after cryopreservation. Theriogenology 1996;46:791–7.
[26] Alghamdi AS, Troedsson MH, Xue JL, et al. Effect of seminal plasma concentration and various extenders on postthaw motility and glass wool-Sephadex filtration of cryopreserved stallion semen. Am J Vet Res 2002;63:880–5.
[27] Weiss S, Janett F, Burger D, et al. The influence of centrifugation on quality and freezability of stallion semen. Schweiz Arch Tierheilkd 2004;146:285–93.
[28] Cochran JD, Amann RP, Froman DP, et al. Effects of centrifugation, glycerol level, cooling to 5C, freezing rate and thawing rate on the post-thaw motility of equine sperm. Theriogenology 1984;22:25–38.
[29] Volkmann DH. Acrosomal damage and progressive motility of stallion semen frozen by two methods in 0.5-milliliter straws. Theriogenology 1987;27:689–98.
[30] Revell SG, Pettit MT, Ford TC. Use of centrifugation over iodixanol to reduce damage when processing stallion sperm for freezing [abstract 92]. In: Proceedings of the Joint Meeting of the Society for the Study of Fertility. Cambridge, UK: Journals of Reproduction and Fertility, Ltd.; 1997. p. 38.
[31] Ecot P, Decuadro-Hansen G, Delhomme G, et al. Evaluation of a cushioned centrifugation technique for processing equine semen for freezing [abstract 18]. Anim Reprod Sci 2005;89:245–8.
[32] Vidament M, Ecot P, Noue P, et al. Centrifugation and addition of glycerol at 22C instead of 4C improve post-thaw motility and fertility of stallion spermatozoa. Theriogenology 2000;54:907–19.
[33] Knop K, Hoffmann N, Rath D, et al. Effects of cushioned centrifugation technique on sperm recovery and sperm quality in stallions with good and poor semen freezability [abstract 36]. Anim Reprod Sci 2005;89:294–7.
[34] Mortimer D. Sperm preparation methods. J Androl 2000;21:357–66.
[35] Rodriguez-Martinez H, Larsson B, Pertoft H. Evaluation of sperm damage and techniques for sperm clean-up. Reprod Fertil Dev 1997;9:297–308.
[36] Bangham AD, Hancock JL. A new method for counting live and dead spermatozoa [letter]. Nature 1955;176:656.
[37] Wikland M, Wik O, Steen Y, et al. A self-migration method for preparation of sperm for in-vitro fertilization. Hum Reprod (Oxf) 1987;2:191–5.
[38] Shamsuddin M, Rodriguez-Martinez H, Larsson B. Fertilizing capacity of bovine spermatozoa selected after swim-up in hyaluronic acid containing medium. Reprod Fertil Dev 1993;5:307–15.
[39] Sieme H, Martinsson G, Rauterberg H, et al. Application of techniques for sperm selection in fresh and frozen-thawed stallion semen. Reprod Domest Anim 2003;38:134–40.

[40] Choi YH, Love CC, Varner DD, et al. Equine blastocyst development after intracytoplasmic injection of sperm subjected to two freeze-thaw cycles. Theriogenology 2006;65:808–19.
[41] Saacke RG. Morphology of the sperm and its relationship to fertility (cattle mainly). In: Proceedings of the Third National Association of Animal Breeders Technical Conference on Artificial Insemination Reproduction. Columbia (MO): National Association of Animal Breeders; 1970. p. 17.
[42] Trokey DE, Merilan CP. Effect of added cold shocked cells upon the viability of pony stallion spermatozoa. Theriogenology 1982;18:723–5.
[43] Stubbings RB, Wosik CP. Glass wool versus swim-up separation of bovine spermatozoa for in vitro fertilization [abstract]. In: Bondioli K, Greve T, Wilmut I, editors. Proceedings Annual Conference International Embryo Transfer Society, Bournemouth: UK 1991;35:276.
[44] Crabo BG, Loseth KJ, Weidel L. Trapping of morphological types of bull spermatozoa by Sephadex/glass wool filters. In: Proceedings of the 12th International Congress on Animal Reproduction, The Hague, The Netherlands; 1992. p. 423–5.
[45] Graham EF, Graham JK. The effect of whole ejaculate filtration on the morphology and the fertility of bovine semen. J Dairy Sci 1990;73:91–7.
[46] Anzar M, Graham EF. Effect of filtration on post-thaw quality of bull semen. Theriogenology 1995;43:439–49.
[47] Samper JC, Hellander JC, Crabo BG. Relationship between the fertility of fresh and frozen stallion semen and semen quality. J Reprod Fertil 1991;(Suppl 44):107–14.
[48] Parish JJ, Krogenaes A, Susko-Parrish JL. Effect of bovine sperm separation by either swim-up or Percoll method on success of in vitro fertilization and early embryonic development. Theriogenology 1995;44:859–69.
[49] Macpherson ML, Blanchard TL, Love CC, et al. Use of a silane-coated silica particle solution to enhance the quality of ejaculated semen in stallions. Theriogenology 2002;58:317–20.
[50] Mendes JOB Jr, Burns PD, De La Torre-Sanchez JF, et al. Effect of heparin on cleavage rates and embryo production with four bovine sperm preparation protocols. Theriogenology 2003;60:331–40.
[51] Carnevale EM, Maclellan LJ, Coutinho da Silva MA, et al. Comparison of culture and insemination techniques for equine oocyte transfer. Theriogenology 2000;54:981–7.
[52] Coutinho da Silva MA, Carnevale EM, Maclellan LJ, et al. Oocyte transfer in mares with intrauterine or intraoviductal insemination using fresh, cooled, and frozen stallion semen. Theriogenology 2004;61:705–13.
[53] Morris LHA, Hunter RHF, Allen WR. Hysteroscopic insemination of small numbers of spermatozoa at the uterotubal junction of preovulatory mares. J Reprod Fertil 2000;118:95–100.
[54] Nie GJ, Johnson KE, Wenzel JGW. Pregnancy outcome in mares following insemination deep in the uterine horn with low numbers of sperm selected by glass wool/Sephadex filtration, Percoll separation or absolute number. Anim Reprod Sci 2003;79:103–9.
[55] Leao KM, Alvarenga MA, Landim-Alvarenga FC, et al. Improvement of motility, longevity and viability of frozen stallion sperm selected by discontinuous Percoll density gradient [abstract 25]. Anim Reprod Sci 2001;68:342–3.
[56] Chen M, Bongso A. Comparative evaluation of two density gradient preparations for sperm separation for medically assisted conception. Hum Reprod 1999;14:759–64.
[57] Soderlund B, Lundin K. The use of silane-coated silica particles for density gradient centrifugation in in vitro fertilization. Hum Reprod 2000;15:857–60.
[58] Ahmad Z, Anzar M, Shahab M, et al. Sephadex and Sephadex ion-exchange filtration improves the quality and freezability of low-grade buffalo semen ejaculates. Theriogenology 2003;59:1189–202.

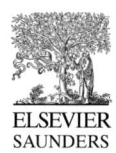

Collection and Freezing of Epididymal Stallion Sperm

Jason E. Bruemmer, MS, PhD

Department of Animal Sciences, Equine Reproduction Laboratory, Animal Reproduction and Biotechnology Laboratory, Colorado State University, 3194 Rampart Road, Fort Collins, CO, 80523 USA

In the event of catastrophic injury, death, or even elective castration, stallion sperm capable of fertilization can be harvested from the cauda epididymides [1,2] and frozen for future use [2], thereby salvaging valuable genetics. The timing and, often, location of the castration or postmortem tissue harvest are not always appropriate for sperm collection and preservation. Little is known regarding the survival and fertility of frozen-thawed epididymal stallion sperm, although the first successful pregnancy resulted from frozen semen collected from the epididymis [2]. Since then, most research has focused on procedures using ejaculated semen. Procedures for the collection or shipment of the epididymides and subsequent sperm cell harvest and cryopreservation are discussed.

Harvesting of epididymides

Collection of sperm from the epididymides requires cannulation of the epididymides or surgical removal. In our laboratory, we have successfully collected sperm via cauda epididymal aspiration from anesthetized and standing stallions. Although this means of sperm harvest is certainly possible, few cells are collected when compared with collection after epididymal removal and are of little value in postmortem situations. The two caudal epididymides of a normal, sexually rested, adult stallion should contain 54 × 10^9 sperm or approximately 61% of the sperm in the excurrent duct system [3]. Therefore, we concluded that the most efficient means of obtaining the greatest number of sperm requires surgical removal of the epididymides, granted that this is for a single and final collection. To accomplish this, both testes and their associated epididymides should be collected using

E-mail address: jason.bruemmer@colostate.edu

0749-0739/06/$ - see front matter © 2006 Elsevier Inc. All rights reserved.
doi:10.1016/j.cveq.2006.08.007   vetequine.theclinics.com

standard surgical castration procedures. It is imperative that the cauda epididymides and as much of the ductus deferens as possible remain intact. Suture material should be used to ligate the ductus deferens as high as possible to prevent loss of sperm cells, because fertile sperm can be isolated from both regions [4]. If possible, castration should be performed before euthanasia, because the effects of euthanasia compounds on sperm viability have yet to be determined. Stallions may be castrated while anesthetized, because the effects of halothane seem to be negligible [5]. Each testis and associated epididymis should then be rinsed with sterile saline and placed in a clean container, such as a rectal sleeve or plastic bag. The sample can be processed immediately or shipped to an appropriate facility for sperm collection and cryopreservation.

Shipping epididymides

The testis and epididymides should be placed in a passive cooling device designed for the shipment of cooled semen and sent to a reproductive referral center that offers the service of collecting and freezing epididymal sperm or processed by a practitioner at an appropriate facility. When shipping, make certain that the coolant source has been added. Sperm from many species, including dogs [6], human beings [7], deer [8], and goats [9], have been processed and successfully frozen after at least 24 hours of storage at 5°C. Results of previous research suggest that sperm harvested from stallion tissues after storage for 24 hours at 5°C remain viable [10,11] and, in some cases, comparable to freshly processed ejaculated samples [12].

Harvesting sperm from epididymides

On arrival at the appropriate laboratory facility, each epididymis should be dissected free of the testis (Fig. 1). The tail and ductus deferens are then isolated (Fig. 2), and spermatozoa can be collected using one of two methods: the float-up method (Fig. 3) or the retrograde flush technique (Fig. 4.)

In the float-up method, the cauda epididymides and proximal ductus deferens are incised in 12 to 15 locations and suspended in semen extender (approximately 5 mL), and sperm are allowed to float into the extender for 10 minutes [13]. Our laboratory has had better success than that reported [13] when the epididymides are flushed in a retrograde fashion. We routinely collect 15 to 20 billion sperm after a retrograde flush as opposed to the 4 to 5 billion [13] reported using the float-up method. This technique requires the use of a commercial semen extender or clear modified Tyrode's medium (approximately 10 mL per epididymis; see Fig. 4). Briefly, the tubules of the vas deferens and caudal epididymides are dissected free of the fascia, usually working distally from the vas deferens toward the corpus epididymis.

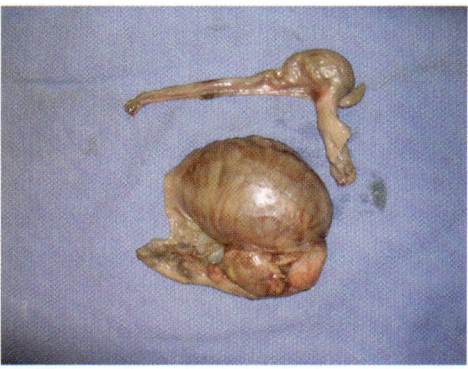

Fig. 1. Epididymis and proximal ductus deferens removed from the testes.

Termination of dissection occurs when the tubule of the cauda becomes indistinguishable from that of the corpus or at least until it is easily visualized. Either a blunt 16-gauge needle or fire-polished glass pipette is attached to a syringe containing flush medium. The needle or pipette is placed into the lumen of the previously ligated vas deferens while the caudal epididymis is suspended in a beaker or 50-mL conical tube (see Fig. 4). The most distal end of the caudal epididymis (ideally the previous site of union with the corpus) is nicked to allow sperm collection. The flush may require a certain amount of pressure; thus, care should be taken to ensure that the tissue does not slip off the end of the needle or pipette.

The concentration of the recovered sperm is determined via a hemacytometer when using cryopreservation media or spectrophotometrically after collection in a clear Tyrode's type medium. Epididymal sperm are then diluted to 200×10 cells/mL [6] or 400×10 cells/mL [6] in a freezing extender and frozen using standard techniques [14]. The type of extender used is based on the history of the stallion. The type of freezing extender best suited for

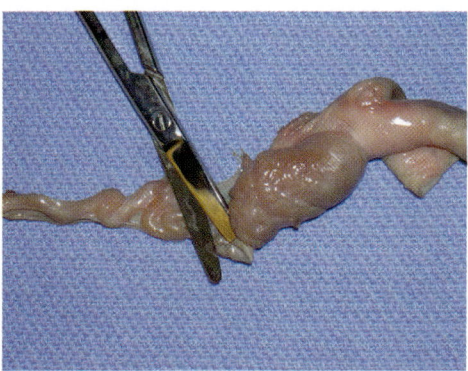

Fig. 2. Isolation of cauda epididymis and proximal ductus deferens.

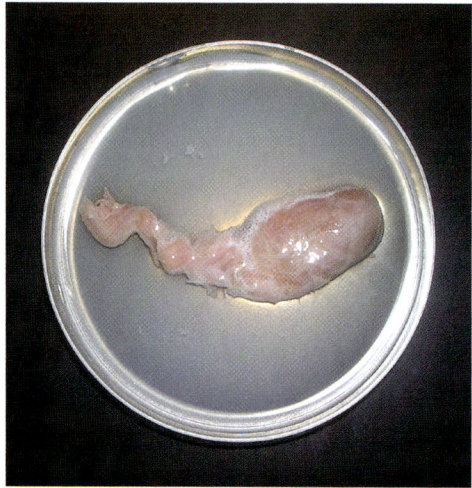

Fig. 3. Float-up collection of ductus deferens and epididymis.

survival of cryopreserved epididymal sperm matched that of ejaculated sperm from a given stallion [10]. If sperm from a given stallion had not been frozen previously, we would suggest that the sample be split, with half frozen in each of the two most common and commercially available extenders (EZ-Freezin MFR5 or EZ-Freezin LE; Animal Reproduction Systems, Chino, California).

Seminal plasma harvested from a stallion of proven fertility can also be added to the sample. Typical additions range from 0.5 mL per 1.6 billion sperm [10] to 5% vol/vol [13,15]. It has been hypothesized that fertility is increased by exposing epididymal sperm to seminal plasma before freezing.

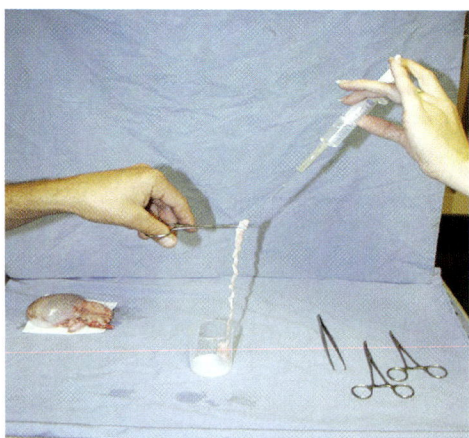

Fig. 4. Retrograde collection method.

Postthaw motility parameters may [15,16] or may not [10,13] be affected; postthaw motility parameters of epididymal sperm were enhanced in the presence of seminal plasma in some studies [15,17], whereas others were unable to duplicate these results [10]. Fertility trials have yet to be conducted using epididymal spermatozoa with and without seminal plasma. Future research should focus on whether and when seminal plasma should be added to epididymal sperm.

Results

Five to 25 breeding doses, consisting of 800×10^6 sperm per dose, are typically obtained from a given stallion. Frozen epididymal sperm harvested from stallions on the premise or cooled and shipped have been used to obtain pregnancies. Again, the first equine pregnancy generated using frozen sperm was obtained using frozen-thawed epididymal sperm [13,15]. Pregnancies and live foals have been produced by using conventional artificial insemination [2] and assisted reproductive techniques, such as low-dose hysteroscopic insemination [18] and intracytoplasmic sperm injection (E.M. Carnevale, DVM, PhD, Colorado State University, Equine Reproduction Laboratory unpublished data, 2005).

Summary

The ability to harvest and preserve epididymal sperm from a stallion after simple elective castration, a catastrophic injury, or severe acute illness and subsequent death has been realized, allowing for the preservation of genetics that would have been lost otherwise. Currently, the care taken to collect the testes and epididymides properly, coupled with proper packaging and shipping, could make the greatest contribution to salvaging viable sperm. As advances in assisted reproductive techniques continue, more offspring may be obtained from stored epididymal sperm from valuable stallions.

References

[1] Johnson L, Amann RP, Pickett BW. Maturation of equine epididymal spermatozoa. Am J Vet Res 1980;41:1190–6.
[2] Barker CAV, Gandier JCC. Pregnancy in the mare resulted from frozen epididymal spermatozoa. Can J Comp Vet Med Vet Sci 1957;21:45–51.
[3] Amann RP, Thompson DL Jr, Squires EL, et al. Effects of age and frequency of ejaculation on sperm production and extragonadal reserves in stallions. J Reprod Fertil Suppl 1979;27:1–6.
[4] Amann RP. Functional anatomy of the adult male. In: McKinnon AO, Voss, JL, editors. Equine reproduction. Philadelphia: Lea & Febiger; 1992. p. 645–57.
[5] Schulman ML, Gerber D, Nurton J, et al. Effects of halothane anesthesia on the cryopreservation of epididymal spermatozoa in pony stallions. Equine Vet J 2003;35:93–5.
[6] Marks SL, Dupus J, Mickelsen WD, et al. Conception by use of postmortem epididymal semen extraction in a dog. J Am Vet Med Assoc 1994;204:1639–40.

[7] Sharma RK, Padron OF, Thomas AJ, et al. Factors associated with the quality before and after thawing of sperm obtained by microsurgical epididymal aspiration. Fertil Steril 1997; 68:626–31.
[8] Zomborsky Z, Zubor T, Toth J, et al. Sperm collection from shot red deer stags (Ervus elaphus) and the utilization of sperm frozen and subsequently thawed. Acta Vet Hung 1999;47: 263–70.
[9] Blash S, Melican D, Gavin W. Cryopreservation of epididymal sperm obtained at necropsy from goats. Theriogenology 2002;54:899–905.
[10] Bruemmer JE, Reger H, Zibinski G, et al. Effect of storage at 5°C on the motility and cryopreservation of stallion epididymal spermatozoa. Theriogenology 2002;58:405–7.
[11] James AN, Green H, Hoffman S, et al. Preservation of equine sperm stored in the epididymis at 4°C for 24, 48, 72 and 96 hours. Theriogenology 2002;58:401–4.
[12] Bruemmer JE, Moore A, Squires EL. Freezing epididymal sperm from transported testicles. Havemeyer Foundation Workshop Monograph Series 2003;15:61–2.
[13] Cary JA, Madill S, Farnsworth K, et al. A comparison of electroejaculation and epididymal sperm collection techniques in stallion. Can Vet J 2004;45:35–41.
[14] Squires EL, Pickett BW, Graham JK, et al. Cooled and frozen stallion semen. Fort Collins (CO): Animal Reproduction and Biotechnology Laboratory, Bulletin No. 9. 1999.
[15] Stout TAE, Morris LHA, Li X. The effect of seminal plasma on the motility and cryopreservability of horse epididymal sperm. In: Allen WR, Wade JF, editors. Proceedings of the Havemeyer Foundation Workshop. Lopuszna, Poland: European Equine Gamete Group. 1999. p. 5–6.
[16] Volkmann DH, Gerber D, Erb HN. Comparison between freezability of ejaculated and epididymal stallion sperm [abstract]. Anim Reprod Sci 2001;68:340.
[17] Aurich JE, Kuhne A, Hoppe H, et al. Seminal plasma affects membrane integrity and motility of equine spermatozoa after cryopreservation. Theriogenology 1996;58:791–7.
[18] Morris L, Tiplady C, Allen WR. The in vivo fertility of cauda epididymal spermatozoa in the horse. Theriogenology 2002;58:643–6.

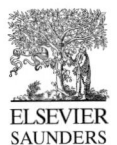

Sperm Morphology in Stallions: Ultrastructure as a Functional and Diagnostic Tool

D.N. Rao Veeramachaneni, BVSc, MScVet, PhD[a],*,
Carol L. Moeller, MS[a], Heywood R. Sawyer, PhD[b]

[a]*Animal Reproduction and Biotechnology Laboratory, Department of Biomedical Sciences, College of Veterinary Medicine and Biomedical Sciences, Colorado State University, Fort Collins, CO 80523–1683, USA*
[b]*Department of Medical Education and Public Health, College of Health Sciences, University of Wyoming, Laramie, WY 82071–3432, USA*

One of the most common laboratory practices in the assessment of potential fertility is evaluation of morphologic features of spermatozoa in seminal ejaculates by light microscopy. Although light microscopy is an important and useful component of most routine breeding soundness evaluations of healthy stallions, use of light microscopy alone limits the inherent utility of a seminal sample in identifying disease conditions contributing to infertility. For example, the structural integrity of the plasma membrane and important organelles (acrosome, mitochondria, and nucleus) pivotal to fertilization and normal progression of embryo development cannot be critically discerned using only light microscopy.

In recent years, a variety of biochemical tests have been developed to assess the functional status of the plasma membrane and sperm organelles. Although the structural integrity of the plasma membrane over the sperm head can be assayed by simple dye exclusion tests using a light microscope and such stains as eosin [1], more efficient flow cytometric techniques using fluorescent nucleic acid stains, such as SYBR-14, in combination with propidium iodide are now available [2]. Likewise, although the integrity of the acrosomal membrane can be assayed using fluorescently labeled lectins, such as *Pisum sativum* and peanut agglutinins, that bind to acrosomal

---

This work was supported by the Research Council of the College of Veterinary Medicine and Biomedical Sciences, Colorado State University.
* Corresponding author.
  E-mail address: d_n_rao.veeramachaneni@colostate.edu (D.N.R. Veeramachaneni).

contents [3], a more efficient technique using the acrosomal probe Lyso-Tracker Green DND-26, which identifies living spermatozoa with intact acrosomes [4], has been developed. Similarly, to evaluate mitochondrial membrane potential, a mitochondria-specific fluorescent probe, JC-l, has been developed [5,6]. More recently, the importance of sperm chromatin packaging and the impact of fragmentation of sperm DNA on fertilization and normal embryonic development have been recognized, and a variety of assays have been developed to evaluate sperm nuclear integrity. These assays include the sperm chromatin structure assay (SCSA) [7], sperm chromatin dispersion assay (Halosperm kit, INDAS Laboratories, Madrid, Spain) [8], and terminal deoxynucleotidyl transferase-mediated–deoxyuridine triphosphate nick end labeling assay (TUNEL), all of which detect fragmentation or breakage of DNA strands. Because of their nature, biochemical functional analyses must be performed individually [6,9] on freshly ejaculated spermatozoa. If evaluation of the functional status of multiple spermatozoal components (eg, plasma membrane, organelles, chromatin) becomes necessary in certain clinical situations, the time constraint between semen collection and evaluation, labor, and cost involved may be prohibitive in routine veterinary practice.

Herein, using a fixed semen sample, we describe a relatively simple morphologic procedure that facilitates critical evaluation of the plasma membrane and multiple organelles simultaneously. We also present examples of morphologic correlates of these structural components that indicate functional impairment. Furthermore, this procedure can be useful in the identification of existing degenerative and inflammatory conditions in the reproductive tract by enabling characterization of exfoliated cells in the seminal ejaculate. For detailed background information, the reader is referred to treatises dealing with morphologic evaluation of spermatozoa of various species at light and electron microscopic levels [10–14] and those that describe histologic [15] and histopathologic evaluation of the testis [16].

Processing of seminal ejaculates

We have presented detailed procedures for processing equine seminal ejaculates for light and transmission electron microscopy elsewhere [13,17]. Briefly, gel-free semen (5 mL) is fixed in a 10-mL cacodylate-buffered 6% glutaraldehyde. The fixed samples are centrifuged, the supernatant is poured off, and the pellet is suspended in sodium cacodylate buffer (0.1 M). An aliquot of the suspension (100 μL) is added to distilled water (1 mL) in a glass vial. A wet smear is freshly prepared by placing a drop of this suspension on a glass slide and placing a coverslip for differential interference contrast (Nomarski) microscopy. A dry smear is also prepared by placing a large drop on a glass slide and distributing the fluid evenly with the tip of a Pasteur pipet. The slide is placed on a heating block at 80°C, stained with toluidine blue, and coverslips are mounted using Poly-mount (Polysciences, Warrington, PA) for bright field microscopy.

The remaining suspension is washed once more as indicated previously, the supernatant is poured off, and the pellet is processed for transmission electron microscopy. The pellet is postfixed in a solution of 1% osmium tetroxide in cacodylate buffer (0.1 M) and centrifuged. Osmicated pellets are dehydrated through a graded series of ethanol, rinsed in propylene oxide, and embedded in Poly/Bed 812 (Polysciences, Warrington, Pennsylvania). For characterization of exfoliated cells using light microscopy, 1-μm thick sections are cut, placed on glass slides, and stained with toluidine blue. For ultrastructural evaluation of spermatozoa and other cellular components using transmission electron microscopy, approximately 80-nm thin sections are cut, mounted on 300-mesh nickel grids, and stained with uranyl acetate and lead citrate.

Light microscopic evaluation of seminal preparations

A light microscope equipped with a planapochromatic ×100 oil immersion objective and a universal condenser (1.4 numeric aperture) that enables bright field and differential interference contrast microscopy (Nikon Microphot FXA, Nikon, Inc., Melville, New York) is used. Toluidine blue–stained smears (bright field microscopy) and unstained wet smears (differential interference contrast microscopy) complement each other by compensating for deficits inherent to these procedures (eg, artifacts associated with smear preparation, resolution of subtle defects), and thus enhance critical evaluation. The microscope is interfaced with a computerized imaging system (ImagePro, version 5.0 Image Pro, Silver Spring, Maryland) and a data collection spreadsheet (Microsoft Excel, Redmond, Washington). Two hundred spermatozoa from each of the wet and toluidine blue–stained smears are classified into normal or abnormal categories. The abnormal categories include defects associated with the acrosome, nucleus, middle piece, principal piece, terminal piece, and entire flagellum; retained cytoplasmic droplets at a proximal (neck) or distal (annulus) position; and diffuse residual cytoplasm. Heads without tails (detached); multiple heads or tails; and miscellaneous forms, such as such as the unique "diadem" and "dag" defects [10], are also enumerated. For each sperm, all defects associated with any of these structural components are individually recorded (Fig. 1). Formulae embedded in the spreadsheet compute the percentage of normal spermatozoa, spermatozoa with a single defect, and spermatozoa with multiple defects. Thus, the total number of sperm abnormalities could exceed 100%, but the total number of normal plus abnormal spermatozoa always equals 100%. The presence of any prematurely exfoliated germ cells or other discernible somatic cells is documented. This approach, with assignment of abnormalities to individual structural components of sperm and assimilation of their collective incidence, facilitates assessment of the severity of damage and identification of the origin of defect(s), pinpointing the phase in spermatogenesis or posttesticular sperm maturation that is affected.

A Individual Sperm Scores

Sperm #	Normal	ACR	NCL	FLG	MP	PP	TP	PD	DD	RC	TLH	MHT	MISC	Single	Multiple
1	1													0	0
2		1												1	0
⋮															
199		1		1										0	1
200			1		1			1						0	1
%															

B Summary

%	Normal	ACR	NCL	FLG	MP	PP	TP	PD	DD	RC	TLH	MF	MISC	Single	Multiple
Wet Smear															
Dry Smear															
Average															

ACR acrosome: missing, ruffled, knobbed/cystic
NCL nucleus: variations in size and shape, multi-headed, malformed
FLG flagellum: entire tail—coiled, coiled around head, thin
MP mid-piece: abaxial, reflected, swollen, thin
PP principal piece: bent, swollen, thin
TP terminal piece: flayed, looped
PD proximal droplet
DD distal droplet
RC residual cytoplasm (other than PD or DD)
TLH tail-less (detached) head
MHT multiple heads and/or tails
MISC miscellaneous: unique defects such as "Diadem", "Dag" etc.

Single sperm having only one defect
Multiple sperm having multiple defects

Record the presence of:
    Premature germ cells: spermatids, spermatocytes
    Epithelial cells: excurrent ducts, accessory glands, urinary tract
    Cell debris, bacteria, macrophages, RBC, WBC

Fig. 1. (*A, B*) Data collection sheet for evaluation of a wet smear (using differential interference contrast microscopy) and a toluidine blue–stained dry smear (using bright field microscopy) of seminal preparations. Two hundred sperm from each preparation (400 sperm per ejaculate) are critically evaluated, assigning defects to individual structural components of sperm. Data are entered into a computerized spreadsheet that computes the percentage of normal sperm, abnormal sperm with a single defect, and abnormal sperm with multiple defects. RBC, red blood cell; WBC, white blood cell.

Using bright field optics, 1-μm thick sections of sperm pellets stained with toluidine blue are also examined for identification and characterization of various cell types (eg, epithelial cells from excurrent ducts and accessory sex glands, urothelium, bacteria, cells of hematologic origin).

Transmission electron microscopic evaluation of seminal preparations

In most so-called "idiopathic" cases of infertility, subtle lesions of the plasma membrane, acrosome, nuclear chromatin, and mitochondria are not uncommon. Using a transmission electron microscope (JEOL-1200EX JEOL USA, Inc., Peabody, Massachusetts), thin sections stained with uranyl acetate and lead citrate are evaluated for ultrastructural defects in these spermatozoal organelles. Although transmission electron microscopic examination does not permit quantification of morphologic defects, it elucidates light microscopic findings in characterizing the lesions, such as defective plasma membranes and prematurely reacted acrosomes (Fig. 2), incomplete condensation and breakage of chromatin (Fig. 3), and swollen degenerate mitochondria (Fig. 4). The use of transmission electron microscopy also facilitates the identification of cellular components other than spermatozoa that are often present in abnormal seminal ejaculates, such as the pathogens, leukocytes, denuded cells, and cellular debris (Fig. 5) from reproductive organs resulting from various disease conditions.

Indicators of common clinical aberrations and possible etiology

The ability to identify what is otherwise dubbed as "debris" at the light microscopic level often provides information that might have valuable diagnostic and prognostic potential. For example, incomplete condensation of chromatin (see Fig. 3B) or apoptosis of spermatozoal nuclei leads to breakage of chromatin, resulting in flocculent aggregates that are not discernible by light microscopy (see Fig. 3A), and is often ignored. A variety of etiologic factors, such as exposure to environmental toxicants and oxidative stress, are known to cause sperm DNA fragmentation. Damage to sperm mitochondria as seen in Fig. 4D is also induced by a variety of etiologic agents,

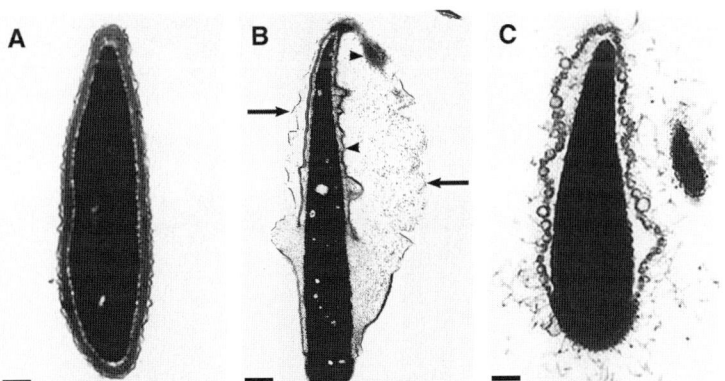

Fig. 2. Transmission electron micrographs of sagittal sections of equine spermatozoal heads. (*A*) Normal sperm head with condensed chromatin tightly enveloped by the acrosome and outer plasma membrane. (*B*) Abnormal sperm head with nuclear vacuolations, a dysplastic acrosome (*arrowheads*), and a swollen disrupted plasma membrane (*arrows*). (*C*) Acrosome-reacted sperm head. Note the acrosomic vesicles resulting from fusion of the inner and outer acrosomal membranes. Normally, an acrosome reaction takes place in the female reproductive tract in the vicinity of the ovum. A premature acrosome reaction as sperm is ejaculated indicates an altered milieu in seminal plasma. Scale bar: 0.25 μm.

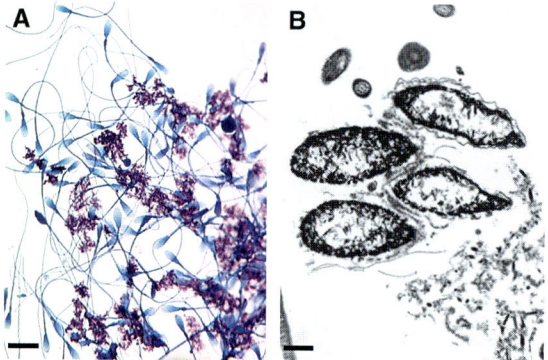

Fig. 3. Chromatin clumps resulting from breakage of incompletely condensed equine spermatozoal nuclei. (*A*) Toluidine blue–stained dry smear. Note the darkly stained clumps of chromatin, which are commonly ignored as debris. (*B*) Transmission electron micrograph of four incompletely condensed spermatozoal nuclei with ruptured plasma membranes. Note the flocculent chromatin fragments in the lower right corner. A variety of environmental factors can cause impaired chromatin condensation and breakage. Scale bars: (*A*) 10 µm, (*B*) 1 µm.

including physical factors like sudden changes in temperature. Such structural changes reflect impaired ATP production and, consequently, sperm motility.

Seminiferous epithelium is sensitive to a wide variety of environmental and endogenous factors, and insults are manifested as a spectrum of

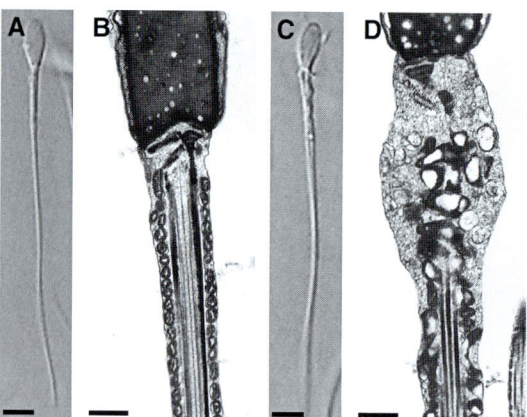

Fig. 4. Mitochondria in the midpieces of equine spermatozoa. Photomicrographs of spermatozoa show normal (*A*) and abnormal (*C*) midpieces. Transmission electron micrographs of normal (*B*) and abnormal (*D*) mitochondria in midpieces. In *D*, note the conspicuous swelling of mitochondria compacting the cristal matrix to an electron-dense band in the periphery of the mitochondria. These are the terminal stages of mitochondrial degeneration. This midpiece also has retained a proximal cytoplasmic droplet. A variety of toxicants can cause mitochondrial lesions and dysfunction. Scale bars: (*A, C*) 10 µm, (*B, D*) 0.5 µm.

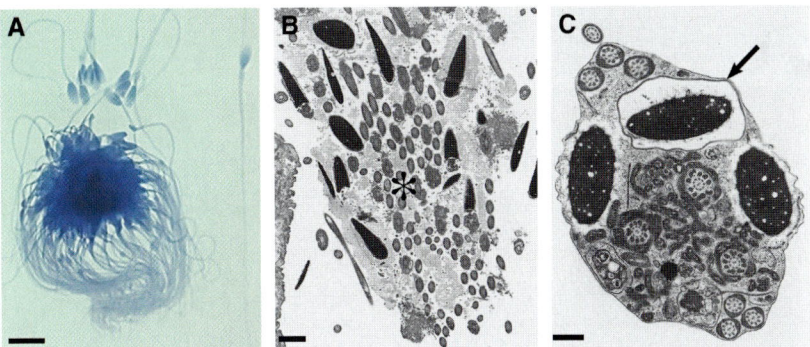

Fig. 5. Denuded seminiferous epithelium with fragments of Sertoli cells containing a cohort of elongated spermatids. (*A*) Photomicrograph of an exfoliated apical portion of seminiferous epithelium with embedded and elongated spermatids that can be mistaken for spermatozoal agglutination. (*B, C*) Exfoliated fragments of seminiferous epithelium seen in transmission electron micrographs provide evidence that such clusters are degenerate. (*B*) Note cross sections of spermatozoal tails cut at various levels (*); compare with proteinaceous aggregate in the center of agglutinated spermatozoa in Fig. 6C. (*C*) Dysplastic acrosome (*arrow*) and nuclear vacuolations are seen. These lesions and ultimate denudation of portions of the seminiferous epithelium result from degenerative changes in the testis. Scale bars: (*A*) 10 μm, (*B*) 1 μm, (*C*) 0.5 μm.

degenerative lesions ranging from prematurely shed spermatids to exfoliation of aggregates of germinal epithelium. In severe instances, exfoliation of fragments of Sertoli cells can occur (see Fig. 5). The degeneration and repair processes in seminiferous epithelium impair spermiogenesis, resulting in such lesions as those seen in Figs. 2 through 5. The presence of prematurely acrosome-reacted spermatozoa as seen in Fig. 2C indicates an altered milieu in seminal fluid that typically results from an inflammatory process in the reproductive tract. Immune disorders, rupture, and loss of integrity of seminiferous tubules or excurrent ducts resulting in sperm granulomatous reactions often produce autosperm antibodies, which result in aggregation of ejaculated spermatozoa as seen in Fig. 6.

Once established, some of these lesions continue to manifest over a lifetime. In this respect, acrosomal dysgenesis, characterized by the sharing of an acrosome by two or more spermatozoa (Fig. 7), warrants special mention. Sperm nuclear-acrosomal defects identical to those encountered in subfertile or infertile stallions can be experimentally induced in rabbits by developmental exposure to industrial chemical contaminants found commonly in drinking water [18], cosmetic nebulizers, and plasticizing chemicals (eg, phthalate esters) [19] that are found ubiquitously in the environment as well as in agricultural pesticides, such as vinclozolin [20]. Interestingly, we found that several stallions manifested similar types of nuclear acrosomal defects consistently over a 5- to 6-year period of observation, indicating that these defects are inducible and perpetuating; it is likely that a permanent epigenetic change had been induced in some but

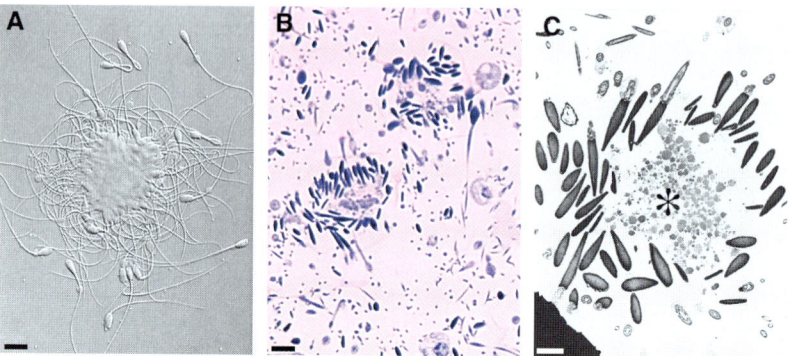

Fig. 6. Spermatozoal agglutination. (*A*) Differential interference contrast (Nomarski) micrograph of agglutinated spermatozoa in a wet smear. (*B*) Bright-field micrograph of a thick section of pelleted cells stained with toluidine blue shows two aggregates of agglutinated spermatozoa. (*C*) Transmission electron micrograph of agglutinated spermatozoa. Note a proteinaceous core (∗) in all aggregates. Usually, spermatozoal agglutination occurs after immune disorders, resulting in the formation of autosperm antibodies. Scale bars: (*A, B*) 10 μm, (*C*) 1 μm.

not all stem spermatogonia or Sertoli cells. Perhaps these horses had been unwittingly exposed to pollutants similar to those we tested in rabbits. Idiopathic infertility in the stallion may not be that hard to explain after all.

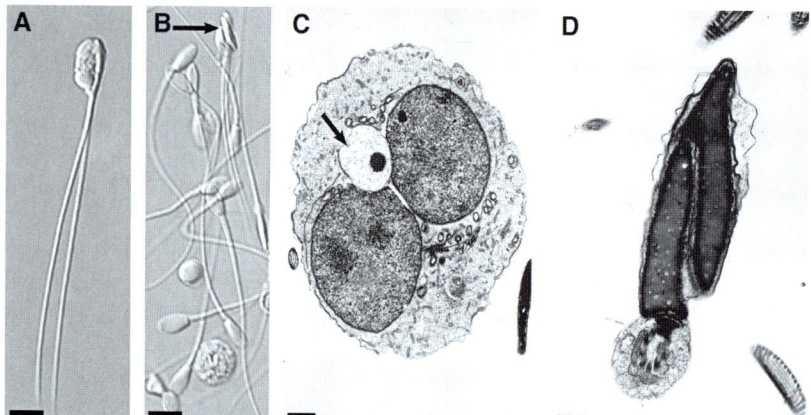

Fig. 7. Acrosomal dysgenesis with shared acrosomes. (*A, B*) Differential interference contrast micrographs of two conjoined spermatozoa with malformed heads. Note the presence of a dysplastic acrosome (*arrow*) shared between the two spermatozoal heads. (*C, D*) Transmission electron micrographs show morphogenesis of conjoined spermatozoa with a shared acrosome. As the two adjacent round spermatids differentiate, they share a common acrosomic vesicle (*arrow*) (*C*), which spreads around both spermatoidal nuclei as they condense and elongate (*D*), resulting in conjoined spermatozoa. These unique defects seem to result from developmental exposure to a variety of environmental pollutants. Scale bars: (*A, B*) 10 μm, (*C, D*) 0.5 μm.

Summary

Conventional light microscopic evaluation of a seminal ejaculate does not fully avail potential indicators of functional impairment in spermatozoal organelles. The technique of critical quantitative evaluation of morphologic features of individual structural components of spermatozoa at a light microscopic level in conjunction with critical qualitative evaluation of spermatozoal organelles at an ultrastructural level, as described in this article, is a valuable clinical tool. Compared with a battery of sperm function assays used in human andrology clinics, this relatively less expensive and simple technique is an efficient functional and diagnostic tool.

References

[1] Dott HM, Foster GC. A technique for studying the morphology of mammalian spermatozoa which are eosinophilic in a differential 'live-dead' stain. J Reprod Fertil 1972;29:443–5.
[2] Garner DL, Johnson LA, Yue ST, et al. Dual DNA staining assessment of bovine sperm viability using SYBR-14 and propidium iodide. J Androl 1994;15:620–9.
[3] Farlin ME, Jasko DJ, Graham JK, et al. Assessment of Pisum sativum agglutinin in identifying acrosomal damage in stallion spermatozoa. Mol Reprod Dev 1992;32:23–7.
[4] Thomas CA, Garner DL, DeJarnette JM, et al. Fluorometric assessments of acrosomal integrity and viability in cryopreserved bovine spermatozoa. Biol Reprod 1997;56:991–8.
[5] Gravance CG, Garner DL, Baumber J, et al. Assessment of equine sperm mitochondrial function using JC-1. Theriogenology 2000;53:1691–703.
[6] Thomas CA, Garner DL, DeJarnette JM, et al. Effect of cryopreservation of bovine sperm organelle function and viability as determined by flow cytometry. Biol Reprod 1998;58: 786–93.
[7] Evenson DP, Jost LK, Marshall D, et al. Utility of the sperm chromatin structure assay as a diagnostic and prognostic tool in the human fertility clinic. Hum Reprod 1999;14:1039–49.
[8] Fernandez JL, Muriel L, Goyanes V, et al. Simple determination of human sperm DNA fragmentation with an improved sperm chromatin dispersion test. Fertil Steril 2005;84:833–42.
[9] Kirk ES, Squires EL, Graham JK. Comparison of in vitro laboratory analyses with the fertility of cryopreserved stallion spermatozoa. Theriogenology 2005;64:1422–39.
[10] Barth AD, Oko RJ. Abnormal morphology of bovine spermatozoa. Ames (IA): Iowa State University Press; 1989.
[11] Holstein AF, Roosen-Runge EC, Schirren C. Illustrated pathology of human spermatogenesis. Berlin: Grosse Verlag; 1988.
[12] Seed J, Chapin RE, Clegg ED, et al. Methods for assessing sperm motility, morphology, and counts in the rat, rabbit, and dog: a consensus report. ILSI Risk Science Institute Expert Working Group on Sperm Evaluation. Reprod Toxicol 1996;10:237–44.
[13] Veeramachaneni DNR, Sawyer HR. Use of semen as biopsy material for assessment of health status of the stallion reproductive tract. Vet Clin North Am Equine Pract 1996;12:101–10.
[14] Zamboni L. The ultrastructural pathology of the spermatozoon as a cause of infertility: the role of electron microscopy in the evaluation of semen quality. Fertil Steril 1987;48:711–34.
[15] Russell LD, Ettlin RA, Sinha-Hikim AP, et al. Histological and histopathological evaluation of the testis. Clear Water (FL): Cache River Press; 1990.
[16] McEntee K. Reproductive pathology of domestic mammals. New York: Academic Press; 1990.
[17] Veeramachaneni DNR, Moeller CL, Pickett BW, et al. On processing and evaluation of equine seminal samples for cytopathology and fertility assessment: the utility of electron microscopy. J Equine Vet Sci 1993;13:207–15.

[18] Veeramachaneni DNR, Palmer JS, Amann RP. Long-term effects on male reproduction of early exposure to common chemical contaminants in drinking water. Hum Reprod 2001;16: 979–87.
[19] Higuchi TT, Palmer JS, Gray LE Jr, et al. Effects of dibutyl phthalate in male rabbits following in utero, adolescent, or post-pubertal exposure. Toxicol Sci 2003;72:301–13.
[20] Veeramachaneni DNR, Palmer JS, Amann RP, et al. Disruption of sexual function, FSH secretion, and spermiogenesis in rabbits following developmental exposure to vinclozolin, a fungicide. Reproduction 2006;131:805–16.

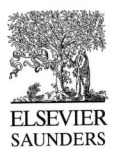

Advanced Insemination Techniques in Mares

Lee Morris, BVSc, DVSc

EquiBreed Ltd, 673 State Highway 1, RD 4, Cambridge 2351, New Zealand

Artificial insemination has been used successfully in the horse since 1322, when semen from an Arabian stallion was recovered from the vagina of a recently mated mare, transported in camel milk, and deposited into the vagina of another mare to produce a foal [1]. Interest in artificial insemination was reignited during the late nineteenth century and early twentieth century in Britain. The Russians and Chinese then seized on this method of expanding their national herds and used artificial insemination in more than 600,000 mares between 1930 and 1960 [1]. Since then, semen collection, handling, and conventional artificial insemination techniques have been refined and described in detail [2,3].

To overcome the variability in fertility among stallions for fresh, chilled, or frozen semen [4], the minimum recommended number of spermatozoa contained within a conventional insemination dose is generally greater than 300×10^6 progressively motile spermatozoa for fresh semen [5–8] and greater than 200×10^6 progressively motile spermatozoa for frozen semen [3]. It has been shown that conventional transcervical insemination of mares with 100×10^6 or less spermatozoa results in unsatisfactory pregnancy rates per cycle [9,10]. Furthermore, provided the inseminate contains an adequate number of spermatozoa, acceptable pregnancy rates have been reported after conventional insemination of mares with semen at rates as little as 0.6 mL [11] or as much as 120 mL [12]. Nevertheless, it has also been demonstrated that pregnancy rates in mares [13] and sperm survival rates in vitro are optimized when extended equine spermatozoa are maintained at concentrations between 25 and 50×10^6 total spermatozoa per milliliter [14].

Despite the high numbers and specific concentrations of spermatozoa required for optimal fertility, it has been demonstrated that most of the ejaculate is effectively and rapidly evacuated from the uterus through the relaxed

---

E-mail address: lee@equibreed.co.nz

estrous cervix [15]. Indeed, only a small proportion of the ejaculate remains on the uterine side of the papillae of each uterotubal junction [16], and few spermatozoa are observed within the oviduct at different stages of the estrous cycle in mares [17,18]. Based on uterine lavage studies, sperm migration from the uterus into the oviduct takes less than 4 hours [19]. This process of sperm transport through the mare's uterus serves as a selective gradient that results in huge losses of spermatozoa [16], regardless of the concentration of the original inseminate [20]. Recently, Troedsson and colleagues [21] demonstrated that components within seminal plasma modulate sperm transport and effectively protect viable spermatozoa from phagocytosis during the uterine phase of sperm transport. At the same time, components within the seminal plasma enhance chemotaxis and facilitate the removal of dead spermatozoa by phagocytosis [21]. Once within the oviduct, the fertilizing population of spermatozoa may be further protected from any inflammation or phagocytosis associated with postbreeding endometritis [22]. Consequently, this preferential selection of viable spermatozoa during sperm transport results in high proportions ($>90\%$) of morphologically normal spermatozoa in the oviduct, even when mares have been inseminated with ejaculates containing greater than 85% morphologically abnormal spermatozoa [16].

Knowledge of the presence of a sperm reservoir at the uterotubal junction [16] and the low numbers of spermatozoa present in the oviduct that result in normal fertilization and pregnancy rates [23] enables us to exploit low numbers of sex-preselected spermatozoa, cryopreserved epididymal spermatozoa, and the limited doses of frozen semen that are available from individual stallions. The advantages of reducing the distance the spermatozoa have to travel in the uterus by depositing them closer to the oviduct have been evaluated in sheep [24], pigs [25,26], and human beings [27]. Similarly, in mares, a number of methods designed to deposit spermatozoa closer to the site of fertilization have evolved in recent years, which include deep uterine insemination [28], hysteroscopic insemination [29], gamete intrafallopian transfer (GIFT) [30], and intrafollicular insemination [31].

Deep uterine insemination

Buchanan and coworkers [28] developed a deep uterine insemination technique to deposit low numbers of spermatozoa closer to the uterotubal junction. This insemination method involves guiding an insemination pipette through the uterine lumen by manipulation of the pipette per rectum until its tip is visualized by ultrasound or palpated in the cranial part of the uterine horn. Several different types of flexible pipettes (Minitube Universal Insemination Pipette and Gun, Minitube, Landshut, Germany [32]); IMV Flexible Equine Catheter, 007356,30 IMV Technologies, Cedex, France [33]) or the rigid disposable implant gun (Disposable Insemination gun, B6-3650; Continental Plastic, Delaver, Wisconsin [34]) have been used for this insemination method. The insemination dose is typically loaded into a 0.25- or 0.5-mL straw, which is inserted into the pipette. Buchanan and coworkers [28] achieved 35% pregnancy rates in mares inseminated with 25×10^6 sex-preselected spermatozoa in 1 or 0.2 mL by deep uterine insemination with a rigid pipette. In this study, a high embryonic loss rate (38%) was observed between days 16 and 60, which may have been associated with inflammation caused by passing the relatively inflexible insemination pipette along the uterine lumen during insemination. Since then, it has been demonstrated that deep uterine insemination of 20 or 200×10^6 frozen spermatozoa with a flexible pipette is not detrimental to uterine health [35]. In an attempt to improve the efficacy of the deep uterine insemination method, Nie and Johnson [36] inseminated mares with 1×10^6 spermatozoa that had been filtered through a glass wool/Sephadex column. Their pregnancy results were disappointingly low (7%–19%) and may reflect the possibility that less than 1×10^6 spermatozoa actually reached the uterotubal junction.

Hysteroscopic insemination

The uterotubal papilla, or the gateway to the oviduct, is readily visualized during hysteroscopy [29,37]; consequently, it is possible to use this technology to deposit small numbers of spermatozoa directly onto this papilla close to the sperm reservoir in the mare [16]. The hysteroscopic insemination technique involves aspiration of a small volume (<250 μL) of the inseminate into a catheter (V-EFIS-2-200; COOK, Eight Mile Plains, Australia) that has been inserted into the working channel of a Pentax EPM 3000 videoendoscope (Slough Berkshire, United Kingdom), which is 1.6 m in length and 12 mm in outer diameter. The tip of the scope is passed through the cervix and into the uterus. The uterine lumen is insufflated with filtered air to facilitate passage of the scope toward the uterotubal junction with minimal trauma. When the uterotubal papilla ipsilateral to the ovary containing the dominant preovulatory follicle is visualized, the catheter is extruded from the tip of the scope. The small volume of spermatozoa is deposited directly onto the papilla, without attempting to catheterize its os. Hysteroscopic insemination is typically performed once at a single fixed time after induction of ovulation. For frozen semen [38], hysteroscopic insemination is performed 32 hours after administration of human chorionic gonadotropin (hCG; Chorulon; Intervet, Milton Keynes, United Kingdom).

Vazquez and colleagues [39] investigated the use of hysteroscopic insemination in an attempt to improve the fertility of subfertile stallions. In their study, three pregnancies were obtained when 10 mares were inseminated hysteroscopically with a 20-μL volume of the inseminate that contained 4×10^6 spermatozoa. In similar studies performed at the same time, Manning and coworkers [40] attempted to cannulate the oviduct hysteroscopically to deposit 1 or 10×10^6 spermatozoa suspended in diluent

(0.16–0.25 mL) into the oviduct. The low pregnancy rates observed in this study may be attributable to the negative effect of excessive insemination volumes within the oviduct or damage to the oviduct during cannulation attempts. It is possible that any attempt to bypass the selective barrier of the uterotubal junction may be detrimental to fertility.

Morris and colleagues [29] inseminated mares hysteroscopically with 10, 5, 1, 0.5, 0.1, or 0.001 $\times$ 10^6 motile spermatozoa suspended in Tyrode's medium (0.03–0.15 mL). The fresh semen was prepared for insemination after centrifugation through a discontinuous Percoll (Sigma-Aldrich, Castle Hill, NSW, Australia) density gradient. High per cycle conception rates of greater than 60% were achieved in the mares inseminated with 10, 5, or 1 $\times$ 10^6 spermatozoa. Hysteroscopic insemination with 0.5 $\times$ 10^6 or less motile spermatozoa began to approach the limit of fertilization success, however. These doses represent 1/500th of the accepted minimum recommended dose of 500 $\times$ 10^6 spermatozoa used for conventional uterine body insemination in the mare [3].

Hysteroscopic insemination of commercially available frozen-thawed semen may increase the potential number of doses of frozen semen from particular stallions. Nevertheless, variability in the fertility of frozen-thawed semen observed among commercially available stallions [4] remained evident when a volume (0.5–1 mL) of frozen-thawed semen containing 50 to 100 $\times$ 10^6 spermatozoa was deposited onto the uterotubal junction hysteroscopically within 6 hours of ovulation and compared with the per cycle pregnancy rates obtained after conventional insemination with frozen-thawed semen from the same stallions in a commercial breeding program [41]. Morris and colleagues [38] demonstrated that similarly high pregnancy rates (>55% per cycle) can be obtained after insemination of frozen spermatozoa: n of only 0.5 mL (14 $\times$ 10^6) from two fertile stallions when inseminated only once, hysteroscopically or conventionally, at 32 hours after induction of ovulation with hCG.

In an attempt to simulate the in vivo selection process for morphologically normal spermatozoa, some studies have processed fresh spermatozoa through density gradients to enhance selection of those with intact plasma membranes [29,42]. In these studies, this step was performed during the centrifugation process to concentrate the fresh spermatozoa for insemination. Similarly, frozen-thawed ejaculated [43] and epididymal [44] spermatozoa have been washed through density gradients to remove those damaged by the cryopreservation process. No beneficial effect of this treatment was observed on the fertility of low numbers of frozen-thawed ejaculated or epididymal spermatozoa, however.

It has also been observed that the incidence of postbreeding endometritis after hysteroscopic insemination is negligible. Indeed, only 1% of mares inseminated hysteroscopically with fresh spermatozoa [29] and 3.5% of mares inseminated hysteroscopically with frozen-thawed spermatozoa had ultrasonographic evidence of intrauterine fluid accumulation after insemination [38]. Therefore, it is apparent that this is a minimally invasive method of insemination in normal mares. Sieme and coworkers [45] observed a significant interaction between mare fertility and insemination technique, such that hysteroscopic insemination produced lower pregnancy rates in problem mares than in normal mares and conventional insemination produced higher pregnancy rates in problem mares than in normal mares.

Rigby and colleagues [46] compared the fertility of deep uterine with hysteroscopic insemination of 5×10^6 fresh spermatozoa suspended in diluent (200 µL). There were no statistically significant differences observed in the pregnancy rates of the mares inseminated hysteroscopically (13 [62%] of 21 mares) or after deep uterine insemination (10 [50%] of 20 mares). The deep uterine insemination method is more practical, less labor-intensive, and easier to perform than the hysteroscopic insemination method, which requires two or three people. This concept was reinforced when no differences in fertility were observed in mares inseminated hysteroscopically or by conventional insemination with 14×10^6 motile frozen-thawed spermatozoa in diluent (0.5 mL) 32 hours after induction of ovulation [38]. In this study, however, once the numbers of spermatozoa were reduced to 3×10^6, hysteroscopic deposition of the spermatozoa directly onto the uterotubal junction produced significantly better pregnancy rates than those obtained by conventional insemination of low numbers of spermatozoa.

Epididymal spermatozoa

The first reported pregnancy from the use of frozen-thawed stallion spermatozoa was in a mare inseminated with epididymal spermatozoa in 1957 [47]. Since then, little has been published on the fertility of epididymal spermatozoa in horses. In sheep, however, it has been shown that the in vivo fertility of cauda epididymal ram spermatozoa only achieved that of ejaculated spermatozoa when it was deposited surgically in the region of the uterotubal junction [48]. Spermatozoa require a period of plasma membrane maturation as they migrate from the caput to the cauda epididymis. During this maturation process, the potential for motility is acquired, albeit suppressed until the time of ejaculation. The reasons for the differences in fertility between epididymal and ejaculated spermatozoa may include the variations in cell surface characteristics and the lower progressive motility of epididymal spermatozoa.

Morris and colleagues [44] inseminated 117 mares with fresh and frozen-thawed epididymal spermatozoa 32 hours after administration of hCG. The mean (±SD) total progressive motility of frozen-thawed epididymal spermatozoa (n = 14) with or without prior exposure to seminal plasma was, respectively, 16.4 ± 5.1% and 20 ± 4.4%. Thus, the simple addition of seminal plasma to epididymal spermatozoa failed to improve its progressive motility to the level of frozen-thawed ejaculated spermatozoa (30.2 ± 8.3%, n = 64). When 200×10^6 fresh epididymal spermatozoa were deposited directly onto the uterotubal papilla hysteroscopically, 45% (9 of 20) mares conceived [44]. These conception rates were reduced substantially when mares were inseminated with similar numbers of frozen-thawed epididymal spermatozoa by conventional (1 [8%] of 13 mares) or hysteroscopic (9 [18%] of 51 mares) insemination. When the frozen-thawed epididymal spermatozoa were processed through sperm Tyrodes albumin lactate pyruvate (TALP), 29% (7 of 24 mares) per cycle conception rates were obtained after hysteroscopic insemination with only 5 to 10×10^6 spermatozoa. No mares conceived (0 of 9 mares) when inseminated hysteroscopically within 6 hours after ovulation with 200×10^6 frozen-thawed epididymal spermatozoa.

Sex-sorted spermatozoa

Since the production of the first live offspring from sex-sorted spermatozoa [49], there have been many developments in the fluorescence-activated cell separation (FACS) procedures that separate X- and Y-chromosome–bearing spermatozoa based on their difference in DNA content. This difference in DNA content is 3.7% in the stallion [50]. The purity of the sorted sperm population can be adjusted to select greater than 90% of X- or Y-sperm populations. The fastest and most accurate sort rates are achievable when only the X-sperm population is selected because of the larger size of the X-chromosome than the Y-chromosome [51] Perhaps the smaller total difference in DNA between X- and Y-chromosome–bearing spermatozoa in stallions (3.7%) compared with rams (4.2%) contributed to lower reported sort rates of 1000 spermatozoa per second for stallions [42] compared with 4000 to 5000 spermatozoa per second for rams [52]. Once sorting is completed, the stallion spermatozoa are centrifuged to provide 20 to 67×10^6 spermatozoa per milliliter for insemination [53,54].

The low number of spermatozoa available after sorting requires that this technology be combined with advanced methods of insemination. Pregnancies have been obtained from many different methods of insemination with sex-sorted spermatozoa, including surgical oviductal insemination of only 50,000 spermatozoa [30], deep uterine insemination of 25×10^6 spermatozoa [28], and hysteroscopic insemination of 5 to 20×10^6 spermatozoa [42,53,54]. Indeed, insemination of 50×10^3 sex-sorted X-bearing spermatozoa directly into the oviduct produced the first foal from sex-sorted spermatozoa [55]. When the insemination dose of spermatozoa approaches the limits of the estimated population of the sperm reservoir [29], it has been shown that hysteroscopic insemination of a small volume of spermatozoa provides better pregnancy rates than deep uterine insemination [38,54]. After hysteroscopic insemination, it is possible to obtain satisfactory pregnancy rates with 5×10^6 fresh [42] or 20×10^6 stored [54] sex-sorted stallion spermatozoa.

To optimize the fertility of frozen sex-sorted spermatozoa, Lindsey and coworkers [54] investigated the effects of three different extenders on post-thaw motility over time and found that FR5 was the preferred extender. In this trial, sorted spermatozoa were frozen with 2.5% glycerol in 0.25-mL straws over liquid N_2 vapor. The pregnancy rate after insemination of the sorted frozen-thawed spermatozoa was low (13%), however, and significantly less than the pregnancy rate obtained with similarly small numbers of nonsorted frozen-thawed spermatozoa (38%). Currently, further studies are underway to improve the freezability of sex-sorted spermatozoa [56].

The ability to achieve satisfactory pregnancy rates after hysteroscopic insemination with low numbers of fresh or stored sex-sorted spermatozoa but not with frozen-thawed sorted spermatozoa suggests that physiologic questions about the timing of insemination and the ability of these frozen-thawed cells to bind to the oviduct or oocyte at the appropriate time are yet to be answered. The cryopreservation of sex-sorted spermatozoa and their effects on sperm membrane physiology at different stages, before and after sorting, warrant further investigation so that damaging effects of centrifugation, incubation, and dilution can be minimized and protective diluents can be developed [57].

Oviductal insemination

The ability to produce pregnancies after surgical deposition of low numbers of spermatozoa directly into the equine oviduct answers a multitude of questions about sperm-oocyte interactions. Carnevale and colleagues [58] achieved conception rates of 67% (12 of 18 mares) after GIFT of an oocyte with 2 to 5×10^5 fresh spermatozoa. The success of GIFT demonstrates that complete capacitation can occur in the oviduct in the absence of a uterine phase of sperm transport. Similarly, there were no significant differences in the pregnancy rates observed in mares inseminated conventionally with 1×10^9 fresh spermatozoa (17 [65%] of 26 mares) and in mares that were inseminated directly into their oviduct (12 [55%] of 22 mares) with only 2×10^5 fresh spermatozoa [59]. These studies also reveal that gamete transfer into the oviduct contralateral to the recipient's impending ovulation can result in normal fertilization of the transferred oocyte in the absence of follicular fluid, which would usually be released during ovulation. Furthermore, failure of the recipient's own oocyte to undergo fertilization demonstrates that there is no significant retrograde transport of spermatozoa from the contralateral oviduct through the uterus and into the oviduct ipsilateral to ovulation.

The fertility of chilled (4 [13%] of 31 mares) or frozen-thawed (1 [8%] of 12 mares) spermatozoa when used in oviductal insemination was less than the fertility of the same amount (2×10^5 fresh spermatozoa). It is speculated that the reduced fertility of chilled or frozen-thawed spermatozoa is attributable to the presence of extenders, which may interfere with the binding of spermatozoa to the oviduct or oocyte [60].

Intrafollicular insemination

Pregnancies have not yet been obtained in mares after insemination of spermatozoa directly into a preovulatory follicle [31]. To investigate the value of this insemination method in more detail, Parlevliet and coworkers [61] evaluated spermatozoa recovered from preovulatory follicles after intrafollicular insemination of 50 or 500×10^6 spermatozoa and found that all the spermatozoa had undergone a spontaneous acrosome reaction. Similarly, Leão and colleagues [62] did not produce any pregnancies after insemination of 20×10^6 frozen-thawed spermatozoa directly into preovulatory follicles in 20 mares. The results of these equine studies may shed some light on the poor efficacy of intrafollicular inseminations observed in human infertility programs [63].

Summary

Different methods of advanced in vivo insemination are constantly emerging to improve the fertility of stallions and the different types of spermatozoa (fresh, chilled, frozen, epididymal, and sex-sorted) that are now available. As technology advances, spermatozoa that are currently not capable of fertilization in conventional circumstances may become fertile if deposited at different sites within the reproductive tract and at different times with respect to ovulation.

References

[1] Allen WR. The development and application of the modern reproductive technologies to horse breeding. Reprod Domest Anim 2005;40:310–29.
[2] Squires EL, Pickett BW, Graham JK, et al. Cooled and frozen semen. Bulletin no. 9. Fort Collins (CO): Animal Reproduction and Biotechnology Laboratory, Colorado State University; 1999.
[3] Pickett BW, Voss JL, Squires EL, et al. Collection, preparation and insemination of stallion semen. Bulletin no. 10. Fort Collins (CO): Animal Reproduction and Biotechnology Laboratory, Colorado State University; 2000.
[4] Boyle MS. Assessing the potential fertility of frozen stallion semen. In: Allen WR, Wade JF, editors. Havemeyer Foundation monograph series no. 1. Newmarket, UK: R & W Publications Ltd; 1999. p. 13–6.
[5] Householder DD, Pickett BW, Voss JL, et al. Effect of extender, numbers of spermatozoa and hCG on equine fertility. Equine Vet Sci 1981;1:9–13.
[6] Pickett BW, Voss JL. The effect of semen extenders and sperm number on mare fertility. J Reprod Fertil Suppl 1975;23:95–8.
[7] Gahne S, Gånheim A, Malmgren L. Effect of insemination dose on pregnancy rate in mares. Theriogenology 1998;49:1071–4.
[8] Vidament M, Dupere AM, Julienne P, et al. Equine frozen semen freezability and fertility field results. Theriogenology 1997;48:907–17.
[9] Pace MM, Sullivan JJ. Effect of timing of insemination, numbers of spermatozoa and extender components on the pregnancy rate in mares inseminated with frozen stallion semen. J Reprod Fertil Suppl 1975;23:115–21.

[10] Voss JL, Wallace RA, Squires EL, et al. Effects of synchronisation and frequency of insemination on fertility. J Reprod Fertil Suppl 1979;27:257–61.
[11] Allen WR, Bowen JM, Frank CJ, et al. The current position of AI in horse breeding. Equine Vet J 1976;8:72–4.
[12] Bedford SJ, Hinrichs K. The effect of insemination volume on pregnancy rates of pony mares. Theriogenology 1994;42:571–8.
[13] Rowley HS, Squires EL, Pickett BW. Effect of insemination volume on embryo recovery in mares. J Equine Vet Sci 1990;10:298–300.
[14] Varner DD, Blanchard TL, Love CL, et al. Effects of semen fractionation and dilution ratio on spermatozoal motility parameters. Theriogenology 1987;28:709–23.
[15] Katila T, Sankari S, Mäkelä O. Transport of spermatozoa in the genital tracts of mares. J Reprod Fertil Suppl 2000;56:571–8.
[16] Scott MA, Liu IKM, Overstreet JW, et al. The structural morphology and epithelial association of spermatozoa at the uterotubal junction: a descriptive study of equine spermatozoa in situ using scanning electron microscopy. J Reprod Fertil Suppl 2000;56:415–21.
[17] Parker WG, Sullivan JJ, First NL. Sperm transport and distribution in the mare. J Reprod Fertil Suppl 1975;23:63–6.
[18] Boyle MS, Cran DG, Allen WR, et al. Distribution of spermatozoa in the mare's oviduct. J Reprod Fertil Suppl 1987;35:79–86.
[19] Brinsko SP, Varner DD, Blanchard TL. The effect of uterine lavage performed four hours post insemination on pregnancy rate in mares. Theriogenology 1991;35:1111–9.
[20] Fiala SM, Pimental CA, Gregory RM, et al. Does equine sperm concentration influence the sperm migration to the oviducts. Anim Reprod Sci 2005;89:261–4.
[21] Troedsson MHT, Desvousges A, Alghamdi AS, et al. Components in seminal plasma regulating sperm transport and elimination. Anim Reprod Sci 2005;89:171–86.
[22] Bader H. An investigation of sperm migration into the oviducts of the mare. J Reprod Fertil Suppl 1982;32:59–64.
[23] Morris LHA, Hunter RHF, Tiplady CA, et al. Low numbers of spermatozoa in the equine oviduct are compatible with fertilization. In: Morris LHA, Foster L, Wade JF, editors. Havemeyer Foundation monograph series no. 6. From epididymis to embryo. Newmarket, UK: R & W Publications Ltd; 2001. p. 30–1.
[24] Lightfoot RJ, Salamon S. Fertility of ram spermatozoa frozen by the pellet method. I. Transport and viability of spermatozoa within the genital tract of the ewe. J Reprod Fertil 1970;22:385–98.
[25] Krüger C, Rath D, Johnson LA. Low dose insemination in synchronised gilts. Theriogenology 1999;52:1363–73.
[26] Martinez EA, Vazquez JL, Vazquez JM, et al. Successful low dose insemination by a fiberoptic endoscope technique in the sow [abstract]. Theriogenology 2000;53:201.
[27] Byrd W, Bradshaw K, Carr B, et al. A prospective randomized study of pregnancy rates following intrauterine and intracervical insemination using frozen donor sperm. Fertil Steril 1990;53:521–7.
[28] Buchanan BR, Seidel GE Jr, McCue PM, et al. Insemination of mares with low numbers of either unsexed or sexed spermatozoa. Theriogenology 2000;53:1333–44.
[29] Morris LHA, Hunter RHF, Allen WR. Hysteroscopic insemination of small numbers of spermatozoa at the uterotubal junction of preovulatory mares. J Reprod Fertil 2000;118:95–100.
[30] McCue PM, Fleury JJ, Denniston DJ, et al. Oviductal insemination of mares. J Reprod Fertil 2000;56:499–502.
[31] Eilts BE, Pinto CRF, Paccamonti DL, et al. Transvaginal intrafollicular sperm cell injection with concomitant artificial insemination in the cyclic mare. Theriogenology 2002;58:631–3.
[32] Minitube Universal Insemination Pipette and Gun. Available at: http://www.minitube.com. Accessed October, 2006.

[33] Flexible Equine Catheter IMV, 007356,30. Available at: http://www.imv-technologies.com. Accessed October, 2006.
[34] Disposable Insemination guns, B6–3650. Continental Plastic, USA. Available at: http://www.continentalplastic.com. Accessed October, 2006.
[35] Güvenc K, Reilas T, Katila T. Effect on insemination dose and site on uterine inflammatory response of mares. Theriogenology 2005;63:2504–12.
[36] Nie GJ, Johnson KE. Pregnancy rate in mares following insemination with a low-dose of progressively motile or filtered sperm cells deep in the uterine horn. In: Proceedings of the Equine Symposium and Society for Theriogenology Annual Conference [abstract]. Nashville (TN): Society of Theriogenology and The American College of Theriogenologists; 2000. p. 303.
[37] Bracher V, Allen WR. Videoendoscopic examination of the mare's uterus. I. Findings in normal fertile mares. Equine Vet J 1992;24:274–8.
[38] Morris LH, Tiplady CA, Allen WR. Pregnancy rates in mares after a single fixed-time hysteroscopic insemination of low numbers of frozen-thawed spermatozoa onto the uterotubal junction. Equine Vet J 2003;35:197–201.
[39] Vazquez JJ, Medina V, Lui IK, et al. Non-surgical utero-tubal insemination in the mare. In: Proceedings of the Annual Meeting Society for Theriogenology. Nashville (TN): Society for Theriogenology; 1998. p. 82–3.
[40] Manning ST, Bowman PA, Fraser LM, et al. Development of hysteroscopic insemination of the uterine tube in the mare. In: Proceedings of the Annual Meeting Society for Theriogenology. Nashville (TN): Society for Theriogenology; 1998. p. 84–5.
[41] Morris LHA, Allen WR. An overview of low dose insemination in the mare. Reprod Domest Anim 2002;37:206–10.
[42] Lindsey AC, Morris LH, Allen WR, et al. Hysteroscopic insemination of mares with low numbers of nonsorted or flow cytometrically sorted spermatozoa. Equine Vet J 2002;34: 128–32.
[43] Alvarenga MA, Leao KM. Hysteroscopic insemination of mares with low number of frozen-thawed spermatozoa selected by Percoll gradient. Theriogenology 2002;58:651–3.
[44] Morris LH, Tiplady CA, Allen WR. The in vivo fertility of caudal epididymal spermatozoa in the horse [abstract]. Theriogenology 2002;58:643–6.
[45] Sieme H, Schafer T, Stout TA, et al. The effects of different insemination regimes on fertility of mares. Theriogenology 2003;60:153–64.
[46] Rigby SL, Lindsey AC, Brinsko SP, et al. Pregnancy rates in mares following hysteroscopic or rectally-guided utero-tubal insemination with low sperm numbers [abstract]. In: Proceedings of the Third International Symposium on Stallion Reproduction [abstract]. Fort Collins (CO): Colorado State University; 2001. p. 49.
[47] Barker CAV, Gandier JCC. Pregnancy in a mare resulting from frozen epididymal spermatozoa. Can J Comp Med 1957;21:47–51.
[48] Fournier-Delpech S, Colas G, Courot M, et al. Epididymal sperm maturation in the ram: motility, fertilizing ability and embryonic survival after uterine artificial insemination in the ewe. Ann Biol Anim Bioch Biophys 1979;19:597–605.
[49] Johnson LA, Flook JP, Hawk HW. Sex preselection in rabbits: live birth from X and Y sperm separated by DNA and cell sorting. Biol Reprod 1989;41:199–203.
[50] Welch GR, Johnson LA. Sex preselection: laboratory validation of the sperm sex ratio of flow sorted X- and Y-sperm by sort reanalysis for DNA. Theriogenology 1999;52: 1343–52.
[51] Johnson LA, Welch GR. Sex preselection: high speed flow cytometric sorting of X- and Y-sperm for maximum efficiency. Theriogenology 1999;52:1323–41.
[52] Hollinshead FK, O'Brien JK, Maxwell WMC, et al. Production of lambs of predetermined sex after the insemination of ewes with low numbers of frozen-thawed sorted X- or Y-chromosome bearing spermatozoa. Reprod Fertil Dev 2002;14:503–8.

[53] Lindsey AC, Schenk JL, Graham JK, et al. Hysteroscopic insemination of low numbers of flow sorted fresh and frozen thawed stallion spermatozoa. Equine Vet J 2002;34:121–7.
[54] Lindsey AC, Varner DD, Seidel GE Jr, et al. Hysteroscopic or rectally guided, deep uterine insemination of mares with spermatozoa stored 18h at either 5°C or 15°C prior to flow cytometric sorting. Anim Reprod Sci 2005;85:125–30.
[55] Schmid RL, Kato H, Herickhoff LA, et al. Fertilization with sexed equine spermatozoa using intracytoplasmic sperm injection and oviductal insemination. In: Proceedings of the Seventh International Symposium on Equine Reproduction. Pretoria, South Africa; 1998. p. 139–40.
[56] Buss H, Clulow J, Sieme H, et al. Improvement of the freezability of sex-sorted stallion spermatozoa. Anim Reprod Sci 2005;89:315–8.
[57] Morris LHA. Challenges facing sex-preselection of stallion spermatozoa. Anim Reprod Sci 2005;89:147–59.
[58] Carnevale EM, Maclellan LJ, Coutinho da Silva MA, et al. Equine sperm-oocyte interaction: results after intraoviductal intrauterine inseminations of recipients for oocyte transfer. Anim Reprod Sci 2001;68:305–14.
[59] Coutinho da Silva MA, Carnevale EM, Maclellan LJ, et al. Effect of time of oocyte collection and site of insemination on oocyte transfer in mares. J Anim Sci 2002;80:1275–9.
[60] Coutinho da Silva MA, Carnevale EM, Maclellan LJ, et al. Oocyte transfer in mares with intrauterine or oviductal insemination using fresh, cooled and frozen stallion semen. Theriogenology 2004;61:705–13.
[61] Parlevliet JM, Lynn JW, Eilts BE, et al. Failure of embryo development after intrafollicular insemination in the horse: due to the sperm viability? In: Havemeyer Foundation Workshop. Proceedings of the Sixth International Symposium on Equine Embryo Transfer [abstract]. Newmarket, UK: R&W Publications Ltd. 2004. p. 25.
[62] Leão KM, Alvarenga MA, Puolli-Filho JN. Factors involved in failure of transvaginal intrafollicular insemination in mares. In: Havemeyer Foundation Workshop. Proceedings of the Sixth International Symposium on Equine Embryo Transfer [abstract]. Newmarket, UK: R&W Publications Ltd. 2004. p. 26.
[63] Nuojua-Huttunen S, Tuomivaara L, Juntunen K, et al. Intrafollicular insemination for the treatment of infertility. Hum Reprod 1995;10:91–3.

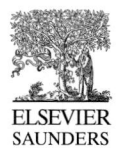

Breeding-Induced Endometritis in Mares

Mats H.T. Troedsson, DVM, PhD

Department of Large Animal Clinical Science, College of Veterinary Medicine, University of Florida, Gainesville, FL 32610–0136, USA

Endometritis is a common cause of infertility in broodmares [1]. In the past, the condition was believed to be exclusively the result of bacterial contamination of the uterus. Treatment strategies were focused on preventing bacteria from entering the uterus and on treating mares with signs of endometritis with antibiotics. Hughes and Loy [2] demonstrated that young reproductively sound mares had natural resistance to an experimentally induced infection. They concluded that local components of uterine defense mechanisms were responsible for the effective and rapid clearance of an infection in mares with natural resistance to uterine infection. Mares that failed to clear the uterus from an infection naturally were classified as susceptible to persistent endometritis [2]. More recent research on uterine defense mechanisms has increased our understanding of the pathophysiology of equine endometritis. Additional causative agents have been identified, and we have learned to separate uterine infections and a physiologic breeding-induced endometritis resulting from uterine exposure to semen.

Pathophysiology of breeding-induced endometritis

Transport of spermatozoa from the equine uterus to the oviduct is completed within 4 hours after breeding [3], and only a small portion of the ejaculated or inseminated spermatozoa reach the oviduct [4]. The rapid transport of spermatozoa to the oviduct coincides with increased uterine activity [5,6]. Increased myometrial contraction is also responsible for sperm elimination from the uterus through the cervix shortly after breeding. Not all excess spermatozoa are removed through this mechanism, however, and other uterine clearance mechanisms are necessary. Because a specific

E-mail address: troedsson@mail.vetmed.ufl.edu

immune response with a memory would be detrimental to fertility during a subsequent breeding, elimination of spermatozoa needs to be achieved by a combination of innate immune reactions and mechanical clearance. This mechanism involves a cascade of inflammatory reactions. In vitro and in vivo studies suggest that when equine spermatozoa enter the uterus, they activate complement in uterine secretion [7–10]. The cleavage of factor C5 into C5a and C5b triggers a chemotactic signal to polymorphonuclear neutrophils (PMNs), resulting in an influx of PMNs into the uterine lumen [9,11–13]. Activated PMNs bind to spermatozoa in the presence of complement factor C3b and complement-independent mechanisms [14]. The nature of this binding is unknown, but recent data suggest that it is mediated by the extrusion of DNA from PMNs forming neutrophil extracellular traps (NETs) and a traditional ligand receptor binding [15,16]. After binding, the spermatozoa are phagocytosed by the PMNs. During the activation of PMNs, prostaglandin $F_{2\alpha}$ ($PGF_{2\alpha}$) is released from the cell membrane by the metabolism of arachidonic acid via the cyclooxygenase pathway. In addition to being an inflammatory mediator, $PGF_{2\alpha}$ causes contraction of smooth muscle, including the myometrium [17]. Uterine contractions are believed to remove accumulated fluid and harmful inflammatory products from the uterus [13]. Once these products are removed from the uterine lumen, the inflammation subsides and the uterine environment returns to its normal state. Breeding-induced uterine inflammation is a physiologic reaction to semen, and it seems to be a normal process by which sperm is eliminated from the mare's reproductive tract. The reaction is probably necessary for normal survival and development of an embryo. A failure of the uterine defense mechanisms to eliminate an antigen and inflammatory products from the uterus effectively results in persistent endometritis. In approximately 15% of broodmares, the system fails and the initial physiologic inflammation becomes a pathologic problem, with a detrimental effect on fertility [18–20]. It is currently believed that a failure of mechanical aspects of the uterine defense system is the major contributor in the development of persistent endometritis. Using intrauterine inoculations of a combination of radioactive-labeled microspheres and bacteria, impaired uterine clearance was demonstrated in mares susceptible but not resistant to persistent endometritis [21,22]. Studies using scintigraphic measurements of uterine clearance of radioactive colloids further defined a delayed physical clearance in susceptible mares [23]. Using electromyography to register myometrial activity, it was observed that the impaired uterine clearance in susceptible mares was caused by reduced myometrial activity in response to the inflammation [24]. The mechanism of impaired myoelectrical activity in susceptible mares is still not fully understood, however. Using an in vitro model to study myometrial activity, it was suggested that mares susceptible to delayed uterine clearance had an intrinsic contractile defect of the myometrium [25]. A recent study found that susceptible mares had an increased uterine accumulation of nitric oxide in the uterine lumen 13 hours after insemination

[26]. Nitric oxide mediates smooth muscle relaxation, and the authors offered this effect as a possible explanation for myoelectrical activity below baseline between 6 and 19 hours into an inflammation in susceptible mares. The authors also observed an increased number of inducible nitric oxide synthase (iNOS)-positive mast cells as well as an upregulation of iNOS mRNA in the endometrium of susceptible mares [26]. The presence of mast cells suggests that histamine-mediated vasodilation may be involved in delayed uterine clearance of susceptible mares.

Factors other than impaired uterine contractility that can predispose to delayed uterine clearance include anatomic abnormalities of the reproductive tract. Mares with delayed uterine clearance often have a forward tilt of the uterus over the pelvic brim. This may be a contributing factor in an abnormal accumulation of fluid and inflammatory products after breeding. A failure of the cervix to relax during estrus or insufficient lymphatic drainage may also contribute to delayed clearance [27].

Role of seminal plasma in breeding-induced endometritis

In vitro experiments have shown that seminal plasma has a suppressive effect on complement activation, PMN chemotaxis, and phagocytosis [14,28,29]. A function of seminal plasma may be to act as an inflammatory modulator in the uterus, which could be of importance for the transient nature of breeding-induced endometritis. Although in vivo experiments have shown a PMN influx into the uterine lumen in response to seminal plasma [11,30], the duration of the induced inflammation is consistently of shorter duration when seminal plasma is included in the insemination dose [30,31]. The mechanism by which seminal plasma shortens the duration of breeding-induced endometritis is not clear, but it could be the result of a modulation of inflammatory mediators or a stimulatory effect on myometrial activity [17,32]. The latter possibility may be less likely, because Katila and coworkers [33] reported a suppressive effect of seminal plasma on uterine contractility in horses. Clinical observations suggest that a marked and prolonged breeding-induced endometritis often follows insemination with frozen-thawed semen. It has been suggested that removal of seminal plasma before freezing of semen may contribute to the increased duration of breeding-induced endometritis. It is not clear, however, if the reduction of seminal plasma during preparation for cryopreservation is enough to suppress the modulatory effect of seminal plasma on breeding-induced endometritis [31].

Another function of seminal plasma in breeding-induced endometritis may be to protect spermatozoa from being phagocytosed and destroyed in an inflammatory environment. PMNs are present in the uterine lumen by 0.5 hours after breeding, but sperm transport is not completed until 3 to 4 hours later [3,34]. In addition, when mares are inseminated twice within a 24-hour period, semen from the second insemination is introduced into an inflammatory environment. This environment is detrimental to sperm motion characteristics, and spermatozoa seem to bind to PMNs, forming large clusters of PMN and spermatozoa [35]. Addition of seminal plasma reduces the binding between spermatozoa and inflammatory cells in vitro, and in vivo experiments also support a protective role of seminal plasma from PMN binding and phagocytosis of spermatozoa [36]. Insemination of viable spermatozoa without any seminal plasma into an inflammatory environment 12 hours after a previous insemination with killed spermatozoa was detrimental to fertility, but the fertility was restored to normal levels if seminal plasma was added to the second insemination dose [36]. The results are, however, somewhat conflicting with clinical observations that mares can conceive after artificial insemination with frozen-thawed semen, which often contains less than 5% seminal plasma, also in the presence of an ongoing inflammation from a previous artificial insemination [37,38]. Further investigations on the mechanism by which seminal plasma interferes with binding of spermatozoa to PMNs and determination of the critical amount of seminal plasma that is necessary for suppression of PMN and sperm binding may provide an explanation.

In vitro experiments have demonstrated that the effect of seminal plasma on PMN and sperm binding and phagocytosis is confined to a protein fraction in seminal plasma [14,36]. A subsequent study suggested that the effect of seminal plasma on PMN and sperm binding is specific to viable but not dead spermatozoa [39]. This effect seemed to be confined to a specific low-molecular-weight protein fraction within seminal plasma. It would, of course, be beneficial to fertility if viable spermatozoa were protected from being phagocytosed while the uterus is able to maintain effective sperm elimination of nonviable spermatozoa. Selective protection of viable spermatozoa from binding and phagocytosis by PMNs would increase their survival in a hostile uterine environment and ensure that a sufficient number of spermatozoa reach the oviduct for fertilization.

Role of bacteria in breeding-induced endometritis

Coitus causes bacterial contamination of the uterus [40]. This was previously believed to be the sole source of breeding-induced endometritis, and previous research on the pathophysiology of persistent endometritis has predominantly been performed using bacterial endometritis as a model. The finding that spermatozoa are triggering an inflammatory response in the uterus has shifted the research focus on endometritis from bacterial endometritis to sperm-induced endometritis [9,11,41]. Bacterial endometritis can still be a significant problem in cycling mares with lowered resistance to persistent inflammation and in mares that are bred by natural cover, however. The most common pathogens cultured from the uterus are *Streptococcus zooepidemicus*, *Escherichia coli*, *Pseudomonas aeruginosa*, and *Klebsiella pneumoniae*. One could speculate that an immunosuppressive effect of seminal plasma that protects spermatozoa from being destroyed in the uterus provides contaminating bacteria with an environment that favors adhesion and growth. A recent report suggested that bacterial endometritis contributes to the aggressive postbreeding endometritis in mares bred with frozen-thawed semen [42]. The interaction between bacteria and seminal components in the uterus needs to be studied further.

Diagnosis and management of mares with persistent breeding-induced endometritis

It is essential to understand the difference between physiologic breeding-induced endometritis and the pathologic condition of persistent breeding-induced endometritis. Breeding-induced endometritis may be clinically evident as purulent vaginal discharge during the first 12 hours after breeding. This could be a normal sign of a natural and necessary mechanism to eliminate excess semen from the uterus, and in this case, the condition should not be interfered with. If the mare experiences delayed uterine clearance, however, the horse would benefit from treatment for the condition [19,43,44].

Diagnostically, it may be difficult to identify susceptible mares before breeding. Some mares have free fluid present in the uterine lumen before breeding, but most mares are not diagnosed until after they have been bred. Clearance of charcoal particles from the uterus within 48 hours of inoculation and the use of scintigraphy to measure uterine clearance have been suggested to be useful when identifying mares that are susceptible to persistent breeding-induced endometritis [23,45]. These diagnostic tools may not always be available or practical to the clinician, however, who often has to rely on previous history and clinical findings after breeding to identify individuals that are susceptible to the condition. If susceptibility to persistent breeding-induced endometritis is suspected, the mare should be monitored closely by ultrasonography per rectum 6 to 24 hours after breeding. Resistant mares can retain fluid up to 6 hours after breeding with fresh semen and up to 12 hours after insemination with frozen-thawed semen. If free fluid is present in the uterine lumen after this time, the mare should be considered to have persistent breeding-induced endometritis.

Impaired fertility associated with persistent breeding-induced endometritis may be caused by premature luteolysis or a direct toxic effect on the embryo. Premature luteolysis could be caused by the inflammatory release of $PGF_{2\alpha}$ [46,47]. Preliminary observations in our laboratory suggest that a persistent inflammatory uterine environment 5 days after fertilization, when the embryo enters the uterus, is incompatible with survival of the embryo.

Management of mares susceptible to persistent breeding-induced endometritis should include limited uterine exposure to semen and bacteria and assisting the uterus to physically clear contaminants and inflammatory products after breeding. Preexisting uterine infections should be resolved before the mare is bred. Exposure to semen should be limited to a single breeding per cycle, if possible. This can be accomplished by closely monitoring follicular development and hormonal treatment to induce ovulation of mature follicles. Physical clearance can be assisted by the use of uterotonic drugs. Oxytocin or $PGF_{2\alpha}$ treatment 4 to 8 hours after breeding has been shown to aid in uterine clearance, resulting in improved pregnancy rates in susceptible mares [18,19,43,44]. Care must be taken with regard to the timing of $PGF_{2\alpha}$ treatment. Recent reports have demonstrated that $PGF_{2\alpha}$ can cause a delay in the formation of a functional corpus luteum (CL) when administered within 2 days after ovulation [47–50]. This was associated with pregnancy failure in two of the reports [47,48]. Large-volume uterine lavage 6 to 24 hours after breeding also effectively assists the uterus in clearing fluid and inflammatory products [51]. Because sperm transport to the oviduct is completed within 4 hours after breeding, uterine lavage between 6 and 24 hours after breeding does not have a negative effect on fertility [3]. Manual dilation of the cervix in mares with poor cervical dilation may help these mares to clear the uterus from fluid more effectively.

It is important for the clinician to keep in mind that a transient inflammatory response to semen is normal and required for normal fertility. Postbreeding treatments of these mares are most likely not to improve fertility and may even cause further contamination and interfere with pregnancy. Only 10% to 15% of all broodmares develop a pathologically persistent form of breeding-induced endometritis [20]. Attention should be given to identify and manage these mares appropriately to optimize the reproductive efficiency.

References

[1] Traub-Dargatz JL, Salman MD, Voss JL. Medical problems of adult horses, as ranked by equine practitioners. J Am Vet Med Assoc 1991;198:1745–7.
[2] Hughes JP, Loy RG. Investigations on the effect on intrauterine inoculation of Streptococcus zooepidemicus in the mare. Proc Am Assoc Equine Pract 1969;15:289–92.
[3] Brinsko SP, Varner DD, Blanchard TL. The effect of uterine lavage performed four hours post-insemination on pregnancy rates in mares. Theriogenology 1991;35:1111–91.
[4] Scott MA, Liu IKM, Overstreet JW. Sperm transport to the oviducts: abnormalities and their clinical implications. Proc Am Assoc Equine Pract 1995;41:1–2.
[5] Katila T, Sankari S, Mäkelä O. Transport of spermatozoa in the reproductive tracts of mares. J Reprod Fertil 2000;56(Suppl):571–8.
[6] Troedsson MHT, Liu IKM, Crabo BG. Sperm transport and survival in the mare: a review. Theriogenology 1998;50:807–18.
[7] Asbury AC, Schultz KT, Klesius PH, et al. Factors affecting phagocytosis of bacteria and neutrophils in the mares uterus. J Reprod Fertil 1982;32(Suppl):151–9.
[8] Troedsson MHT, Liu IKM, Thurmond M. Immunoglobulins (IgG and IgA) and complement (C3) concentrations in uterine secretion following an intrauterine challenge of Streptococcus zooepidemicus in mares susceptible to versus resistant to chronic uterine infection. Biol Reprod 1993;49:502–6.
[9] Troedsson MHT, Steiger BN, Ibrahim NM, et al. Mechanisms of sperm induced endometritis in the mare [abstract]. Biol Reprod 1995;52(Suppl):307.
[10] Watson ED, Stokes CR, Bourne FJ. Cellular and humoral mechanisms in mares susceptible and resistant to persistent endometritis. Vet Immunol Immunopathol 1987;16:107–21.

[11] Kotilainen T, Huhtinen M, Katila T. Sperm induced leukocytosis in the equine uterus. Theriogenology 1994;41:629–36.
[12] Rozeboom KJ, Troedsson MHT, Crabo BG. Artificial insemination induces a post-mating inflammatory response in gilts [abstract]. J Anim Sci 1998;76(Suppl 1):71.
[13] Troedsson MHT. Uterine clearance and resistance to persistent endometritis in the mare. Theriogenology 1999;52:461–71.
[14] Dahms BJ, Troedsson MHT. The effect of seminal plasma components on opsonisation and PMN-phagocytosis of equine spermatozoa. Theriogenology 2002;58:457–60.
[15] Alghamdi AS, Foster DN. Seminal DNAse frees spermatozoa entangled in neutrophil extracellular traps (NETs). Biol Reprod 2005;73:1174–81.
[16] Brinkman V, Reichard U, Goosmann C, et al. Neutrophil extracellular traps kill bacteria. Science 2004;203:1532–5.
[17] Troedsson MHT, Liu IKM, Ing M, et al. Smooth muscle electrical activity in the oviduct and the effect of oxytocin PGF2α, and PGE2 on the myometrium and the oviduct of the cycling mare. Biology reproduction monograph 1. Equine reproduction VI. Ann Arbor (MI): Society for the Study of Reproduction, Inc. Edward Brothers, Inc.; 1995. p. 439–52.
[18] Pycock JF, Newcombe JR. Relationship between intraluminal uterine fluid, endometritis, and pregnancy rate in the mare. Equine Pract 1996;18:19–22.
[19] Rasch K, Schoon H-A, Sieme H, et al. Histomorphological endometrial status and influence of oxytocin on the uterine drainage and pregnancy rates in mares. Equine Vet J 1996;28: 455–60.
[20] Zent WW, Troedsson MHT. Post breeding uterine fluid accumulation in a normal population of Thoroughbred mares: a field study. Proc Am Assoc Equine Pract 1998;44:64–5.
[21] Evans MJ, Hamer JM, Gason LM, et al. Factors affecting uterine clearance on inoculated materials. J Reprod Fertil 1987;35(Suppl):327–34.
[22] Troedsson MHT, Liu IKM. Uterine clearance of non-antigenic markers (Cr^{51}) in response to a bacterial challenge in mares potentially susceptible and resistant to chronic uterine infection. J Reprod Fertil 1991;44(Suppl):283–8.
[23] LeBlanc MM, Neuwirth L, Asbury AC, et al. Scintigraphic measurement of uterine clearance in normal mares and mares with recurrent endometritis. Equine Vet J 1994;26: 109–13.
[24] Troedsson MHT, Liu IKM, Ing M, et al. Multiple site electromyography recordings of uterine activity following an intrauterine bacterial challenge in mares susceptible and resistant to chronic uterine infection. J Reprod Fertil 1993;99:307–13.
[25] Rigby SL, Barhoumi R, Burghardt RC, et al. Mares with delayed uterine clearance have an intrinsic defect in myometrial function. Biol Reprod 2001;65:740–7.
[26] Alghamdi AS, Foster GN, Troedsson MHT. Nitric oxide levels and nitric oxide synthase expression in uterine samples from mares susceptible and resistant to persistent breeding-induced endometritis. Am J Reprod Immunol 2005;53(5):230–7.
[27] LeBlanc MM, Johnson RD, Calderwood Mays MB, et al. Lymphatic clearance of India ink in reproductively normal mares and mares susceptible to endometritis. Biology reproduction monograph 1. Equine reproduction VI. Ann Arbor (MI): Society for the Study of Reproduction, Inc. Edward Brothers, Inc.; 1995. p. 501–6.
[28] Troedsson MHT, Lee C-S, Franklin R, et al. Post-breeding uterine inflammation: the role of seminal plasma. J Reprod Fertil 2000;56(Suppl):341–9.
[29] Troedsson MHT, Alghamdi AS, Mattisen J. Equine seminal plasma protects fertility of spermatozoa in an inflamed uterine environment. Theriogenology 2002;58:453–6.
[30] Fiala SM, Pimentel CA, Steiger K, et al. Effect of skim milk and seminal plasma uterine infusions in mares. Theriogenology 2002;58:491–4.
[31] Troedsson MHT, Loseth K, Alghamdi AM, et al. Interaction between equine semen and the endometrium: the inflammatory response to semen. Anim Reprod Sci 2002;68:273–8.
[32] Crane LH, Martin L. Postcopulatory myometrial activity in the rat as seen videolaparoscopy. Reprod Fertil Dev 1991;39:297–310.

[33] Katila T, Portus BJ, Reilas T. The effect of seminal plasma on uterine inflammation and contractility in mares [abstract]. In: Proceedings of the 15th International Congress on Animal Reproduction. Bella Horizonte–MG, Brazil: Brazilian College for the Study of Reproduction; 2004. p. 392.

[34] Katila T. Onset and duration of uterine inflammatory response of mares after insemination with fresh semen. Biology reproduction monograph 1. Equine reproduction VI. Ann Arbor (MI): Society for the Study of Reproduction, Inc. Edward Brothers, Inc.; 1995. p. 515–7.

[35] Alghamdi AS, Troedsson MHT, Laschkewitsch T, et al. Uterine secretion from mares with post-breeding endometritis alters sperm motion characteristics in vitro. Theriogenology 2001;55:1019–28.

[36] Alghamdi AS, Foster DN, Troedsson MHT. Equine seminal plasma reduces sperm binding to polymorphonuclear neutrophils and improves fertility of fresh semen inseminated into inflamed uteri. Reproduction 2004;127:593–600.

[37] Metcalf ES. The effect of post-insemination endometritis on fertility of frozen stallion semen. Proc Am Assoc Equine Pract 2000;46:330–1.

[38] Squires EL, Reger HP, Maclellan LJ, et al. Effect of time of insemination and site of insemination on pregnancy rates with frozen semen. Theriogenology 2002;58:655–8.

[39] Troedsson MHT, Alghamdi AS, Desvousges A, et al. Components in seminal plasma regulating sperm transport and elimination. Anim Reprod Sci 2005;89:171–86.

[40] Kenney RM, Bergman RV, Cooper WL, et al. Minimal contamination techniques for breeding mares: techniques and preliminary findings. Proc Am Assoc Equine Pract 1975;21:327–36.

[41] Troedsson MHT, Crabo BG, Ibrahim NM, et al. Mating-induced endometritis: mechanisms, clinical importance, and consequences. Proc Am Assoc Equine Pract 1995;41:11–2.

[42] Maloufi F, Pierson R, Otto S, et al. Mares susceptible or resistant to endometritis have similar endometrial echographic and inflammatory cell reactions at 96 hours after infusion with frozen semen and extender. Proc Am Assoc Equine Pract 2002;48:51–7.

[43] LeBlanc MM. Oxytocin—the new wonder drug for treatment of endometritis? Equine Vet Educ 1994;6:39–43.

[44] Pycock JF. Assessment of oxytocin and intrauterine antibiotics on intrauterine fluid and pregnancy rates in the mare. Proc Am Assoc Equine Pract 1994;40:19–20.

[45] LeBlanc MM, Asbury AC, Lyle SK. Uterine clearance mechanisms during the early postovulatory period in mares. Am J Vet Res 1989;6:864–7.

[46] Neely DP, Kindahl H, Stabenfeldt GH, et al. Prostaglandin release pattern in the mare: physiological, pathophysiological, and therapeutic responses. J Reprod Fertil 1979;27(Suppl):181–9.

[47] Troedsson MHT, Ohlgren AF, Ababneh M, et al. Effect of periovulatory prostaglandin $F_2\alpha$ on pregnancy rates and luteal function. Theriogenology 2001;55:1891–9.

[48] Brendemuehl JP. Effect of oxytocin and cloprostenol on luteal formation, function and pregnancy rates in mares. Theriogenology 2002;58:623–6.

[49] Gunthle LM, McCue PM, Farquhar VJ, et al. Effect of prostaglandin administration postovulation on corpus luteum formation in the mare. In: Proceedings of the Society of Theriogenology Annual Conference, San Antonio, TX. Nashville (TN): Society of Theriogenology; 2000. p. 139.

[50] Nie GJ, Johnson KE, Wenzel JGW, et al. Effect of periovulatory ecbolics on luteal function and fertility. Theriogenology 2002;58:461–3.

[51] Troedsson MHT, Scott MA, Liu IKM. Comparative treatments of mares susceptible to chronic uterine infection. Am J Vet Res 1995;56:468–72.

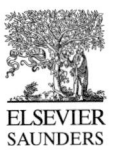

Management of Postfixation Twins in Mares

Karen E. Wolfsdorf, DVM

Hagyard Equine Medical Institute, 4250 Iron Works Pike, Lexington, KY 40511, USA

The establishment and loss of twins after 35 days of gestation often result in a mare that is barren for a year and the associated economic loss. The birth of twins has been documented as occurring in 1% to 2% of the equine population [1], with twinning accounting for 6% to 30% of abortions in the mare [2–4]. Abortion or stillbirth resulted in 64.5% of twin conceptuses that were maintained for 8 months or longer, with only 14% of surviving foals reaching the second week of neonatal life [2]. In another study, only 11% of 130 mares carrying twins produced viable foals, and only 38% of these mares produced viable foals the next year [5]. When twins are present, gestation proceeds normally until the conceptuses begin to compete for uterine space or placenta. With or without mummification, death of one fetus leads to abortion, usually between 5 and 9 months of gestation [6]. Lactation commonly occurs after one foal dies and causes premature mammary gland development [6]. If one or both foals are born alive, the mare may require assistance. Surviving foals are usually weaker, more susceptible to infection, and slower to develop than singletons. To avoid the potentially disastrous outcomes with twin fetuses, veterinarians have used various management practices, such as not breeding mares with two dominant follicles, breeding mares after the second ovulation, or short cycling mares that ovulate two follicles [7–9]. These strategies result in the loss of valuable estrous cycles during the breeding season, leading to a decreased number of pregnancies and increased economic loss [7]. Fortunately, with the use of ultrasound and an increased understanding of the mechanisms involved in twinning, better approaches to breeding management and twin reduction been developed [10–12].

Although pregnancies can be diagnosed with ultrasound as early as 9 days after ovulation, twin pregnancies are optimally detected between days 13 and 15 of gestation when the embryonic vesicles are still mobile

E-mail address: kwolfsdorf@hagyard.com

and two embryonic vesicles can be imaged [13–15]. Natural twin reduction does not occur before day 11, and it is negligible between days 11 and 15 [8,14,16]. Therefore, twin pregnancies that are detected during the mobility phase (days 9–15) are best managed by manually crushing one embryonic vesicle [6]. The smaller vesicle or the vesicle that needs the least amount of uterine manipulation is preferentially destroyed [17]. Survival rates of the remaining vesicle exceed 90% [5,17].

After fixation of the embryonic vesicles between 16 and 17 days of gestation, the success rate of reducing the twins to a viable singleton varies tremendously among procedures. No procedure is considered to be consistent or successful enough to be the optimal solution. The following section focuses on the options available to practitioners after fixation of twin fetuses has occurred and reviews the viability of each procedure.

Natural reduction and the deprivation theory

Biologic or natural reduction occurs when excess embryos are eliminated and one viable embryo continues to develop [18]. The surviving embryonic vesicle continues to grow and develop normally in appearance, with the only potential difference from a singleton pregnancy being vesicle orientation. Orientation can be defined as rotation of the embryonic vesicle so that the embryo proper is on the ventral aspect of the vesicle and the thickest portion of the wall of the conceptus, assuming a ventral position. This is hypothesized to be a function of disproportionate strength of the yolk sac wall and thickening and encroachment of the dorsal uterine wall on the conceptus [18]. The actual mechanism of natural reduction is not known [19]. Whether twin embryonic vesicles fix unilaterally (in the same uterine horn) or bilaterally (in different uterine horns) affects the incidence of natural reduction. Ginther [7,18] presented landmark research in 1982 and 1984 in which it was suggested that close apposition of the embryonic vesicles seemed to result in compression of the vesicles against each other; subsequently, contact between the endometrial and trophoblastic surfaces of the vesicles was lost. Most unilateral reductions occurred before day 26, potentially because the yolk sac is not efficient as a nutrient purveyor. Ginther [20] determined the overall incidence of natural reduction resulting in a single conceptus to be 64%. Although 83% to 89% of twins with unilateral fixation naturally reduced to a singleton, only 4% of twins with bilateral fixation reduced to a singleton. In this study, Ginther [20] did not include mares that lost both conceptuses, which would result in 17 (77%) of 22 mares naturally losing one or both of the twin conceptuses. The probability of natural reduction decreases as gestational age increases to day 40, with 53% of unilateral reductions occurring before day 20 and 82% occurring before day 30 [14,19]. When twins were present at examinations between 40 and 42 days of gestation, only 6% of the pregnancies terminated in the birth of one foal, 31% resulted in two foals, and 63% resulted in the loss of both fetuses [7]. Factors that seem to influence natural reduction are relative orientation of the embryonic vesicles, synchronicity of the ovulatory follicles, and size disparity between the vesicles. If a vesicle has the embryo proper adjacent to another vesicle, it is more likely to be reduced than if the embryo proper is in contact with the endometrium; in addition, if asynchronous ovulations occur and one embryonic vesicle is larger, it can impede the movement and growth of the smaller, leading to a higher likelihood of reduction.

Manual reduction after fixation

Manual reduction is preferentially and most successfully performed before fixation of the embryonic vesicles. If twin conceptuses are observed after fixation, manual reduction can be attempted; however, manual reduction of unilaterally fixed twins is difficult without damaging both conceptuses. If the vesicles can be separated, 90% of unilateral twins can be manually crushed between days 17 and 20 [11,21]. An attempt at manual reduction of bilateral twins between days 16 and 40 is a necessity if abortion at a later stage of gestation is to be avoided. Seventy-five percent of bilateral twins may be successfully reduced to a singleton pregnancy by crushing one vesicle before 30 days of gestation. With bilateral twins of gestational age longer than 35 days, however, there is a greater risk of abortion at a later stage if a vesicle is crushed [8,11], potentially because fluid released from the crushed vesicle gets between the chorioallantois and endometrium and causes loss of contact [22]. Manual manipulation transrectally, damaging without rupturing of one of the vesicles between 28 and 42 days, resulted in 28% of the mares having a single viable foal [20].

Dietary manipulation

The increased incidence of twins in Thoroughbred mares, as opposed to other breeds, has been postulated to be caused by environmental factors, such as more intensive methods of husbandry, especially high nutritional levels [2,9]. Merkt and colleagues [9] reduced the food intake of mares with early twins in an attempt to cause the death of one conceptus. Forty-one Thoroughbred mares in which twin pregnancies were diagnosed between 3 and 7 weeks by rectal palpation were treated. Treatment included complete removal of oats, concentrates, or alfalfa so that only grass hay was offered. Mares on pasture were kept indoors during the night or even for part of the day without additional feeding. Nursing mares were less severely fasted because of energy drain by milk production. Full feed was resumed when a single conceptus was identified, usually within 2 to 4 weeks. Mares were palpated once weekly. Most of the mares (63%) delivered a single foal, 1 mare delivered live twins, and the remaining mares aborted in late term. The researchers concluded that dietary restriction may be helpful in the management of twins in Thoroughbred mares, resulting in approximately a 60% chance of the mare producing a single foal [9]. Unfortunately, no comparisons were made in the study between the treated mares and mares that did not have their feed restricted. Therefore, the extent to which natural reduction of the twins may have occurred without feed restrictions is not known.

Surgical removal of one conceptus

Pascoe and Stover [22] described a surgical technique for the removal of one twin conceptus through a ventral midline approach. Operations were performed between 41 and 65 days of gestation. Five of eight mares with bilateral fixation delivered a single foal, and none of seven mares with unilateral fixation produced a viable foal. Failure of unilateral twin reduction was attributed to the disruption of the remaining chorioallantois during surgical removal of the selected chorioallantois, reducing oxygen and nutrient supplies and resulting in death of the remaining fetus [22]. Through histologic evidence, the researchers demonstrated that villous formation had not occurred in either chorion when the two chorions were in apposition; however, fibrin bands and small vessel anastomoses were present between the two surfaces [22].

Transvaginal ultrasound-guided twin reduction

Various procedures have been described for the reduction of twin conceptuses to a singleton using transvaginal ultrasound-guided aspiration [23,24]. In general, a 5- or 7.5-MHz transvaginal transducer is placed in the vaginal fornix. An 18-gauge needle is guided through the vaginal and uterine walls and into the conceptus. The fluid within the yolk sac or allantois is aspirated with suction from a syringe or pump. Success of the procedure has varied, when performed between 20 and 71 days of gestation. Reduction occurred in 33% of unilateral and 75% of bilateral twins [23]. When the procedure was performed on unilateral twins on day 36 or earlier, 40% of mares had a viable singleton 10 days later; in contrast, only 10% of mares had a viable singleton when aspirations occurred after day 36 [23]. In subsequent studies, 31% of unilateral twin reductions produced live foals, with all successful procedures being performed before 35 days of gestation [24]. In other reports, 0% to 9% of unilateral twin reductions resulted in the delivery of a single foal, depending on gestational age, and 25% of bilateral twin reductions resulted in the birth of a single viable foal [25]. In most cases, if death of the remaining twin occurred, it was noted between 10 and 14 days after the procedure; however, some mares aborted 3 to 9 months later [25]. Results of these studies suggest that transvaginal ultrasound-guided twin reductions are best performed before day 35 of gestation [26]. Recently, however, the procedure was reportedly performed by Mari and coworkers [27] on 24 Standardbred mares with 21 unilateral and 3 bilateral conceptuses. Aspirations were performed on 20 mares between 16 and 25 days of gestation and on 4 mares between 40 and 55 days of pregnancy. Viable foals resulted for 14 (70%) of the 20 mares, with unilateral twins reduced between 16 and 25 days of gestation. Success during this period has been attributed to the ability to stabilize the pregnant horn easily per rectum, allowing one of the vesicles to be imaged and penetrated without difficulty [27]. Because of the technical prowess needed in performing this procedure, a variety of factors influence its success and limitations. These factors include day of gestation at the time of reduction, unilateral versus bilateral fixation because of close proximity of the fetuses and associated membranes, operator experience so as to avoid damaging the adjacent vesicle or traumatizing the uterus, and leakage of fluid from the aspirated vesicle causing separation of placental membranes from the endometrium [25,26]. Gestational age was not discussed in the previous study, and the author believes that it needs to be mentioned. The period of time, 16 to 25 days of gestation, during which the procedure needed to be performed for a high success rate is the period of gestation during which natural reduction occurs at a similar rate. Because natural reduction is far less invasive, performing transvaginal ultrasound-guided twin reduction does not seem to be of practical use for unilateral twins during this early stage of gestation.

Craniocervical dislocation

Craniocervical dislocation is described as the dislocation of the first cervical vertebrae from the cranium, disrupting the ligamentous attachments and severing the spinal cord. This new procedure can be performed using transrectal or transabdominal techniques between 60 and 110 days of gestation to produce a single foal [28]. The basis for this procedure is to eliminate one twin before placental formation is complete, allowing the remaining fetus to use the entire endometrial surface for nutrient and oxygen exchange and to grow to its full potential.

Transrectal manipulations have been performed between 60 and 90 days of gestation. The mare is restrained in stocks or twitched in the doorway. Sedation using detomidine hydrochloride (detomidine HCl; 10–20 mg/kg) can be administered intravenously as needed. After sedation, however, the uterus may relax and the fetuses may move cranially in the abdomen and out of reach. Relaxation of the smooth muscle in the uterus and rectum can be achieved by the intravenous administration of propantheline bromide (30 mg); this allows easier identification and manipulation of the fetuses. To help inhibit prostaglandin release, flunixin meglumine (1 mg/kg) is administered intravenously before the procedure. The smaller fetus or the fetus that has less contact with the endometrium and minimal space to grow is preferentially reduced. This fetus is usually identified in the more cranial aspect of the uterine horn in unilateral twins. Once the identified fetus is located, the head must be isolated by finding the dome-shaped head and palpating the mandible or moving caudally and locating the cervical vertebrae. Craniocervical dislocation is performed by stabilizing the head between the thumb and forefinger and bending the head from side to side. This damages the ligaments attaching the head and neck (Fig. 1A). Dislocation is then created by placing the thumb at the base of the cranium and applying pressure proximal and dorsally (see Fig. 1B). A distinctive pop is felt if dislocation is achieved, and the thumb and forefinger can be placed in the space created between the head and neck. Mares should be placed on altrenogest (0.088 mg/kg/d) for 3 to 4 weeks. After craniocervical dislocation, death with loss of the fetal heartbeat is usually evident within 24 hours to 1 week. Fetal viability should be evaluated 1 week later and every 2 weeks for a month to establish normal growth of the continuing fetus and demise of the other.

If transrectal reduction cannot be achieved, a surgical procedure can be used. To date, this procedure has been used for twins between the gestational ages of 58 and 110 days. Transabdominal ultrasound is used to identify the horn in which the most viable fetus is located, as determined by fetal size and by the fetus that has the greatest surface area for attachment to the endometrium. A standing flank laparotomy is performed ipsilateral to the horn containing the fetus that has been identified for reduction. Operative medications include propantheline bromide (30 mg administered intravenously), flunixin meglumine (1 mg/kg administered intravenously), procaine penicillin G, and gentamicin sulfate (6.6 mg/kg administered intravenously). Propanthentheline bromide is essential for relaxing and preventing uterine contractions while finding and manipulating the fetus. While the mare is

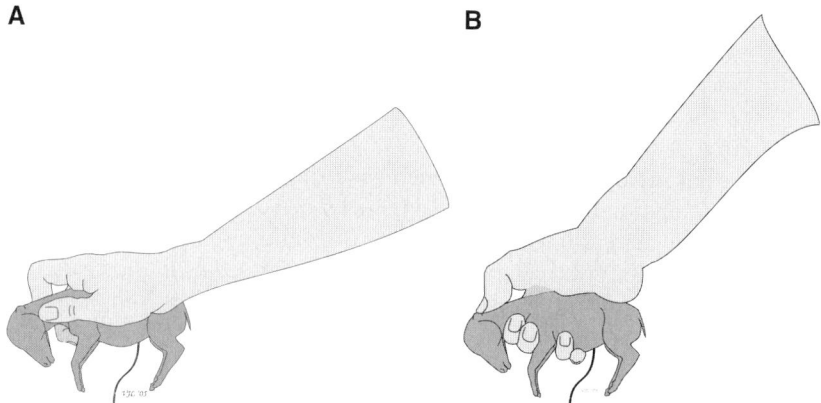

Fig. 1. (*A*) During craniocervical dislocation, the head is stabilized between the thumb and forefinger before bending from side to side to damage the ligamentous attachments. (*B*) Dislocation is achieved by placing the thumb on the base of the cranium and applying pressure.

standing, a flank incision is made ipsilateral to the uterine horn containing the fetus that has been identified for reduction. Identification of the preferred uterine horn is not always possible because of fetal movements and imaging capabilities. If this occurs, we prefer to make an incision on the right flank of the mare, allowing more access to the reproductive tract without intestinal interference. The uterus is located within the abdominal cavity with one arm, and the twin is isolated as described for transrectal dislocations. Craniocervical dislocation is performed by manipulating the fetus through the uterus, without incising or invading the uterine lumen. The flank incision is then routinely closed. With this technique, death of the manipulated twin may not be evident until 24 hours to 7 weeks. For 2 days after surgery, mares receive flunixin meglumine, procaine penicillin G, and gentamicin sulfate. After this time, sulfamethoxazole/trimethoprim tablets (24 mg/kg) are administered orally twice daily for 1 week and altrenogest (0.088 mg/kg) is administered orally once daily for 1 month.

The ultimate success of this procedure is still to be determined. To date, eight sets of twins have been reduced with transrectal manipulations, with gestation lengths between 55 and 90 days. Five (63%) of the eight mares delivered a single fetus of normal size. Three mares aborted both fetuses between 30 and 60 days after the procedure was performed. No viable heartbeat was observed in the reduced fetus between 1 and 3 weeks after craniocervical dislocation. Unfortunately, the transrectal procedure is technically difficult, and multiple manipulations of the fetus are sometimes necessary before dislocation is achieved. Of the eight mares, three had multiple manipulations of a fetus, and only one of these mares aborted. We have not determined if additional manipulations result in a detrimental effect on the remaining conceptus, however.

Craniocervical dislocations using the surgical procedure have been performed on 16 sets of twins between days 60 and 110. The procedures were performed on 5 mares sufficiently long ago for them to have completed the length of their gestation. Of these mares, 3 have delivered single healthy foals, 1 mare aborted within 30 days of the procedure, and 1 mare was not pregnant at 110 days of gestation (Karen Wolfsdorf, Dwayne Rodgerson, and Richard Holder, unpublished data, 2005). The remaining 11 mares have not completed the length of their gestation. To date, 2 mares have aborted, although in 1 of the sets of twins, one of the conceptuses did not appear normal at the time of reduction. Another mare had two viable fetuses at 9 weeks after the procedure, and at 5 months of gestation, induction of premature parturition was elected. Craniocervical dislocation was revealed to have been complete in the fetus on which the procedure was performed. The remaining mares have ongoing pregnancies with a single fetus. Manipulations were only performed once. Manipulated fetuses lost their heartbeat from 1 to 49 days after the procedure. Re-evaluation of fetal viability is performed with transrectal or transabdominal ultrasonography every 2 weeks until demise of one twin is observed.

Signs of impending death of a fetus include loss of thoracic shape, with the fetus becoming more convex; loss of definition of abdominal organs; and irregular weak heartbeats (Fig. 2). Placentas from mares delivering singleton foals have a small sack attached to the allantoic surface (Fig. 3). The nonviable fetus is marsupialized, forming a small pouch, with a stalk protruding from the allantoic surface. This pouch contains the mummified fetal bones. Examination of the chorionic surface reveals minimal evidence that a twin was present, with microvilli present along the entire attachment of the placenta.

Craniocervical dislocation could have advantages when compared with other procedures for reducing postfixation twins. Results of this procedure may have a better outcome than those of transcutaneous ultrasound-guided reductions, in which a large percentage of single foals have been undersized and weak (Johanna Reimer, personal communication, 2001). Outcomes of the different procedures may be affected by the time of reduction. Other procedures have not been successful at the stage of gestation (60–110 days) in which craniocervical dislocations are performed. Transcutaneous ultrasound-guided reductions are done later in gestation than craniocervical dislocations, and placental function and growth may be limited when twin reductions occur later in gestation. When performing craniocervical dislocations at a later stage of gestation than transvaginal ultrasound-guided aspirations, the uterus is not punctured with a needle and fluid does not leak from the reduced conceptus, potentially disrupting the fetal membranes of the remaining conceptus. Consequently, oxygenation and nutrition exchange of the remaining conceptus can be compromised [22,25]. Concurrently, not transversing the abdomen and entering the lumen of the uterus reduces the chance of bacterial contamination resulting in placentitis.

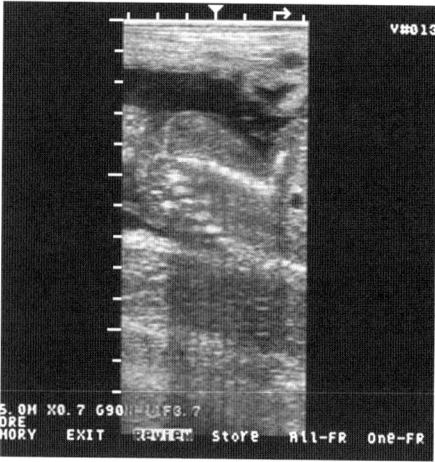

Fig. 2. Ultrasound image of a fetus undergoing fetal death after craniocervical dislocation.

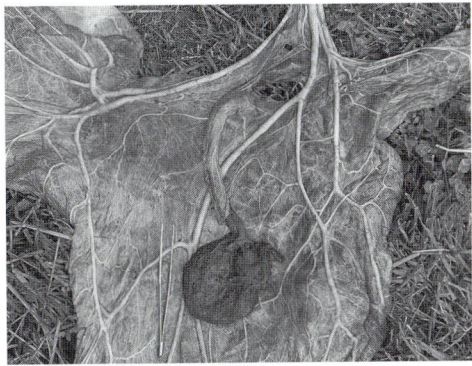

Fig. 3. Placenta from a mare after craniocervical dislocation to eliminate one twin. The sac attached to the allantoic surface contains the remnants of the fetus that died after craniocervical dislocation.

Disadvantages of craniocervical dislocation mostly pertain to isolation of the fetus. When the mare is at this stage of gestation, identifying the correct fetus within the uterus is similar to "bobbing for apples." It is absolutely imperative that the uterus is relaxed enough for identification of fetal anatomy. No documented evidence is available at this time of gestation regarding the extent of trauma or prostaglandin release that occurs with manipulation of the fetus through the uterus, although previous studies have demonstrated that 20 minutes of uterine manipulation is necessary for significant prostaglandin release [17]. The procedure is relatively rapid from isolation of the fetus to craniocervical dislocation; therefore, severe inflammation should not result, but proficiency and time of manipulations may affect the outcome. The incision site of the flank laparotomy heals with few complications. If a seroma or cellulitis develops, the incision can be opened on the ventral end and drained. Scarring was minimal, and all the mares' incisions healed normally. The duration of time that the manipulated fetus survives is inconsistent, and an explanation is unknown [28].

If the existing singleton pregnancies continue to term after craniocervical dislocation, the surgical procedure results in a 69% (11 of 16 mares) success rate. This would be a higher success rate than that of other procedures and would make this procedure a viable alternative for twin reduction after fixation.

Transcutaneous ultrasound-guided twin reduction

Transcutaneous ultrasound-guided twin reductions can be performed in mares between 66 and 168 days of gestation. For the procedure, the mare is tranquilized with a combination of acepromazine, xylazine hydrochloride, and butorphanol. Fetal locations are determined after the uterus is relaxed and forward [29]. The orientation, position, and size of the twins are determined relative to each other. The most accessible fetus or the smaller fetus is selected for reduction. Routine surgical preparation is performed on the mare's abdomen directly over the fetal heart, and 2% lidocaine is infiltrated. A sterile sleeve is placed over a 3-MHz transducer that is fitted with a biopsy guide. The required length of the spinal needle is determined by the depth of the fetus from the abdominal wall. The biopsy guide allows the needle tip to be introduced through the skin and abdomen in a single motion. In small thrusting motions, the needle is punctured through the uterus and into the fetal heart [26]. Potassium chloride (KCl) is injected into the heart of a fetus. This procedure has resulted in 38% to 40% of mares delivering a normal live foal [25,29]. Subsequent variations of transcutaneous ultrasound-guided twin reductions have included using a 5-MHz transducer and injecting procaine penicillin instead of KCl. The researchers concluded that the procedure is most successful when done between 115 and 130 days of gestation, with 49% of mares delivering a live foal after injection of KCl and 60% of mares having a live foal when procaine penicillin was used [21]. Unfortunately, the success of this procedure depends heavily on the experience of the operator and the prevention of iatrogenic infection or prostaglandin release. Some of the single live foals that are born seem to have some degree of placental insufficiency; they are weak and small at birth and unthrifty. Therefore, the financial investment may result in a foal being born that is of little economic value, especially if it is a colt [25].

Abortion of twins

When other procedures fail to produce a single viable conceptus and endometrial cup formation has occurred, aborting both conceptuses is the last option. Most mares that are carrying twins naturally abort between 7 and 9 months. If natural abortion is allowed to occur, however, the current breeding season is lost and the next breeding season may be affected. In addition, the mares have increased risks for dystocia, cervical tears, retained placentas, and associated complications. Premature induction of parturition between 150 and 180 days of gestation reduces the potential complications associated with abortion of both conceptuses. Although various methods to induce parturition at term have been described, few protocols have been described for the induction of premature parturition [30–34]. In early gestation and before endometrial cup formation, variable doses of prostaglandin have been effective in terminating pregnancy [35,36]. Between 70 and 77 days of gestation, multiple doses of fluprostenol (250–500 µg administered intramuscularly once or twice daily) have resulted in abortion after four to eight injections [37]. Fluprostenol (prostaglandin growth factor-2α [$PGF_{2\alpha}$]) and oxytocin were compared as induction agents during the previable and premature periods of gestation. Fluprostenol, natural $PGF_{2\alpha}$, intramuscular oxytocin, and intravenous oxytocin were ranked, as listed, in order of increasing effectiveness [38]. Oxytocin regimens were used after induction was attempted with fluprostenol, however. Oxytocin treatments comprised intravenous injection of 10 to 20 IU in 5-IU increments every 15 to 20 minutes or 20 to 80 IU administered intramuscularly at intervals from 30 minutes to 20 hours. Because the treatments were so varied, the effectiveness of the different protocols is hard to compare. Unfortunately, different agents for premature induction of parturition have not been studied; therefore, more research is needed in this area. In addition, at the present time, fluprostenol is not commercially available and has been replaced by another analogue of $PGF_{2\alpha}$, cloprostenol. The author's clinical impression is that after administration of cloprostenol by the regimen described, the mare delivers within 4 hours if the delivery is going to be predictable. Cloprostenol has varied results, however, with respect to efficacy and duration to pregnancy termination. Cloprostenol has been used at different doses and frequencies, but the author's preferred regimen is 7.5 µg administered intramuscularly at 20-minute intervals for two doses, with repeated daily injections if parturition has not occurred within 2 hours after the second injection. If repeated dosing is needed, the addition of prostaglandin E_2 (PGE_2; 2–2.5 mg in sterile 0.9% sodium chloride [NaCl] solution, 0.5 mL) on the second day may help to dilate the cervix and hasten delivery.

Summary

At this time, craniocervical dislocation seems to be the most promising method to obtain a single normal foal when twins are detected after fixation. None of the reviewed procedures (natural reduction, dietary restriction, transvaginal and transabdominal ultrasound-guided injections, and craniocervical dislocation) provide a method to unequivocally produce a healthy normal singleton, however. Therefore, at the present time, the best solution is to reduce twins manually early in gestation before mobility has ceased.

Acknowledgments

Dr. Valerie Linse created the diagrams portraying craniocervical dislocation.

References

[1] Ginther OJ. Reproductive biology of the mare. Cross Plains (WI): Equiservices; 1979.
[2] Jeffcott LB, Whitwell KW. Twinning as a cause of neonatal loss in the Thoroughbred. J Comp Pathol 1973;83:91–105.
[3] Roberts SJ. Physiology of the gestational period. In: Veterinary obstetrics and genital diseases. 2nd edition. Ithaca (NY): Woodstock; 1986. p. 81–106.

[4] Giles R, Donahue J, Hong C, et al. Causes of abortion, stillbirth, and prenatal death in horses. J Am Vet Med Assoc 1993;8:1170–5.
[5] Pascoe R. Methods for the treatment of twin pregnancy in the mare. Equine Vet J 1983;15:40–2.
[6] Roberts C. Termination of twin gestation by blastocyst crush in the broodmare. J Reprod Fertil Suppl 1982;32:447–9.
[7] Ginther OJ. Twinning in mares: a review of recent studies. J Equine Vet Sci 1982;2:127–35.
[8] Pascoe RR, Pascoe DR, Wilson MC. Influence of follicular status on twinning rate in mares. J Reprod Fertil Suppl 1987;35:183–9.
[9] Merkt H, Jungnickel S, Klug E. Reduction of early twin pregnancy to a single pregnancy in the mare by dietetic means. J Reprod Fertil Suppl 1982;32:451–2.
[10] Chevalier F, Palmer E. Ultrasonic echography in the mare. J Reprod Fertil Suppl 1982;32:423–30.
[11] Bowman T. Ultrasonic diagnosis and management of early twins in the mare. Proc Am Assoc Equine Pract 1986;32:35–43.
[12] Simpson DJ, Greenwood RES, Ricketts SW, et al. Use of ultrasound echography for early diagnosis in single and twin pregnancies in the mare. J Reprod Fertil Suppl 1982;32:431–9.
[13] Ginther OJ. Ultrasonic imaging and reproductive events in the mare. Cross Plains (WI): Equiservices; 1986. p. 378.
[14] Ginther OJ. Twin embryos in the mare: 1. From ovulation to fixation. Equine Vet J 1989;21:166–70.
[15] Palmer E, Driancourt M. Use of ultrasonic echography in equine gynecology. Theriogenology 1980;13:203–16.
[16] Ginther OJ, Bergfelt DR. Embryonic reduction before Day 11 in mares with twin conceptuses. J Anim Sci 1988;66:1727–31.
[17] Pascoe D, Pascoe R, Hughes J, et al. Comparison of two techniques and three hormone therapies for management of twin conceptuses by manual embryonic reduction. J Reprod Fertil Suppl 1987;35:701–2.
[18] Ginther OJ. Postfixation embryo reduction in unilateral and bilateral twins in mares. Theriogenology 1984;22:213–23.
[19] Ginther O, Griffen P. Natural outcome and ultrasonic identification of equine fetal twins. Theriogenology 1994;41:1193–9.
[20] Ginther OJ. The nature of embryo reduction in mares with twin conceptuses: deprivation hypothesis. Am J Vet Res 1989;50:45–53.
[21] McKinnon A, Rantanen N. Twins. In: Equine diagnostic ultrasonography. Baltimore (MD): Williams & Wilkins; 1998. p. 141–56.
[22] Pascoe DR, Stover SM. Surgical removal of one conceptus from fifteen mares with twin conceptuses. Vet Surg 1989;18:141–5.
[23] Bracher V, Parlevliet J, Pieterse M, et al. Transvaginal ultrasound-guided twin reduction in the mare. Vet Rec 1993;133:478–9.
[24] Jonker F, Parlevliet J, Vos P. Twin reduction in sixteen mares by transvaginal ultrasound-guided puncture of the embryonic vesicle. In: Proceedings of the British Equine Veterinary Association Annual Congress, Volume 34. Fordham, Ely, UK: British Equine Veterinary Association; 1995. p. 49.
[25] Macpherson ML, Reimer JM. Twin reduction in the mare: current options. Anim Reprod Sci 2000;60-61:233–44.
[26] Macpherson ML, Homco LD, Varner DD. Transvaginal ultrasound-guided allocentesis for pregnancy elimination in the mare. Biol Reprod Monogr 1995;1:215–23.
[27] Mari G, Iacono E, Merlo B, et al. Reduction of twin pregnancy in the mare by transvaginal ultrasound-guided aspiration. Reprod Domest Anim 2004;36(6):434–7.
[28] Wolfsdorf K, Rodgerson D, Holder R. How to manually reduce twins between 60-120 days gestation using cranio-cervical dislocation. Proc Am Assoc Equine Pract 2005;51:284–7.

[29] Rantanen NW, Kincaid B. Ultrasound guided fetal cardiac puncture. A method of twin reduction in the mare. Proc Am Assoc Equine Pract 1988;34:173–9.
[30] Alm CC, Sullivan JJ, First NL. Induction of premature parturition by parenteral administration of dexamethasone in the mare. J Am Vet Med Assoc 1974;165(8):721–2.
[31] Hillman RB. Induction of parturition in mares. J Reprod Fertil 1975;23:641–4.
[32] Jeffcott LB, Rossdale PD. A critical review of current methods for induction of parturition in the mare. Equine Vet J 1977;9(4):208–15.
[33] Rossdale PD, Pashen RL, Jeffcott LB. The use of synthetic prostaglandin analogue (Fluprostenol) to induce foaling. J Reprod Fertil 1979;27:521–9.
[34] Klem ME, Kreider JL, Harms PG, et al. Induction of parturition in the mare with prostaglandin F_2a. Theriogenology 1982;42(1):89–96.
[35] Douglas RH, Squires EL, Ginther OJ. Induction of abortion in mares with prostaglandin F_2a. J Anim Sci 1974;39:404.
[36] Kooistra LH, Ginther OJ. Termination of pseudopregnancy by administration of prostaglandin F2a and termination of early pregnancy by administration of prostaglandin F2a or colchicines or by removal of embryos in mares. Am J Vet Res 1976;37:35.
[37] Squires EL, Hillman RB, Pickett BW, et al. Induction of abortion in mares with Equimate: effect on secretion of progesterone, PMSG and reproductive performance. J Anim Sci 1980; 50:490–5.
[38] Leadon DP, Rossdale PD, Jeffcott LB, et al. A comparison of agents for inducing parturition in mares in the pre-viable and premature periods of gestation. J Reprod Fertil Suppl 1982;32: 597–602.

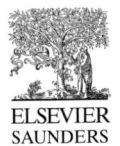

Hormone Profiles and Treatments in the Late Pregnant Mare

J.C. Ousey, MSc, PhD

The Equine Fertility Unit, Department of Veterinary Medicine, University of Cambridge, Mertoun Paddocks, Woodditton Road, Newmarket, Suffolk, CB8 9BH United Kingdom

Delivery of a healthy foal requires the successful coordination of maturational events within the fetal and maternal tissues to ensure the smooth delivery of the fetus from its intra- to extrauterine environment. These events may be identified by hormone changes during the last few weeks of gestation. Delivery itself is characterized by a cascade of endocrine changes that act in an orderly sequence, commencing in the fetus and spreading into the maternal tissues, so that once the fetus has signaled its readiness for birth, the mare can regulate the final timing of delivery. The hormones and the pathways involved in the preparations for birth are still not yet fully understood, because (1) the mare shows few overt signs of first-stage labor and has a rapid expulsive phase of delivery, making if difficult to collect blood samples at key stages during labor; (2) some hormones act in a paracrine fashion within the fetal or uteroplacental (UP) tissues, and thus cannot be detected in the peripheral circulation; and (3) blood sampling from the equine fetus is technically challenging, and the procedure itself may stimulate abnormal hormone responses.

Not surprisingly, there is even less information available about the endocrine events associated with late gestation abortions or preterm birth in mares. Unless the mare is sick or shows premonitory signs, such as "running milk," it often delivers precipitously and unattended. If the insult is chronic and directly affects the fetoplacental unit, the normal endocrine profiles may be disrupted. Monitoring these hormone changes, particularly maternal plasma progestagens, can be useful to identify the degree of fetal or placental dysfunction. Treatment with hormone products is more controversial,

---

This work was funded by the Horserace Betting Levy Board and Thoroughbred Breeders Association.

E-mail address: efu@tesco.net

however, because the physiologic mechanisms involved in abortion and preterm birth are not well understood.

This article reviews the major endocrine changes before normal parturition, describes the hormone changes associated with fetoplacental problems, and discusses some of the hormone treatments that are currently in use or could be used to improve pregnancy outcome.

Hormone changes during late pregnancy and parturition

Progestagens

Progesterone (P4) is one of several progestagens (or progestins) identified by gas-chromatography–mass spectrometry (GC-MS) in pregnant mares' plasma. P4 is only present in the peripheral circulation during the first trimester. From midgestation on, P4 is generally undetectable, at less than 1 ng/mL, whereas the other progestagens assume greater quantitative significance, typically reaching concentrations in the maternal plasma between 5 and 50 ng/mL; by late gestation, concentrations of some progestagens exceed 500 ng/mL [1–3]. Umbilical progestagen concentrations are significantly greater than maternal (uterine) concentrations, because the fetus synthesizes large quantities of pregnenolone (P5; probably derived from the fetal adrenal gland) and other progestagens that are released into the umbilical artery (Fig. 1) [1,4,5]. The P5 is converted into P4 in the placenta and then into 5α-pregane,3,20,-dione (DHP) in the endometrium [6,7]. Most (70%) of the 5α-DHP produced in late gestation is returned to the fetus for further metabolism, while some 5α-DHP (30%) is excreted into the maternal (uterine) circulation along with other progestagens. Compared with other progestagens, there is little P4 in the umbilical circulation. Most P4 remains within the UP tissues, where it can presumably direct steroid metabolism and regulate myometrial activity.

Fetal production of P5 increases in late gestation and, consequently, progestagen concentrations in maternal plasma also increase, typically peaking a few days before parturition and declining on the last day or even hours before birth (Fig. 2). The prepartum rise in progestagens is associated with development of the mare's mammary gland and onset of mammary secretion electrolyte changes, whereas the decline is concurrent with an increase in fetal cortisol. There are quantitative differences in plasma progestagen concentrations between different breeds of horses; for example, ponies show greater individual variation in plasma progestagen concentrations and display a smaller prepartum rise compared with Thoroughbreds (see Fig. 2) [8]. These differences may reflect disparities in maternal and/or fetal size. The individual progestagens identified in maternal plasma are consistent between the different breeds of horses, however [1].

Because there are so many progestagens in maternal plasma, assays using an antibody raised against P4 usually cross-react with one or more of these

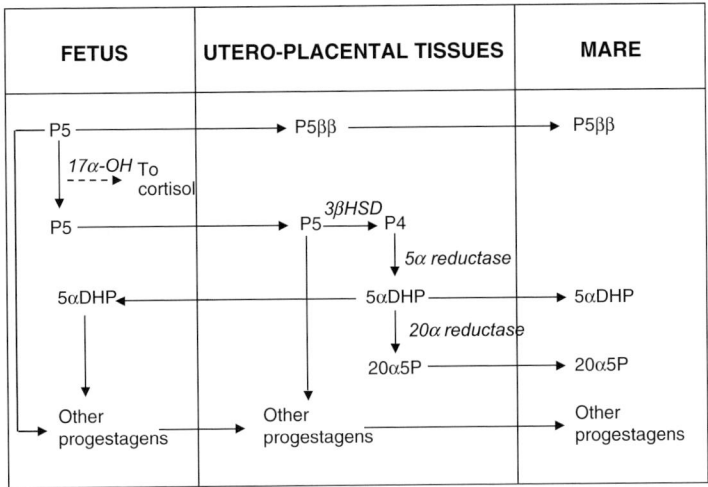

Fig. 1. Simplified diagram showing the progestagen biosynthetic pathway in the fetus, UP tissues, and mare in late gestation. The pathway to cortisol is also shown. 5α-DHP, 5α-pregnane,3,20-dione; P5ββ, pregnanediol; 20α-5P, 20α-hydroxy-5α-pregnan-3-one. Other progestagens include 3β-hydroxy-5α-pregnan-20-one, 5α-pregnane-3β, 20β-diol, 5α-pregnane-3β, 20a-diol, 20α-hydroxyprogesterone, and 20β-hydroxyprogesterone. Enzymes include *3β-hydroxysteroid dehydrogenase (3β-HSD)* and *17α-hydroxylase (17α-OH)*. (*Adapted from* Ousey JC, Forhead AJ, Rossdale PD, et al. Ontogeny of uteroplacental progestagen production in pregnant mares during the second half of gestation. Biol Reprod 2003;69(2):540–8.)

other progestagens; therefore, they are measuring "total progestagens" rather than P4. The actual concentrations of total progestagens measured in mare's plasma in late gestation can vary substantially depending on the cross-reactivity of the antibody (Fig. 3). Consequently, it is essential to know the normal total progestagen concentrations for a particular assay system before one can identify what constitutes a normal level for pregnant mares.

It is generally believed that the role of P4 is to block myometrial activity during pregnancy and that the decline in P4 at birth removes this blockade [9]. In women, however, there is no systemic decline in P4 before delivery [10]. Instead, there is a "functional" P4 withdrawal caused by an increase in the ratio of the progesterone receptor (PR) isoform A compared with PR-B, leading to a suppression in P4 responsiveness within the myometrium [11,12]. In the late pregnant mare, P4 is quantitatively the least important progestagen in maternal and fetal plasma, with no information about its concentration within the UP tissues. In contrast, most other progestagens increase and then decline prepartum. Therefore, it is possible that another progestagen may be biologically active in the mare, for example 5α-DHP, the direct metabolite of P4 [4,13]. The 5α-DHP is produced within the UP tissues but is preferentially directed into the umbilical circulation in late

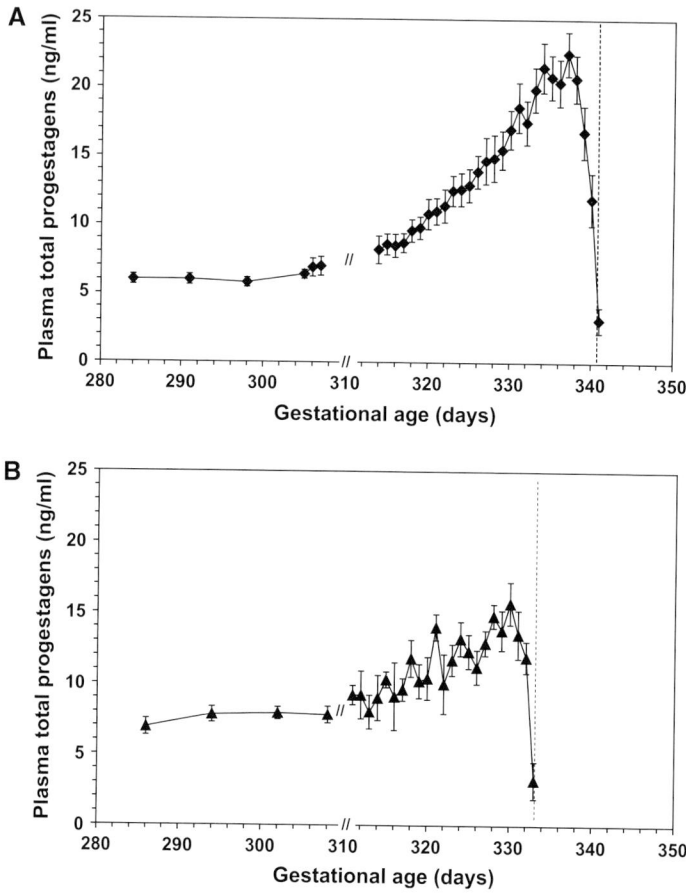

Fig. 2. Mean ± SEM plasma total progestagen concentrations in Thoroughbred (*A*) and pony (*B*) mares during the last 8 weeks prepartum. (*Adapted from* Rossdale PD, Ousey JC, Cottrill CM, et al. Effects of placental pathology on maternal plasma progestagen and mammary secretion calcium concentrations and on neonatal adrenocortical function in the horse. J Reprod Fertil Suppl 1991;44:583; © Society for Reproduction and Fertility, 1991. Reproduced by permission.)

gestation, suggesting that it may play an important role within the fetoplacental tissues [5,6]. Moreover 5α-DHP competes more strongly than P4 for the uterine PR [14]. In vitro studies using myometrial strips from pregnant mares demonstrated that neither P4 nor 5α-DHP prevented oxytocin (OX)-induced contractions of the myometrium, however [15]. Interestingly, the only hormone that was effective at inhibiting myometrial contractility in vitro was the parathyroid-related protein fragment$_{1-34}$, an oncofetal protein that is found in the placenta and is a potent myometrial relaxant in other species [16,17]. Therefore, the current evidence that P4 regulates myometrial quiescence is conflicting.

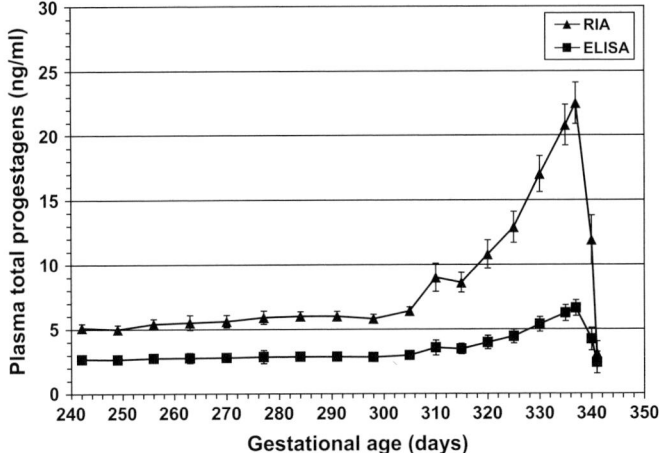

Fig. 3. Total progestagen concentrations in plasma samples from 19 healthy mares in late gestation measured using two different assays specific for P4 but having differing cross-reactions with other progestagens. RIA, radioimmunoassay cross-reaction with 100% P4, 6.2% 5α-DHP, 2% 17α-hydroxyprogesterone, and less than 1% of all other progestagens; ELISA, enzyme-linked immunoassay cross-reaction with 100% P4, 1.6% 5α-DHP, 1% 17α-hydroxyprogesterone, and 0.3% P5.

Estrogens

Estrogens are important for active labor in most animals by promoting the synthesis of prostaglandins (PGs), increasing OX receptor numbers and myometrial gap junctions, and increasing the estrogen/P4 ratio, leading to myometrial contractility [18–20]. The mare differs from most other mammals with respect to estrogen production, because, first, total estrogen concentrations decline rather than increase before parturition and, second, mares produce large quantities of the equine-unique ring B estrogens equilin and equilenin. The estrogens, like the progestagens, are produced by the fetoplacental unit, but they originate from different fetal tissues. The estrogen precursors are produced by the fetal gonads and are aromatized by the placenta. The metabolic pathways for production of the classic phenolic estrogens and the ring B estrogens differ [21]. Estrone and estradiol are produced from dehydroepiandrosterone (DHA), whereas equilin and equilenin are produced from farnesyl pyrophosphate [21,22].

Total estrogen concentrations in maternal blood decline gradually over the last 2 to 3 months prepartum, reaching baseline after delivery [23,24]. Despite this decline, estrogens are essential for labor in the mare, because removing the fetal gonads, and hence the source of DHA, causes not only a dramatic fall in estrogen concentrations but weak myometrial contractions and a significant reduction in maternal plasma prostaglandin $F_{2\alpha}$ metabolite (PGFM) concentrations during labor [24]. These effects were not observed in sham operated controls. In most other species, estrogens increase prepartum, and in nonhuman primates, this rise occurs at night in conjunction with increased uterine electromyographic (EMG) activity. Recently, it has been reported that mares have nocturnal increases in uterine EMG activity during the last week prepartum and that this correlates with a rise in estradiol-17β [25,26]. Therefore, despite the overall decline in peripheral total estrogen concentrations at term in the mare, estradiol-17β may act locally within the UP tissues to promote release of PGs and OX, and thereby stimulate the onset of myometrial contractions, particularly at night, when most mares foal.

Prostaglandins

PGs are clearly involved in labor in mares. Exogenous $PGF_{2\alpha}$ (and OX) is a potent inducing agent throughout pregnancy. $PGF_{2\alpha}$ promotes myometrial contractility by acting on intracellular calcium, whereas PGE_2 promotes cervical relaxation and ripening. They are synthesized by the UP tissues and are present in maternal and fetal plasma and allantoic fluids [27]. These hormones are labile and difficult to measure accurately; therefore, the stable metabolite PGFM is measured more frequently in peripheral plasma. During the second half of pregnancy, plasma PGFM concentrations are low and increase only slightly toward term (2–4 ng/mL); however, during second-stage labor, there is a 50-fold increase in PGFM [19,28]. PGs are rapidly metabolized into inactive metabolites by the enzyme 15-hydroxyprostaglandin dehydrogenase (PGDH). This enzyme is present in the equine maternal endometrium from approximately 150 days of gestation, thus ensuring that PG concentrations remain low during pregnancy [7]. These authors have suggested that P4 produced within the placenta may act in a paracrine fashion to regulate PGDH in the adjacent maternal endometrium. The increase in plasma progestagens that occurs at term inhibits the enzyme 3β-hydroxysteroid dehydrogenase (3B-HSD) causing a decline in P4 synthesis, and thus decreasing PGDH activity and enabling an increase in PG concentrations and onset of myometrial contractility [4].

Oxytocin

OX is a peptide hormone secreted by the posterior pituitary gland. Plasma OX concentrations are low throughout gestation and increase substantially only during labor. Even when blood is sampled from the intercavernous sinus, the blood system draining the pituitary, OX levels remain low until rupture of the allantochorion and peak only during fetal expulsion [28]. In women, OX concentrations are low during labor [29]. It has been suggested that OX may act in a paracrine manner within the UP tissues and that high oxytocin receptor (OR) numbers may be more important than high circulating OX concentrations. Although uterine ORs have not yet been identified in the late pregnant mare, it is likely that they are, in fact, present in high concentrations, as suggested by the marked sensitivity of the uterus to low doses (1 IU) of OX at this time [30,31].

Relaxin

Relaxin is produced by the placental trophoblast cells [32]. Maternal concentrations are high in late gestation and increase again during labor [33]. Postpartum relaxin concentrations diminish gradually with delivery of the placenta but remain elevated if the placenta is retained. Substantial differences in maternal plasma relaxin levels exist between different breeds of horses, which seems to be unrelated to placental size but may reflect differences in physiology between the breeds [34]. Relaxin is thought to contribute to myometrial relaxation; however, paradoxically, relaxin concentrations increase substantially during labor. These high levels may account for a period of myometrial quiescence observed in the 2 to 4 hours before delivery and are probably overcome by the high concentrations of $PGF_{2\alpha}$ that occur during second-stage labor [19].

Cortisol

An increase in fetal cortisol before delivery is essential for maturation of fetal organ systems and for the initiation of parturition in many species [35,36]. In sheep, the rise in fetal cortisol occurs gradually over the last few weeks (15%) of gestation. In contrast in horses, a marked rise in fetal cortisol occurs only within the last 2 to 3 days (1%–2%) of gestation, and this coincides with the decline in total progestagens; this switch from progestagens to cortisol production is achieved via induction of the adrenal enzyme, 17α-hydroxylase [37]. The rise in fetal cortisol is stimulated by increases in fetal plasma corticotropin (adrenocorticotrophic hormone) concentrations, enhanced sensitivity of the adrenal cortex to corticotropin, and a decrease in the cortisol-binding capacity over the last week(s) of gestation [37,38]. The prepartum increase in fetal cortisol seems to occur independently of any changes in maternal plasma cortisol concentrations, although some authors have reported a rise during the last 48 hours [39,40]. Equally, there is no change in uterine glucocorticoid receptor concentrations [14]. The rise in equine fetal cortisol has been correlated with a number of maturational events in fetal tissues. These are summarized in Table 1. Because cortisol is essential for fetal maturation, foals delivered before the rise in fetal cortisol exhibit typical signs of prematurity and usually die from multiorgan failure [41]. They fail to show the normal postnatal increase in plasma cortisol concentrations, and postnatal treatment with hydrocortisone or corticotropin has only limited success in a clinical setting, although administration of depot corticotropin can increase adrenal responsiveness [42]. In contrast, foals born after the normal rise in fetal cortisol are mature and viable and exhibit large increases in plasma cortisol after birth and in response to endogenous or exogenous corticotropin.

Table 1
Maturational effects of the pre-partum cortisol surge on various tissues in the equine fetus

Tissue	Effects
Liver	Deposition of glycogen
	Induction of glucose-6-phosphatase for gluconeogenesis
	Induction of β adrenergic receptors
	Decreased production of cortisol binding globulin
Thyroid	Increase in T3, possibly via induction of hepatic T4 deiodinase
Lung	Indirect evidence for a role in lung maturation
Gut	Indirect evidence for a role in maturation of the gastrointestinal tract
Adrenal	Increased sensitivity to corticotropin hormone (possibly via induction of corticotropin receptors)
	Induction of 17α-hydroxylase for cortisol production
Bone marrow	Increase in leucocytes, particularly neutrophils
Cardiovascular	Increase in blood pressure and plasma angiotensin converting enzyme

Data from [7,41,42,72,83,84].

Endocrine changes associated with fetoplacental problems

Any clinical condition that directly affects the placenta or fetus, for example, placentitis, placental separation, or alteration in umbilical blood flow attributable to a cord pathologic condition, is likely to have disruptive effects on the endocrine capacity of the fetoplacental unit. Maternal signs are manifested only after some time, because the disease process alters endocrine pathways and stimulates inflammatory and immune responses leading to, for example, the onset of premature mammary development or a vaginal discharge. Consequently, the hormone patterns measured by the clinician in the mare's peripheral plasma often reflect the later rather than early stages of a disease process. This section discusses the major hormone patterns that may be used to diagnose fetoplacental dysfunction.

Progestagens

Maternal plasma total progestagen concentrations are useful to predict fetal health. Progestagen production involves the fetal adrenal; therefore, progestagens can provide a measure of fetal stress and fetal adrenocortical activity, which is necessary for postnatal survival of the foal. Three abnormal patterns have been observed in maternal plasma.

The first pattern is when progestagen concentrations are declining rapidly (over a few hours or days) or are already close to zero (Fig. 4). This pattern represents the worst scenario, where there is fetal death or fetal expulsion is imminent. It is an acute condition and has been recorded in cases of maternal stress, uterine torsion, colic, or experimentally induced placentitis when

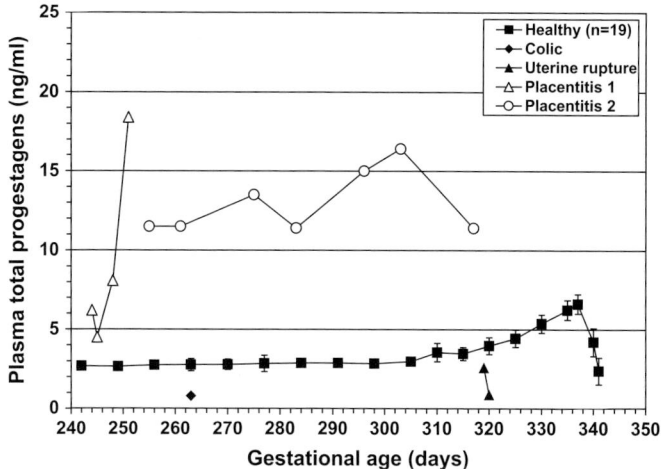

Fig. 4. Plasma total progestagens in 19 normal mares in late gestation, in 2 mares with placentitis (high concentrations), and in 2 mares with colic or uterine rupture (low or declining concentrations).

the mares abort rapidly (ie, within 7 days of infection) [43–45]. Measurement of specific progestagens in maternal plasma has revealed that all the metabolites of P5 and P4 are less than the 95% confidence interval (CI), consistent with failure of the fetus and UP tissues to produce and metabolize progestagens [5].

The second pattern occurs when progestagen concentrations are raised precociously to levels greater than 95% CI for healthy mares of a similar gestation age (see Fig. 4). Such high concentrations are usually found only before spontaneous parturition at term. Maternal plasma total progestagen concentrations may remain elevated for several weeks before delivery, and the foals, if born alive, often have normal or hyperadrenocortical function with raised plasma P5 concentrations, even when delivered before term [8,46,47]. This pattern of high total progestagen concentrations is generally associated with placental pathologic findings. Analysis of specific progestagens by GC-MS has revealed two different profiles associated with different placental problems [5]. The first profile involves unusually high concentrations of nearly all the progestagens and has been observed most frequently in mares with placentitis [8,43,48,49]. This pattern indicates that the fetus and the UP tissues are metabolically active, despite the presence of bacteria or their products within these tissues.

The second profile of high progestagens contains, specifically, elevated concentrations of P4, but concentrations of P5 and several metabolites are normal or low; this profile was found in two mares, one with extensive placental villous poverty (poor or sparsely developed microvilli) and one with placental edema. In these cases, it seems that the placenta was less capable of metabolizing P4 into 5α-DHP and other progestagens, and demonstrates the importance of a functional placental-endometrial complex for the metabolism of progestagens.

The third pattern occurs when maternal plasma total progestagen concentrations fail to show the normal prepartum rise. This pattern is almost exclusively found in mares that are exposed to ergopeptine alkaloids from the endophyte fungus found on tall fescue grass (fescue toxicosis), although it has also been observed in apparently healthy mares with prolonged gestations (J.C. Ousey, MSc, PhD, unpublished observations, 2005) [50]. In mares with fescue toxicosis, prepartum total plasma progestagen concentrations remain low up to parturition; their foals have low cortisol concentrations, indicating suppression of fetal adrenocortical activity and P5 production [50]. Fescue toxicosis is also associated with agalactia and an increased incidence of stillbirth, dystocia, and placental and fetal abnormalities. Administration of the dopamine receptor antagonist domperidone (1.1 mg/kg of body weight administered orally) for 30 days before the expected foaling date improves foal outcome [51].

In general, mares with high total progestagen concentrations are more likely to deliver live foals than those with low concentrations, because there has been some degree of fetal hypothalamo-pituitary-adrenal (HPA) activity. Foals born after these chronic insults often show precocious fetal maturation even when born many weeks before term (Fig. 5) [8,52]. Although

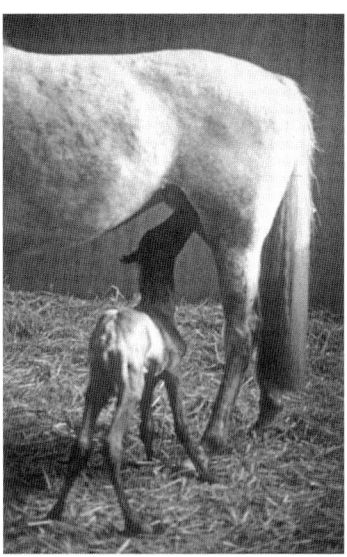

Fig. 5. Thoroughbred foal (body weight of 21 kg) born at 277 days of gestation from a mare with a placental hemorrhage. The mare "ran milk" and had raised plasma progestagens for 3 weeks before delivery. The foal survived with minimal nursing care. (Photograph courtesy of A.J. McGladdery, Newmarket, England.)

an increase in fetal cortisol is advantageous for fetal survival, exposure to high levels of glucocorticoids causes a reduction in fetal body weight at birth [53]. Foals born after placentitis frequently have a low birth weight (typically <35 kg for Thoroughbred foals even when born at term). They may also have poor skeletal development with subsequent limb problems (see Fig. 5). It is not clear whether these low birth weights are caused by exposure to high cortisol concentrations, limited nutrient supplies attributable to reduced placental blood flow, or a combination of the two.

Based on these three progestagen profiles, the data indicate that maternal plasma progestagen concentrations provide a measure not only of placental function but of fetal adrenocortical activity, and thus foal outcome. To monitor progestagen profiles of mares at risk of losing their pregnancies, it is recommended that, initially, three jugular blood samples be collected daily for measurement of total progestagens using an assay that has been well characterized for normal concentrations in late pregnancy. These samples should determine if profiles are increasing or decreasing. Thereafter, regular sampling will enable the clinician to monitor any changes in fetoplacental health.

Estrogens

Because estrogens are produced by the fetoplacental unit, they can provide a measure of fetal viability. In clinical cases of threatened abortion, estrone sulfate (E_1S) concentrations are frequently measured because E_1S is the most abundant estrogen. If the fetus is severely compromised or dead in utero, maternal plasma E_1S concentrations are baseline because of the absence of the C19 precursors secreted by the fetal gonads. In mares with pregnancies compromised by equine herpesvirus-1 infection or severe colic, maternal plasma E_1S concentrations may be normal or transiently decreased [44,54]. Conversely, estrogen concentrations are higher than normal in mares carrying twins [48]. Compared with the adrenal glands, the gonads are unlikely to respond to fetal stress; consequently, it is doubtful that total estrogen concentrations can predict fetal death. For example, in mares induced to abort with PG or its analogue, conjugated estrogen concentrations did not decline until within 5 hours of fetal death [55]. To identify a significant change in E_1S concentrations before fetal death or abortion, it would be necessary to sample mares several times a day, and in most situations, this procedure would have no advantages over a fetal ultrasound or electrocardiographic (ECG) examination.

Prostaglandins

PGs are released in response to inflammation. For example, recent data have shown that mares with experimentally induced placentitis have substantially higher allantoic concentrations of $PGF_{2\alpha}$ and PGE_2 48 hours before delivery compared with healthy mares, although maternal plasma PGFM concentrations were decreased [49,56]. These increases are associated with greater expression of mRNA for the proinflammatory cytokines interleukin-1 and interleukin-8 in placental tissue. Although high concentrations of PGs probably indicate imminent delivery, it is unlikely that they can be used diagnostically because they are rapidly metabolized and their release may be localized within the uterus; thus, changes in PG concentrations may not be apparent in maternal peripheral plasma.

Relaxin

Relaxin should reflect placental function, and preliminary evidence indicates that maternal plasma relaxin concentrations decline before abortion [34,57]. Decreasing levels are associated with poor development of the placental microcotyledons; therefore, it seems that relaxin may be useful as a biologic marker of placental viability provided that suitable equine assays become widely available [32,57].

Cortisol

Maternal cortisol concentrations increase in response to various types of stress. In theory, there is little transplacental transfer of cortisol from the mare to the fetus, because cortisol is converted to inactive cortisone by the placental enzyme 11β-HSD type 2 [58]. Although the fetus is protected from fluctuations in maternal cortisol, fetal levels may still increase in response to a variety of stimuli. For example, 11β-HSD type 2 is not 100% efficient, allowing 10% to 20% of cortisol to cross the placenta in rats, whereas synthetic glucocorticoids completely bypass placental 11β-HSD type 2 [53]. In pigs and mares, elevated maternal cortisol concentrations after corticotropin administration stimulate fetal adrenocortical activity [59,60]. In many species, alterations in UP blood flow or hypoxemia stimulates the fetal HPA axis and fetal cortisol production [61]. Clearly, the equine fetus is not immune to the effects of maternal stress. Measurement of maternal cortisol does not necessarily provide a good marker of fetal health, however [44].

Hormone treatments for mares at risk of preterm birth

There is little empiric evidence that hormone treatments can be used to prevent preterm birth in mares. Yet, the administration of P4 to mares at risk of abortion is widespread, although its use has not been justified. In contrast, experimental work with glucocorticoids to promote fetal maturation in the horse is encouraging, but such treatments are not used routinely as they are in human obstetrics. This section reviews the rationale for various hormone treatments in late gestation and discusses the evidence that is available to support or refute the clinical benefits of such treatments.

Progesterone

Mares that show premonitory signs of threatened abortion or have a history of pregnancy loss may be given P4 treatment in an attempt to delay parturition. The basis for this treatment is the belief that P4 maintains myometrial quiescence. As discussed previously, however, this tenet is complicated by (1) the number of progestagens that are quantitatively important in mares' plasma, (2) information suggesting that 5α-DHP or another progestagen may be biologically active in the pregnant uterus, and (3) the fact that progestagens did not prevent OX-induced myometrial contractions in vitro. The orally active synthetic P4 altrenogest (44 mg) is given daily to mares with signs of impending abortion (eg, premature mammary development, raised plasma progestagen concentrations) in the hope that it may reverse these effects and prolong gestation. The underlying principle for giving P4 is unclear, because plasma progestagen concentrations typically are raised in mares that show these premonitory signs [8,43]. Moreover, it may even be contraindicated, because high progestagen concentrations inhibit the placental enzyme 3β-HSD, which is responsible for producing P4 from P5 and causes a decline in progestagens in vitro and in vivo [62,63]. Blockade of 3β-HSD experimentally actually causes parturition in the pig, sheep, and primate, although not in the mare [4,64,65]. There may be cause for concern with increasing peripheral or tissue concentrations of progestagens, however, particularly in mares that are prone to premature delivery.

Altrenogest acts by binding to the PR but has little effect on endogenous plasma total progestagen concentrations [66]. Specifically, P4 concentrations are unchanged but 5α-DHP and 3β-5P levels may be increased, despite the fact that altrenogest is not metabolized to 5α-pregnanes in the horse [67]. The only scientific evidence that altrenogest prevents abortion in mares is during the first trimester, when it prevented abortion induced by repeated administration of $PGF_{2\alpha}$ (cloprostenol), whereas all the control mares and three of eight mares receiving authentic P4 aborted [68]. Results from clinical practice demonstrate that mares can still abort while receiving altrenogest treatment in the last trimester of pregnancy, however [5]. In women at risk of preterm birth, administration of 17α-hydroxyprogesterone caproate, a metabolite of P4, significantly reduced the incidence of early deliveries, and this was more effective than other reported progestagen treatments [69]. The level of 17α-hydroxyprogesterone is low (0.5 ng/mL) in the plasma of late pregnant mares [3]. Nevertheless, it is possible that a progestagen other than P4 (or synthetic P4) may be more effective at preventing preterm birth in the mare.

Recent findings from a clinical study demonstrated that altrenogest, when given in combination with antimicrobials, pentoxifylline, and nonsteroidal anti-inflammatory drugs (NSAIDs) to 15 mares with placentitis, decreased the incidence of abortion and low birth weight in live-born foals [70]. It is not clear what role, if any, altrenogest plays within this multitreatment approach. Placentitis or intrauterine infection is a complex disease and clearly involves many endocrine pathways. Mares with placentitis have raised progestagen concentrations, increased cytokine and PG concentrations in amniotic fluid, and increased myometrial activity [43]. P4 may exert its effects by interfering with PG production stimulated by proinflammatory cytokines. Certainly, the study of Daels and colleagues [68] demonstrated that the rise in endogenous $PGF_{2\alpha}$ concentrations was inhibited by altrenogest treatment. Furthermore, if altrenogest acts in the same manner as P4 to regulate PG catabolism via PGDH in the placenta (as described previously), this may provide one pathway by which altrenogest could regulate PG synthesis, and hence myometrial activity.

The evidence that progestagen treatment prevents preterm birth in mares is conflicting and can only be resolved by further scientific work.

Glucocorticoids

Administration of synthetic glucocorticoids to pregnant women is used clinically to reduce the incidence of respiratory distress syndrome and cerebral hemorrhage in the neonate, while fetal cortisol infusion in animal species stimulates precocious delivery of mature offspring [37,71]. In the cow and goat, glucocorticoids also induce parturition [20]. Glucocorticoids are rarely used to induce parturition in mares because they are unreliable and because uterotonic agents, such as OX and PGs, are more effective. Research into glucocorticoids as a means of inducing precocious fetal maturation in mares has been limited. Silver and coworkers [72] infused a catheterized pony fetus with $corticotropin_{1-24}$ on day 315 of gestation, before the marked rise in fetal cortisol concentrations, and delivered a mature foal 4.5 days later. Subsequently, Ousey and colleagues [73] injected equine fetuses at 300 days of gestation with depot corticotropin at a dose of 1 mg/d over 3 days using a transabdominal approach and induced delivery of mature viable foals before term (Fig. 6). This technique caused abortion in 33% of mares treated, however. In a second study, maternally administered depot corticotropin (4–5 mg administered intramuscularly) also induced precocious fetal maturation, but this approach was not 100% effective [60]. Limited experience in using corticotropin in clinical cases, where there was little chance of fetal viability without intervention, resulted in a viable foal in one of three mares (Table 2).

There has been a resurgence of interest in the use of synthetic glucocorticoids in pregnant mares. Originally Alm and coworkers [74] used dexamethasone as an inducing agent and showed that dexamethasone at a dose of 100 mg/d administered intramuscularly from 320 days of gestation in Saddlebred mares induced delivery of viable foals within 4 days; gestational length was significantly reduced compared with that of control mares. In contrast, Jeffcott and Rossdale [75] gave dexamethasone at a dose of 100 mg to pony mares close to parturition and caused dystocia and fetal death in

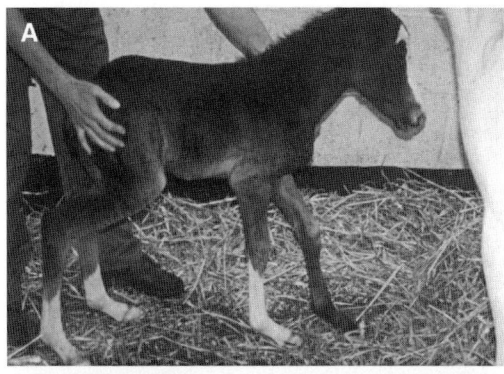
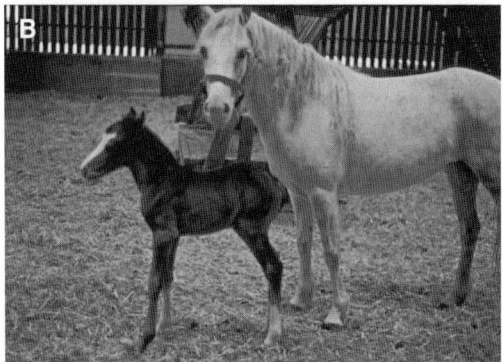

Fig. 6. Pony foal born at 307 days of gestation after three intrafetal injections with corticotropin depot (1 mg) at 300, 301, and 302 days of gestation. The foal was precociously mature but initially required assistance to stand. (*A*) Foal aged 1 hour shows slight laxity of fetlock joints. (*B*) Foal aged 24 hours shows normal fetlock extension.

two of three mares. Despite these adverse results, there are unpublished clinical reports that fetal outcome is improved after dexamethasone (100 mg) administered intramuscularly over 1 to 4 days to mares at risk of premature delivery through illness. This has not been scientifically verified. The author recently repeated the original work of Alm and coworkers [74] in Thoroughbred mares treated at 315 days of gestation with dexamethasone at a dose of 100 mg administered intramuscularly for 3 days; the foals were delivered early but were mature based on a number of clinical and endocrine parameters, and no adverse effects were observed. In contrast, intramuscular administration of betamethasone (12–30 mg) to pregnant mares at 305 to 307 days of gestation, followed by induction of delivery at 320 days, did not induce fetal maturation and resulted in a poor outcome in some foals [76]. The difference in the results between all these studies may partially reflect the gestational age at the time of administration and the degree of fetal HPA activity. Dexamethasone has anti-inflammatory effects that decrease PG production and could disrupt the normal endocrine pathways at

Table 2
Foal outcome in 3 Thoroughbred mares given intra-fetal corticotropin Depot injections in late gestation. All 3 mares were undergoing treatment for clinical conditions that necessitated euthanasia at, or shortly after, delivery

ID	Mare clinical condition	Fetal corticotropin treatment	Foaling	Foal outcome
1	Chronic laminitis	1 mg at 337, 338 & 339 days gestation	Induced with 12 IU oxytocin at 341 days gestation. Milk Ca^{2+} 5.5 mmol/L	Foal had post-natal cortisol rise. Survived with intensive care
2	Eosinophillic Granulomatous Enteritis	1 mg at 368 & 370 days gestation	Spontaneous delivery at 372 days gestation Premature placental separation	Dead on delivery
3	Leg injury. Received long term Phenylbutazone and antibiotics	1 mg at 314, 315 and 316 days gestation	Caesarean section at 331 days	Intensive care, developed joint sepsis. Euthanasia at aged 10 days

parturition if given to mares close to term. Similarly, if fetuses already have some degree of HPA activity, administration of glucocorticoids may have a suppressive effect rather than a stimulatory effect on the fetal adrenal, which may account for poor fetal outcome in some of these studies.

A new role for glucocorticoids is under consideration as a possible treatment to suppress inflammatory responses in mares with placentitis. In human beings and nonhuman primates with intrauterine infections, fetal cortisol levels are increased during preterm labor, and the evidence from mares with placentitis certainly indicates that there is increased fetal adrenocortical activity [8,43,77,78]. It has been suggested that this fetal stress response may have evolved to suppress and modulate the inflammatory responses caused by intrauterine infection. Glucocorticoids are immunosuppressants and act, in part, by blocking genes for the proinflammatory cytokines, which, in turn, can have effects on PG production [78]. The duration of pregnancy in infected nonhuman primates was significantly prolonged after treatment with dexamethasone, indomethacin, and antibiotics compared with antibiotic treatment alone [79]. Studies are currently being performed to test whether a treatment regimen with dexamethasone and antibiotics may be effective in mares with experimentally induced placentitis [80].

These data indicate that glucocorticoids may offer some new treatments for pregnant mares at risk of preterm delivery. Further information is needed about their possible mode of action, however, and refinements need to be made regarding their route of administration, dosages, and gestational age for treatment. Also, the effects of glucocorticoids on long-term health of the fetus may need to be considered [53].

Antiprostaglandins

Administration of the PG synthetase inhibitor meclofenamic acid to pregnant mares after abdominal surgery diminishes the normal postsurgical rise in PGFM and facilitates fetal survival compared with that in untreated mares [27]. Again, interest in PG inhibitors may emerge in the context of suppressing inflammatory responses in mares with placentitis as it has in other animals [79]. Blockade of myometrial activity in mares in second-stage labor is particularly difficult, however. Administration of the cyclooxygenase inhibitor flunixin meglumine (1.1 mg/kg administered twice intravenously) to healthy mares at term failed to prevent or even delay OX-induced delivery. Although plasma $PGF_{2\alpha}$ concentrations were significantly reduced in the treated mares, OX and arginine-vasopressin concentrations were no different from those of untreated controls [81].

Other agents

A number of other treatments may be important to prevent preterm birth in mares. Many of these tocolytic drugs (eg, β-sympathomimetics, calcium channel blockers) that prevent or disrupt myometrial activity are not strictly hormones; therefore, the reader is referred to reviews elsewhere [43,71,82].

Summary

The hormones discussed here are not an exhaustive list of the hormones involved in parturition, but they provide the key elements to the process of parturition in mares at term and preterm. The role of progestagens has been elucidated regarding prepartum changes in healthy mares and in mares at risk of abortion. It is still not known which, if any, progestagen regulates myometrial quiescence, and hence whether exogenous P4 therapy may assist in preventing preterm birth. More information is being gathered, particularly on the endocrine changes associated with placentitis and about exogenous glucocorticoid therapy. At present, progestagen profiles provide the best endocrine test to diagnose fetoplacental health, particularly when used in conjunction with other diagnostic techniques, such as fetal and placental ultrasound examinations.

Acknowledgments

This manuscript was prepared with kind help from Lorraine Palmer and Françoise Hess-Dudan.

References

[1] Holtan DW, Houghton E, Silver M, et al. Plasma progestagens in the mare, fetus and newborn foal. J Reprod Fertil Suppl 1991;44:517–28.
[2] Short RV. Progesterone in blood: IV. Progesterone in the blood of mares. J Endocrinol 1959; 19:207–10.
[3] Holtan DW, Nett TM, Estergreen VL. Plasma progestins in pregnant, postpartum and cycling mares. J Anim Sci 1975;40(2):251–60.
[4] Chavatte P, Holtan D, Ousey JC, et al. Biosynthesis and possible biological roles of progestagens during equine pregnancy and in the newborn foal. Equine Vet J Suppl 1997;24: 89–95.
[5] Ousey JC, Forhead AJ, Rossdale PD, et al. Ontogeny of uteroplacental progestagen production in pregnant mares during the second half of gestation. Biol Reprod 2003;69(2):540–8.
[6] Hamon M, Clarke SW, Houghton E, et al. Production of 5 alpha-dihydroprogesterone during late pregnancy in the mare. J Reprod Fertil Suppl 1991;44:529–35.
[7] Han X, Rossdale PD, Ousey J, et al. Localisation of 15-hydroxy prostaglandin dehydrogenase (PGDH) and steroidogenic enzymes in the equine placenta. Equine Vet J 1995;27(5): 334–9.
[8] Rossdale PD, Ousey JC, Cottrill CM, et al. Effects of placental pathology on maternal plasma progestagen and mammary secretion calcium concentrations and on neonatal adrenocortical function in the horse. J Reprod Fertil Suppl 1991;44:579–90.
[9] Csapo A. Progesterone block. Am J Anat 1956;98(2):273–91.
[10] Elovitz MA, Mrinalini C. Animal models of preterm birth. Trends Endocrinol Metab 2004; 15(10):479–87.
[11] Haluska GJ, Wells TR, Hirst JJ, et al. Progesterone receptor localization and isoforms in myometrium, decidua, and fetal membranes from rhesus macaques: evidence for functional progesterone withdrawal at parturition. J Soc Gynecol Investig 2002;9(3):125–36.
[12] Mesiano S, Chan EC, Fitter JT, et al. Progesterone withdrawal and estrogen activation in human parturition are coordinated by progesterone receptor A expression in the myometrium. J Clin Endocrinol Metab 2002;87(6):2924–30.
[13] Fowden AL, Ousey J, Forhead AJ, et al. Uteroplacental production of 5α-pregnane-3,20-dione (5α-DHP) in pregnant mares. Theriogenology 2002;58:821–4.
[14] Chavatte Palmer P, Duchamp G, Palmer E, et al. Progesterone, oestrogen and glucocorticoid receptors in the uterus and mammary glands of mares from mid- to late-gestation. J Reprod Fertil Suppl 2000;56:661–72.
[15] Ousey JC, Freestone N, Fowden AL, et al. The effects of oxytocin and progestagens on myometrial contractility in vitro during equine pregnancy. J Reprod Fertil Suppl 2000;56: 681–9.
[16] Barri ME, Abbas SK, Care AD. The effects in the rat of two fragments of parathyroid hormone-related protein on uterine contractions in situ. Exp Physiol 1992;77(3):481–90.
[17] Bowden SJ, Emly JF, Hughes SV, et al. Parathyroid hormone-related protein in human term placenta and membranes. J Endocrinol 1994;142(2):217–24.
[18] Egarter CH, Husslein P. Biochemistry of myometrial contractility. Baillieres Clin Obstet Gynaecol 1992;6(4):755–69.
[19] Haluska GJ, Currie WB. Variation in plasma concentrations of oestradiol-17 beta and their relationship to those of progesterone, 13,14-dihydro-15-keto-prostaglandin F-2 alpha and oxytocin across pregnancy and at parturition in pony mares. J Reprod Fertil 1988;84(2): 635–46.
[20] Silver M. Prenatal maturation, the timing of birth and how it may be regulated in domestic animals. Exp Physiol 1990;75(3):285–307.
[21] Pashen RL. Maternal and foetal endocrinology during late pregnancy and parturition in the mare. Equine Vet J 1984;16(4):233–8.
[22] Mostl E. The horse feto-placental unit. Exp Clin Endocrinol 1994;102(3):166–8.

[23] Cox JE. Oestrone and equilin in the plasma of the pregnant mare. J Reprod Fertil Suppl 1975;23:463–8.
[24] Pashen RL, Allen WR. The role of the fetal gonads and placenta in steroid production, maintenance of pregnancy and parturition in the mare. J Reprod Fertil Suppl 1979;27: 499–509.
[25] McGlothlin JA, Lester GD, Hansen PJ, et al. Alteration in uterine contractility in mares with experimentally induced placentitis. Reproduction 2004;127(1):57–66.
[26] O'Donnell LJ, Sheerin BR, Hendry JM, et al. 24-Hour secretion patterns of plasma oestradiol 17beta in pony mares in late gestation. Reprod Domest Anim 2003;38(3): 233–5.
[27] Silver M, Barnes RJ, Comline RS, et al. Prostaglandins in maternal and fetal plasma and in allantoic fluid during the second half of gestation in the mare. J Reprod Fertil Suppl 1979;27: 531–9.
[28] Vivrette SL, Kindahl H, Munro CJ, et al. Oxytocin release and its relationship to dihydro-15-keto PGF2alpha and arginine vasopressin release during parturition and to suckling in post-partum mares. J Reprod Fertil 2000;119(2):347–57.
[29] Mitchell BF, Fang X, Wong S. Oxytocin: a paracrine hormone in the regulation of parturition? Rev Reprod 1998;3(2):113–22.
[30] Camillo F, Marmorini P, Romagnoli S, et al. Clinical studies on daily low dose oxytocin in mares at term. Equine Vet J 2000;32(4):307–10.
[31] Pashen RL. Low doses of oxytocin can induce foaling at term. Equine Vet J 1980;12(2):85–7.
[32] Klonisch T, Hombach-Klonisch S. Review: relaxin expression at the feto-maternal interface. Reprod Domest Anim 2000;35:149–52.
[33] Stewart DR, Kindahl H, Stabenfeldt GH, et al. Concentrations of 15-keto-13, 14-dihydro-prostaglandin F2 alpha in the mare during spontaneous and oxytocin induced foaling. Equine Vet J 1984;16(4):270–4.
[34] Stewart DR, Addiego LA, Pascoe DR, et al. Breed differences in circulating equine relaxin. Biol Reprod 1992;46(4):648–52.
[35] Fowden AL. Endocrine regulation of fetal growth. Reprod Fertil Dev 1995;7(3):351–63.
[36] Liggins GC. The role of cortisol in preparing the fetus for birth. Reprod Fertil Dev 1994;6(2): 141–50.
[37] Fowden AL, Silver M. Comparative development of the pituitary-adrenal axis in the fetal foal and lamb. Reprod Domest Anim 1995;30:170–7.
[38] Cudd TA, LeBlanc M, Silver M, et al. Ontogeny and ultradian rhythms of adrenocorticotropin and cortisol in the late-gestation fetal horse. J Endocrinol 1995;144(2):271–83.
[39] Nathanielsz PW, Rossdale PD, Silver M, et al. Studies on fetal, neonatal and maternal cortisol metabolism in the mare. J Reprod Fertil Suppl 1975;23:625–30.
[40] Silver M, Fowden AL. Prepartum adrenocortical maturation in the fetal foal: responses to ACTH. J Endocrinol 1994;142(3):417–25.
[41] Rossdale PD, Ousey JC, Silver M, et al. Studies on equine prematurity 6: guidelines for assessment of foal maturity. Equine Vet J 1984;16(4):300–2.
[42] Silver M, Ousey JC, Dudan FE, et al. Studies on equine prematurity 2: post natal adrenocortical activity in relation to plasma adrenocorticotrophic hormone and catecholamine levels in term and premature foals. Equine Vet J 1984;16(4):278–86.
[43] LeBlanc MM, Macpherson M, Sheerin P. Ascending placentitis: what we know about pathophysiology, diagnosis and treatment. Proc Am Assoc Equine Pract 2004;50:127–43.
[44] Santschi EM, LeBlanc MM, Weston PG. Progestagen, oestrone sulphate and cortisol concentrations in pregnant mares during medical and surgical disease. J Reprod Fertil Suppl 1991;44:627–34.
[45] van Niekerk CH, Morgenthal JC. Fetal loss and the effect of stress on plasma progestagen levels in pregnant Thoroughbred mares. J Reprod Fertil Suppl 1982;32:453–7.
[46] Houghton E, Holtan D, Grainger L, et al. Plasma progestagen concentrations in the normal and dysmature newborn foal. J Reprod Fertil Suppl 1991;44:609–17.

[47] Rossdale PD, Ousey JC, McGladdery AJ, et al. A retrospective study of increased plasma progestagen concentrations in compromised neonatal foals. Reprod Fertil Dev 1995;7(3): 567–75.
[48] Hoffmann B, Gentz F, Failing K. Investigations into the course of progesterone-, oestrogen- and eCG- concentrations during normal and impaired pregnancy in the mare. Reprod Domest Anim 1996;31:717–23.
[49] Stawicki RJ, Reubel H, Hansen PJ, et al. Endocrinological findings in an experimental model of ascending placentitis in the mare. Theriogenology 2002;58:849–52.
[50] Brendemeuhl JP, Williams MA, Boosinger TR, et al. Plasma progestagen, trioiodo-thyronine and cortisol concentrations in postdate gestation foals exposed in utero to the tall fescue endophyte *Acremonium coenophialum*. Biol Reprod Monogr 1995; 1:53–9.
[51] Cross DL, Redmond LM, Strickland JR. Equine fescue toxicosis: signs and solutions. J Anim Sci 1995;73(3):899–908.
[52] Ousey J, McGladdery A. Clinical diagnosis and treatment of problems in the late pregnant mare. In Pract 2000;22(4):200–7.
[53] Seckl JR. Prenatal glucocorticoids and long-term programming. Eur J Endocrinol 2004;151: U49–62.
[54] Ousey JC, Rossdale PD, Cash RS, et al. Plasma concentrations of progestagens, oestrone sulphate and prolactin in pregnant mares subjected to natural challenge with equid herpes-virus-1. J Reprod Fertil Suppl 1987;35:519–28.
[55] Daels PF, Mahammed HO, Montavon SME, et al. Endogenous prostaglandin secretion during cloprostenol-induced abortion in mares. Anim Reprod Sci 1995;40:305–21.
[56] LeBlanc MM, Giguere S, Brauer K, et al. Premature delivery in ascending placentitis is associated with increased expression of placental cytokines and allantoic fluid prostaglandins E2 and F$_{2\alpha}$. Theriogenology 2002;58:841–4.
[57] Ryan P, Vaala W, Bagnell C. Evidence that equine relaxin is a good indicator of placental insufficiency in the mare. Proc Am Assoc Equine Pract 1998;44:62–3.
[58] Chavatte P, Rossdale PD, Tait AD. 11β-hydroxysteroid dehydrogenase (11β-HSD) in equine placenta. Proc Am Assoc Equine Pract 1995;41:264–5.
[59] Otten W, Kanitz E, Tuchscherer M, et al. Effects of adrenocorticotropin stimulation on cortisol dynamics of pregnant gilts and their fetuses: implications for prenatal stress studies. Theriogenology 2004;61(9):1649–59.
[60] Ousey JC, Rossdale PD, Palmer L, et al. Effects of maternally administered depot ACTH1-24 on fetal maturation and the timing of parturition in the mare. Equine Vet J 2000;32: 489–96.
[61] Challis JRG, Cox DB, Sloboda DM. Regulation of corticosteroids in the fetus: control of birth and influence on adult disease. Semin Neonatol 1999;4:93–7.
[62] Chavatte PM, Rossdale PD, Tait AD. Modulation of 3 beta-hydroxysteroid dehydrogenase (3 beta-HSD) activity in the equine placenta by pregnenolone and progesterone metabolites. Equine Vet J 1995;27(5):342–7.
[63] Schutzer WE, Kerby JL, Holtan DW. Differential effect of trilostane on the progestin milieu in the pregnant mare. J Reprod Fertil 1996;107(2):241–8.
[64] Fowden AL, Silver M. Effect of inhibiting 3β-hydroxysteroid dehydrogenase on plasma progesterone and other steroids in the pregnant mare near term. J Reprod Fertil Suppl 1987;35: 539–45.
[65] Silver M, Fowden AL. Induction of labour in domestic animals: endocrine changes and neonatal viability. In: Kűnzel W, Jensen A, editors. The endocrine control of the fetus. Berlin: Springer-Verlag; 1988. p. 401–11.
[66] Jackson SA, Squires EL, Nett TM. The effect of exogenous progestins in endogenous progesterone secretion in pregnant mares. Theriogenology 1986;25:275–9.
[67] Ousey JC, Rossdale PD, Palmer L, et al. Effects of progesterone administration to mares during late gestation. Theriogenology 2002;58:793–5.

[68] Daels PF, Besognet B, Hansen B, et al. Effect of progesterone on prostaglandin F2 alpha secretion and outcome of pregnancy during cloprostenol-induced abortion in mares. Am J Vet Res 1996;57(9):1331–7.
[69] Meis PJ, Klebanoff M, Thom E, et al. Prevention of recurrent preterm delivery by 17 alpha-hydroxyprogesterone caproate. N Engl J Med 2003;348(24):2379–85.
[70] Troedsson MHT, Zent WW. Clinical ultrasonagraphic evaluation of the equine placenta as a method to successfully identify and treat mares with placentitis. In: Proceedings of a Workshop on the Equine Placenta. Lexington (KY): Kentucky Agricultural Experiment Station. 2003. p. 66–7.
[71] Haram K, Mortensen JH, Wollen AL. Preterm delivery: an overview. Acta Obstet Gynecol Scand 2003;82(8):687–704.
[72] Silver M, Fowden AL, Knox J, et al. Relationship between circulating tri-iodothyronine and cortisol in the perinatal period in the foal. J Reprod Fertil Suppl 1991;44:619–26.
[73] Ousey JC, Rossdale PD, Dudan FE, et al. The effects of intrafetal ACTH administration on the outcome of pregnancy in the mare. Reprod Fertil Dev 1998;10(4):359–67.
[74] Alm CC, Sullivan JJ, First NL. The effect of a corticosteroid (dexamethasone), progesterone, oestrogen and prostaglandin F2alpha on gestation length in normal and ovariectomized mares. J Reprod Fertil Suppl 1975;23:637–40.
[75] Jeffcott LB, Rossdale PD. A critical review of current methods for induction of parturition in the mare. Equine Vet J 1977;9(4):208–15.
[76] Christiansen D, Olsen G, Smith J, et al. The use of betamethasone to advance fetal maturation in the equine. Havemeyer Foundation Monograph Series 2006;19:19–20.
[77] Gravett MG, Haluska GJ, Cook MJ, et al. Fetal and maternal endocrine responses to experimental intrauterine infection in rhesus monkeys [abstract]. Am J Obstet Gynecol 1996;174(6):1725–31.
[78] Gravett MG, Hitti J, Hess DL, et al. Intrauterine infection and preterm delivery: evidence for activation of the fetal hypothalamic-pituitary-adrenal axis. Am J Obstet Gynecol 2000;182(6):1404–13.
[79] Gravett MG. Novel treatment strategies for infection-induced pre-term birth: a non-human primate model [abstract]. Havemeyer Foundation Monograph Series 2006;19:32.
[80] Ryan P, Crouch J, Sykes D, et al. Experimentally induced placentitis in late gestation mares with *streptococcus equi zooepidemicus*: prevention of pre-term birth [abstract]. Havemeyer Foundation Monograph Series 2006;19:35–6.
[81] Vivrette SL, Kindahl H, Munro CJ, et al. Effects of flunixin meglumine on pituitary effluent oxytocin, arginine vasopressin and 15-ketodihydroprostaglandin F2α concentrations and clinical parturient events during oxytocin-induced parturition in mares. Biol Reprod Monogr 1995;1:69–75.
[82] Macpherson ML. Treatment strategies for mares with placentitis. Theriogenology 2005;64(3):528–34.
[83] Forhead AJ, Broughton Pipkin F, Taylor PM, et al. Developmental changes in blood pressure and the rennin-angiotensin system in pony fetuses during the second half of gestation. J Reprod Fertil Suppl 2000;56:693–703.
[84] Fowden AL, Mundy L, Ousey JC, et al. Tissue glycogen and glucose 6-phosphatase levels in fetal and newborn foals. J Reprod Fertil Suppl 1991;44:537–42.

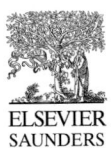

Diagnosis of the Compromised Equine Pregnancy

Stefania Bucca, DVM

The Irish Equine Centre, Johnstown, Naas, County Kildare, Ireland

A compromised equine pregnancy is commonly associated with a high risk of an unfavorable outcome, with maternal, fetal, and neonatal implications. The maternal consequences of a compromised pregnancy may vary from the premature interruption of gestation to reproductive and medical issues, which may interfere with the mare's general health or challenge its ability to carry another pregnancy to term. The impact of maternal or placental disorders on the intrauterine environment generally results in fetal or neonatal compromise that summarizes the effects of one or a combination of three mechanisms: hypoxia, infection, and derangement of in utero development. Fetal compromise may ultimately result in premature or complicated delivery, fetal demise, stillbirth, or abnormalities in neonatal development and behavior. The effects of fetal compromise are dependant on the nature, duration, severity, and stage of gestation of occurrence of the stressful condition.

Perinatal death accounts for the largest percentage of foal mortality, despite our increased ability to treat neonatal disease. Intrauterine disturbance with the restriction of normal development of tissue microstructure provides a potential explanation for some of the findings in the deaths of premature and dysmature foals [1,2]. Fetal growth and development rely on a healthy intrauterine environment and on placental efficiency. Disturbances in the fetomaternal exchange pathways may alter the interchanges of gases, nutrients. and waste products and modify fetal metabolic and endocrine pathways [3]. Maternal health and environment play a major role in the well-being of the intrauterine milieu. Maternal disease, altered gut function, poor or imbalanced nutrition, and the impact of environmental contaminants may profoundly influence fetomaternal communications and critically undermine fetoplacental well-being and development, with immediate and long-term consequences. Abnormal development in utero and diseases of later life may be correlated

E-mail address: stefbucca@hotmail.com

as a result of subtle effects on programming and organogenesis; this has been recently highlighted by Rossdale [4] and opens a new dimension in medical understanding of conditions of the newborn and older individual [5].

Risk factors for the identification of the compromised pregnancy

Mare owners commonly seek veterinary intervention during a periparturient emergency. Difficult deliveries, prolonged gestations, compromised neonates in need of intensive care, overt signs of impending abortion, and sudden increases in abdominal volume represent some of the most common problems requiring veterinary attention in late pregnancy. Under those circumstances, clinicians may have no option but to perform a salvage procedure that often results in the survival of the mare or the neonate. Equine pregnancies at risk of an unfavorable outcome have three problem sources: maternal, placental, and fetal risk factors. Early identification of mares at risk for a compromised pregnancy prompts close supervision of fetomaternal parameters and periparturient events so as to allow for early detection, management, and possible prevention of a perinatal crisis. Furthermore, early recognition of fetal distress signals and abnormal development patterns may help us to understand pathophysiology later in life.

Maternal risk factors are usually readily identified, but the impact on fetal well-being is not clearly quantifiable. Equine fetuses are heavily dependent on the dam's blood glucose and oxygen levels for survival and development [6–8]. Even transient episodes of maternal starvation and hypoxia may have effects on fetal metabolic and endocrine pathways. When nutrient availability is limited, fetal insulin and thyroxine (T_4) decrease and cortisol and prostaglandins increase [9], with a resultant restriction in fetal growth. These endocrine changes are observed whether the fetal supply of substrate is restricted by maternal under nutrition, placental insufficiency, or reduction of uterine or umbilical blood flow [9]. Finally, any condition that affects the thermoregulatory, endocrine, or metabolic state of the mare may influence the uterine circulation, thereby affecting the fetal environment.

Placental risk factors may not be easily recognized, and placental dysfunction represents a diagnostic challenge. Equine placentation requires fetomaternal interdigitation over the entire endometrial surface to optimize fetal development in utero, as illustrated by the inability of most twin conceptuses to be carried to term [10]. Conditions affecting uteroplacental contact and placental efficiency may profoundly influence fetal well-being, development, and survival. Placental edema, placentitis, vasculitis, thrombosis, developmental abnormalities, and umbilical cord obstructions are the most common conditions causing placental dysfunction. Age-related degenerative changes in the endometrium (endometriosis) [11] may also limit placentation by reducing the effective area for fetomaternal exchanges, thereby leading to intrauterine growth restriction (IUGR) of the fetus. Recent stereologic studies of the equine placenta have demonstrated the correlation between foal weight at birth and the balance between fetomaternal contact and placental efficiency in Thoroughbred mares [12]. From this study, it seems that the placenta has the ability to modify its exchange capabilities. The extent and the depth of endometrioplacental contact required to ensure fetal survival to term are not known and cannot be appreciated in vivo. Our ability to diagnose and understand placental dysfunction during gestation is limited by our inability to obtain allantochorion samples safely for histopathologic assessment.

Risk factors of fetal origin include multiple fetuses, congenital abnormalities, infection, prematurity or dysmaturity, fetal malpresentation, and neonatal isoerythrolysis. Some of these conditions may be identified antepartum (ie, detection of twin fetuses by ultrasound in early gestation, blood type screening of dam and stallion to determine the potential for neonatal isoerythrolysis, blood screening for increasing antibody titers during an outbreak of infectious disease, ultrasound assessment of fetal presentation after 9 months of gestation to rule out fetal malpresentation). Other conditions may only be identified after birth.

Finally, some maternal risk factors may develop unexpectedly and trigger an unanticipated perinatal crisis. Examples of these factors would be dystocia, uterine inertia, premature placental separation, and early umbilical cord rupture. In these cases, no previous history can be demonstrated, and they represent challenging veterinary emergencies. Some perinatal problems may not be unpredictable; however, traditionally, the pregnant mare remains without gynecologic supervision during most of middle and late pregnancy. Consequently, subtle signs of fetal distress may not be detected until a crisis precipitates. Ideally, fetoplacental well-being should be monitored throughout gestation by serial collection of a database, including historical, biochemical, and biophysical parameters.

Historical parameters

The past reproductive and medical history of the mare should be collected; this should include all records relevant to previous pregnancies, deliveries, and neonates. The potential risk of recurrence of a medical or reproductive problem should be determined. Concerns should be raised with a past reproductive history of premature delivery, premature separation of the placenta, twin pregnancy, peripartum hemorrhage, development of abdominal hernia or rupture of the prepubic tendon (RPPT) in late gestation, and foal rejection. Medical problems, including chronic laminitis and pelvic injuries, may seriously compromise the successful outcome of a pregnancy.

The recent reproductive and medical history relates more specifically to the current gestation and should be evaluated in detail. Information regarding the status of the endometrium before breeding and after conception, the covering events and modalities, and the type of semen may all be relevant. Results of ultrasound examinations, vaccination history, and blood typing compatibility between the mare and stallion as well as full medical and surgical records should be made available for the complete diagnostic workup of a suspected compromised pregnancy. A full physical examination of the mare should be done, including transrectal palpation of the pelvic contents and laboratory parameters to assess the current health status, when indicated. The environment should be evaluated, including a collective history of the resident equine population. Conditions commonly developing during gestation that increase the risk of an abnormal pregnancy outcome and require in-depth investigation of fetomaternal well-being include severe maternal illness, acute abdominal crisis (eg, gastrointestinal tract conditions, hydroallantois, uterine torsion, uterine rupture, peripartum hemorrhage, abdominal hernia, RPPT), uterine discharge, premature lactation, twinning, and prolonged gestation. Historical parameters related to the postpartum assessment of the dam and neonate include a detailed analysis of the delivery and postfoaling events, colostral quality, and gross and microscopic evaluation of fetal membranes. All these factors may retrospectively identify subtle signs of compromise that may not have been apparent during the course of gestation.

Biochemical parameters

The search for biochemical markers of fetoplacental well-being is the focus of continuing research and speculation. The biochemical parameters most frequently used to assess fetal compromise and predict successful neonatal adaptation include hormonal profiling, electrolyte and immunoglobulin concentrations in mammary secretions, and, occasionally, fetal fluid analysis. Although fetal fluid analysis [13,14] may be useful to measure prostaglandin concentrations, evaluate fetal karyotype, and detect cytologic evidence of infection, amniocentesis and allantocentesis are infrequently performed because they carry a potential degree of risk. Fetal fluid may be collected intrapartum for viral and bacterial culture.

Hormonal profiling

Estrogens and progestagens are the hormonal parameters traditionally evaluated when assessing fetoplacental compromise. Relaxin may be a more reliable indicator of fetoplacental pathologic findings, but the lack of commercially available assays poses major obstacles to its practical application [15]. Prolactin levels at parturition should be evaluated [16] when investigating agalactia, particularly when tall fescue toxicosis is suspected. Plasma hormonal assessment requires multiple sampling for correct interpretation of trends rather than absolute values.

Estrogens

Total estrogen concentrations increase to a variable peak between days 190 and 280 of gestation and fall to baseline values at term [17]. A concentration greater than 1000 ng/mL is considered to be normal. Levels less than 1000 ng/mL are considered to be indicative of fetal distress. Before 300 days of gestation, total estrogens less than 500 ng/mL are commonly associated with a severely compromised or dead fetus, whereas levels between 500 and 800 ng/mL indicate a compromised fetus [18]. Santchi and colleagues [19] concluded from observations on pregnant mares during medical disease that estrone sulfate is not an accurate indicator of fetal viability during late pregnancy.

Progestagens

Placental pathologic findings are strongly correlated with increments in maternal plasma progestagens occurring before day 310 of gestation, when an increase may be caused by approaching parturition [20]. The criteria for interpretation of results should include reference values of the laboratory assay used, breed of mare being tested, and gestational age.

Progesterone (P4) assays that cross-react with pregnanes are often used. Therefore, cross-reactivity is a critical determinant between assays [4]. Ponies usually have lower normal values that increase less and nearer to parturition than those of Thoroughbreds. In the latter breed, however, there is a wide range after 300 days and before parturition. A cutoff of 310 days, before a normal rise in values occurs, represents a practical approach to interpreting abnormal values in Thoroughbreds. Abnormal changes in the dam's progestin profile, such as an abrupt drop or a gradual premature rise, may be diagnostic for fetal stress, such as hypoxia, or mild ischemic events resulting from placentitis or medical or anesthetic compromise. Maternal plasma progestagen concentrations do not change in conditions that directly affect the fetus, such as in herpes virus infection [21].

Concentration of mammary electrolytes

Values at term for calcium (Ca), sodium (Na), and potassium (K) concentrations in mammary secretions (Ca = 30 mmol/L, Na < 20 mmol/L, K > 40 mmol/L) have been identified and related to readiness for birth [22]. Induction of parturition may be safely considered under those circumstances. If these values are approached in the period before 310 days of gestation, this may indicate fetoplacental problems in the presence of other abnormal parameters.

Colostral specific gravity

Foals are born without any immune protection, because immunoglobulins do not cross the equine placenta [23]. The immune protection of the foal during the first 4 to 8 weeks after birth is usually conferred by the ingestion of maternal colostrum at birth. Mare's colostrum should be evaluated for IgG content at parturition to assess one of the possible risks for failure of passive transfer. Colostral specific gravity is related to IgG concentration, and values greater than 1.060 indicate adequate IgG content. Colostral density may be measured with a colostrometer [24] or with a sugar or alcohol refractometer, which provides an easier and more accurate estimate for colostral quality.

Biophysical parameters

Fetal electrocardiography, ultrasonography, and Doppler ultrasonography represent the available technologies to obtain a biophysical assessment of the equine pregnancy.

Fetal ultrasonography is the most reliable and accessible technology because it may be used efficiently to assess fetal growth, presentation, activity, and mobility throughout gestation utilizing combined transrectal and transabdominal approaches [25,26]. Qualitative and quantitative assessment of fetal fluid, multiple fetuses, integrity, and combined thickness of the uteroplacental unit can be evaluated using ultrasound. Normal reference values for fetoplacental parameters from midgestation to term have been established for light-breed mares [27,28]. A comprehensive range of parameters aiming at assessing fetoplacental well-being may include fetal presentation, fetal heart rate (FHR) and rhythm (Fig. 1), fetal activity and size, fetal stomach measurements, uteroplacental thickness, fluid depth, and presence of multiple fetuses.

Fetal presentation

Variability of fetal presentation decreases as gestation advances [28,29] (Fig. 2). After 9 months of gestation, adequate size and positioning of the

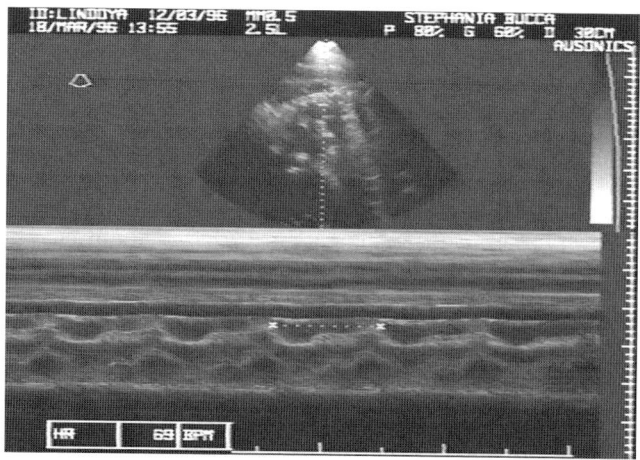

Fig. 1. FHR in a term fetus using M-mode over the cardiac area, with the mare facing toward the right of the sonogram.

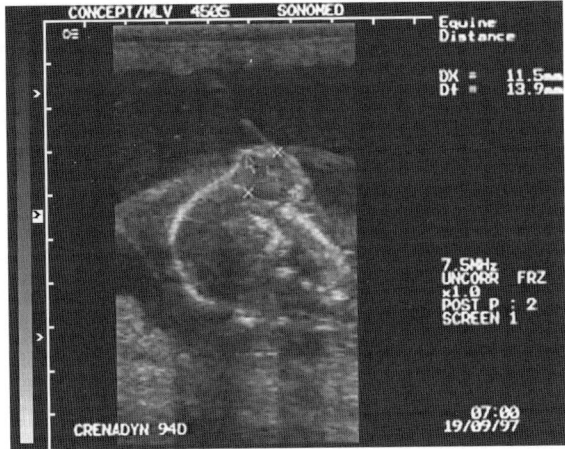

Fig. 2. Anterior fetal presentation and orbital measurements at 94 days of gestation. The right side of the sonogram is cranial.

hind limbs within the pregnant horn prevent further rotation of the fetus over its short axis. Detecting a fetus in posterior presentation (Fig. 3) in the last 2 months of pregnancy therefore indicates that delivery is going to occur that way, when fetal size reflects gestational age. Provisions should be made to assist the delivery of a fetus in posterior presentation. Ultrasound detection of fetal hind limbs in a flexed or extended position may aid the clinician in determining the proper course of action (assisted vaginal

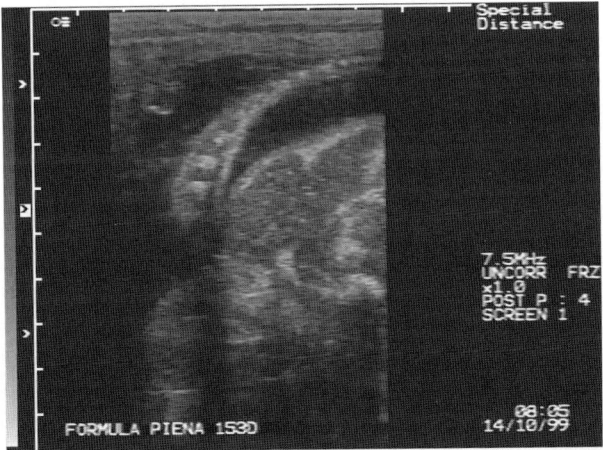

Fig. 3. Posterior fetal presentation at 153 days of gestation. The right side of the sonogram is cranial.

delivery or cesarean section). Associated risk factors of chronic umbilical compression, a dilated or hypotonic bladder, and hind limb angular deformity may be anticipated under these circumstances. Fetal transverse presentation warrants close supervision of foaling, because complicated deliveries often result, particularly when the fetus lies in a dorsocaudal position.

Fetal heart rate and rhythm

FHR and FHR variability represent two of the most sensitive indicators of fetal well-being. FHR declines as gestation progresses. FHR variations depend on a functional central nervous system (CNS) and occur in response to environmental alterations and fetal activity. Associated with movements in normal equine fetuses, FHR accelerations of 25 to 40 beats per minute (bpm) for approximately 30 seconds are frequently detected [25]. Tachycardia [30] or a large range of FHRs may indicate excessive fetal stress and could be brought on by painful maternal systemic problems. Bradycardia [25,26,30], inappropriate FHR for gestational age, or lack of heart rate variation suggests CNS depression, probably attributable to hypoxia, and possible impending fetal demise. Asystole may be detected by transabdominal ultrasound in association with an immobile fetus. Equine fetal cardiac rhythm is usually regular, and cardiac arrhythmias [31] are commonly associated with a negative outcome.

Fetal activity

Fetal activity is a reflection of CNS function, with depressed CNS function resulting in decreased activity. Activity is required to ensure satisfactory muscular development and skeletal joint function and to promote successful postnatal adaptation. Dormant (inactive) phases are observed in fetuses of all ages but are more common in late gestation [32], where they can last up to 60 minutes or longer on occasion. Therefore, caution should be used when interpreting fetal activity, and reassessments are advisable. Lack of fetal movement has been associated with a negative outcome; however, sudden bouts of excessive activity followed by abrupt cessation have also been recorded in fetuses that subsequently died [33].

Fetal size

In the horse, fetal growth depends on adequate placental development. In a normal pregnancy, fetal size and placental surface area are correlated [12]. Structures that have been measured sequentially to estimate fetal size include aortic [27,28,34] and orbital diameters [27,28,35]. Fetal aortic diameter (Fig. 4) is significantly correlated with neonatal foal weight as well as girth and hip height in normal pregnancies, whereas orbital size offers only a rough estimate of trends in fetal growth. Disrupted patterns of growth indicate IUGR, and possible causes should be investigated.

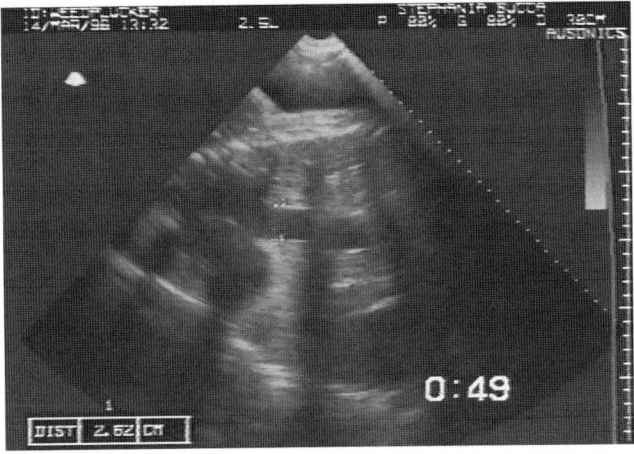

Fig. 4. Fetal aortic diameter in a term fetus. Measurements are taken in systole as the aorta emerges from the heart from leading edge to leading edge. The mare is facing toward the right of the sonogram.

Stomach and bladder measurements

Stomach measurements are easily obtained and increase as gestation advances [28]. A direct correlation between stomach size and fetal swallowing activity has been demonstrated [36,37]. Fetal swallowing represents one of the mechanisms regulating the volume of amniotic fluid and requires integrity of anatomic structures and neurologic pathways of the fetal upper digestive tract. The fetal bladder should be measured when a mechanical obstruction of umbilical flow is suspected in the amniotic portion of the cord. Chronic bladder distention may be associated with umbilical cord pathologic findings, particularly in the colt, because of its longer urethra. Doppler ultrasonography may assist in the diagnosis of abnormal umbilical cord flow, and more normal data should be generated by the widespread application of this technology throughout gestation and in different breeds [38].

Uteroplacental thickness and contrast

An average combined thickness of the uteroplacental unit has been reported for different stages of gestation and areas of the allantochorion, including the cervical pole [28]. Transrectal echography has been used to diagnose placentitis of the cervical pole [39,40]. No structural distinction should normally be detected on ultrasound between the allantochorion and uterine wall. Allantochorial edema may become apparent in term pregnancies close to delivery time (Fig. 5). Abnormally thick or thin uteroplacental units have been associated with a poor fetal outcome. Not all mares at risk of premature labor exhibit changes in the ultrasound appearance of a diseased placenta. Sheerin and coworkers [41] demonstrated that

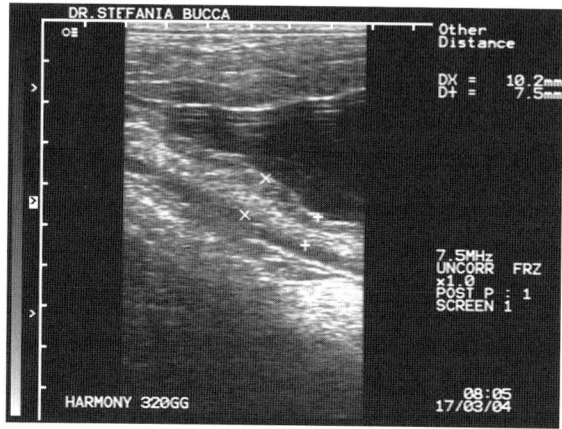

Fig. 5. Combined thickness of the uteroplacental unit at the cervical pole in a term mare with mild diffuse edema of the allantois. The right side of the sonogram is cranial.

only 60% of experimentally infected mares had ultrasound evidence of placental thickening or separation before delivery. Large areas, where uteroplacental contact is lost, are also associated with a negative fetal outcome.

Fetal fluid depth

Fetal fluid depths have been recorded for different gestational stages using transabdominal ultrasonography [28]. Assessment of fetal fluid depth may be possible only when the fetus is not in contact with the abdominal wall. Full appreciation of intrauterine contents is limited by ultrasound penetration and the inability to explore the uppermost fluid accumulations efficiently. Excessive collection of fetal fluids may be caused by hydramnios and hydroallantois, which are uncommon pathologic conditions of advanced pregnancy in horses. Hydramnios [36,37] invariably causes fetal demise, with little repercussion on the mare's health and reproductive performance. Hydroallantois [42] may result in fetal growth restrictions and malaise; associated negative maternal consequences include abdominal distention causing colic and difficult deambulation, abdominal hernia or RPPT, rupture of the uterus, uterine inertia, dystocia, retained placenta, and cardiocirculatory collapse at parturition.

Multiple fetuses

Multiple fetuses may be detected by ultrasound at all stages of gestation using a combined transrectal and transabdominal approach. Twin or multiple fetuses are a natural model of IUGR in the horse because of competition between the two placentae for attachment to the endometrium. This results in preterm delivery, full-term delivery of undersized dysmature individuals, or abortion of twins after the fetal death of one.

Equine biophysical profile

An equine biophysical profile has been developed [30], adapted from a human model, using dynamic ultrasound techniques in pregnancies from 298 days of gestation to term. Six ultrasound parameters are included, chosen in relation to their ability to predict the delivery of an abnormal foal. These parameters are FHR, aortic diameter, fetal activity level, uteroplacental thickness, uteroplacental contact, and maximal allantoic fluid depth. Each parameter is given a score value ranging from 0 to 2. Normalcy scores for these six variables are summed to give a biophysical profile value that ranges from 0 to 12. The results of a study by Reef and colleagues [30] indicated that a biophysical profile score of 8 or less ensures a negative fetal outcome. A maximal score does not ensure a positive outcome, however, because unpredictable events may occur. These are events that could not realistically be predicted by a biophysical profile (ie, uterine inertia, premature placental separation at birth). Limitations of this biophysical profile relate to the fact that its applicability has only been verified in late-gestation or term pregnancies.

Summary

Identification of a compromised pregnancy in the mare requires the exhaustive collection of a database that includes past and recent reproductive and medical histories and a variety of parameters indicating fetal distress and possibly suggesting neonatal compromise. Judicious interpretation of findings and serial recording of data throughout gestation may help in the early detection of abnormal fetomaternal exchange pathways. Some sources of compromise may be identified, and the impact on fetomaternal well-being may be calculated. Appropriate preventive or corrective measures may then be implemented to minimize the risks of an unfavorable outcome.

References

[1] Sibbons PD, Ansari T, Beech DJ, et al. Microanatomical defects in kidneys, lungs, brain, phrenic nerve, and diaphragm, in SIDS infants—a stereological study. Third International Workshop on Equine Perinatology: Comparative Aspects. Equine Vet J 1998;30: 458.

[2] Ansari T, Beech D, Sibbons PD, et al. Pilot investigation into microanatomical defects associated with IUGR in the horse and other domestic animals. Third International Workshop on Equine Perinatology: Comparative Aspects. Equine Vet J 1998;30:458–9.

[3] Fowden AL, Li J, Forehead AJ, et al. Hormones as nutritional signals during intrauterine development. Third International Workshop on Equine Perinatology: Comparative Aspects. Equine Vet J 1998;30:468.

[4] Rossdale PD. Milne lecture: the maladjusted foal: influences of intrauterine growth retardation and birth trauma. In: Proceedings of the 50th Annual Convention of the American Association of Equine Practitioners. Lexington (KY): American Association of Equine Practitioners; 2004. p. 75–126.

[5] Barker DJ. The fetal and infant origins of adult disease. London: British Medical Journal Books; 1992.
[6] Comline RS, Silver M. PO2, PCO2 and PH levels in the umbilical and uterine blood of the mare and ewe. J Physiol 1970;209:587–609.
[7] Fowden AL. Comparative aspects of fetal carbohydrate metabolism. Equine Vet J 1997; 24(Suppl):19–25.
[8] Evans JW. Effects of fasting, gestation, lactation and exercise on glucose turnover in horses. J Anim Sci 1971;33:1001–4.
[9] Fowden AL. Pancreatic endocrine function and carbohydrate metabolism in the fetus. In: Albrecht EB, Pepe G, editors. Perinatal endocrinology. Ithaca (NY): Perinatal Press; 1985. p. 71–90.
[10] Jeffcott LB, Whitwell KE. Twinning as a cause of fetal and neonatal loss in the thoroughbred mare. J Comp Pathol 1973;83:91–105.
[11] Kenny RM. Proceedings of the John P. Hughes International Workshop on Equine Endometritis. Equine Vet J 1993;25:184–7.
[12] Wilscher S, Allen WR. The effects of maternal age and parity on placental and fetal development in the mare. Equine Vet J 2003;35:476–83.
[13] McGladdery AJ, Ousey JC, Rossdale PD. Amniotic and allantoic fluid concentrations of PGE_2 and $PGF_{2\alpha}$ in the mare during late pregnancy [abstract]. In: Proceedings of Havemeyer Foundation International Workshop: Disturbances in Equine Fetal Maturation: Comparative Aspects. Naples (FL); 1992. p. 45.
[14] Schmidt AR, Williams MA, Carleton CL, et al. Evaluation of trans-abdominal ultrasound-guided amniocentesis in the late gestational mare. Equine Vet J 1991;23:261–5.
[15] Ryan P, Vaala W, Bagnell C. Evidence that equine relaxin is a good indicator of placental insufficiency in the mare. In: Proceedings of the 44th Annual Convention of the American Association of Equine Practitioners. Lexington (KY): American Association of Equine Practitioners; 1998. p. 62–3.
[16] Chavatte P. Lactation in the mare. Equine Vet Educ 1997;9(2):62–7.
[17] Cox JE. Oestrone and equilin in the plasma of the pregnant mare. J Reprod Fertil 1975; 23(Suppl):463–8.
[18] Riddle WT. Preparation of the mare for normal parturition. In: Proceedings of the 49th Annual Convention of the American Association of American Practitioners. Lexington (KY): American Association of Equine Practitioners; 2003. p. 1–5.
[19] Santchi EM, LeBlanc MM, Western PG. Progestagen, oestrone sulphate and cortisol concentrations in pregnant mares during medical and surgical disease. J Reprod Fertil 1991; 44(Suppl):627–34.
[20] Rossdale PD, Ousey JC, Cottrill CM, et al. Effects of placental pathology on maternal plasma progestagen and mammary secretion Ca concentrations and on neonatal adrenocortical function in the horse. J Reprod Fertil 1991;44:579–90.
[21] LeBlanc MM, Macpherson M, Sheerin P. Ascending placentitis: what we know about pathophysiology, diagnosis and treatment. In: Proceedings of the 50th Annual Convention of the American Association of Equine Practitioners. Lexington (KY): American Association of Equine Practitioners; 2004. p. 127–43.
[22] Paccamonti DL. Milk electrolytes and induction of parturition. Pferdeheilkunde 2001;17(6): 616–8.
[23] Jeffcott LB. Some practical aspects of the transfer of passive immunity to newborn foals. Equine Vet J 1974;6:445–51.
[24] LeBlanc MM. Colostrometer: method evaluating immunoglobulin content in mare colostrums. Presented at the Equine Neonatal Research Conference. Gainesville (FL), 1984.
[25] Adams-Brendemuhel CS, Pipers FS. Antepartum evaluation of the equine fetus. J Reprod Fertil 1987;35(Suppl):565–73.
[26] Pipers FS, Adams-Brendemuhel CS. Techniques and application of transabdominal ultrasonography in the pregnant mare. J Am Vet Med Assoc 1984;185:766–71.

[27] Renaudin CD, Gillis CL, Tarantal AF, et al. Evaluation of equine fetal growth from day 100 of gestation to parturition, by ultrasonography. J Reprod Fertil Suppl 2000;56:651–60.
[28] Bucca S, Fogarty U, Collins A, et al. Assessment of feto-placental well-being in the mare from mid-gestation to term: transrectal and transabdominal ultrasonographic features. Theriogenology 2005;64:542–57.
[29] Ginther OJ, Griffin PG. Equine fetal kinetics; presentation and location. Theriogenology 1993;40:1–11.
[30] Reef VB, Vaala WE, Worth LT, et al. Ultrasonographic assessment of fetal well-being during late gestation: development of an equine biophysical profile. Equine Vet J 1996;28:200–8.
[31] Yamamoto K, Yasuda J, Too K. Arrhythmias in newborn thoroughbred foals. Equine Vet J 1992;24:169–73.
[32] Fraser AF, Keith NW, Hastie H. Summarised observations on the ultrasonic detection of pregnancy and fetal life in the mare. Vet Rec 1973;92:20–1.
[33] Fraser AF, Hastie H, Callicott RB, et al. An exploratory ultrasonic study on quantitative fetal kinesis in the horse. Appl Anim Ethics 1975;1:395–404.
[34] Reimer JM. Use of transcutaneous ultrasonography in complicated latter-middle to late gestation pregnancies in the mare: 122 cases. In: Proceedings of the 43rd Annual Convention of the American Association of Equine Practitioners. Lexington (KY): American Association of Equine Practitioners; 1997. p. 259–61.
[35] McKinnon AO, Squires EL, Pickett BW. In: Equine reproductive ultrasonography. Animal reproductive laboratory bulletin 04. Fort Collins (CO): Colorado State University; 1988. p. 31–40.
[36] Wintour EM, Barnes A, Brown AJ, et al. The role of deglutition in the production of hydramnios. Theriogenology 1977;8:160.
[37] Bucca S, Romano G. Un caso di idramnios in una fattrice in gestazione avanzata. Ippologia 2000;11:35–8.
[38] McGladdery AL, Ousey JC, Rossdale PD. Serial Doppler ultrasound studies of the umbilical artery during equine pregnancy. In: Proceedings of the Third Conference of the International Veterinary Perinatology Society, 1993. p. 37.
[39] Renaudin CD, Troedsson MHT, Gillis CL. Transrectal ultrasonographic evaluation of the normal equine placenta. Equine Vet Educ 1999;11:75–6.
[40] Renaudin CD, Liu IKM, Troedsson MHT, et al. Transrectal ultrasonographic diagnosis of ascending placentitis in the mare: a report of two cases. Equine Vet Educ 1999;11:69–74.
[41] Sheerin PC, Morris S, Kellerman A, et al. Diagnostic efficiency of transrectal ultrasonography and plasma progestin profiles in identifying mares at risk of premature delivery. In: Proceedings of the Focus on Equine Reproduction Meeting. Lexington (KY): American Association of Equine Practitioners; 2003. p. 22–3.
[42] Oppen TV, Bartmann CP. Two cases of hydroallantois in the mare. Pferdeheilkunde 2001; 17(6):593–6.

Diagnosis and Treatment of Equine Placentitis

Margo L. Macpherson, DVM, MS

Department of Large Animal Clinical Sciences, College of Veterinary Medicine, University of Florida, PO Box 100136, Gainesville, FL 32667, USA

Placentitis is a leading cause of fetal and neonatal death in horses. A study in more than 3500 mares revealed that one third of pregnancy losses attributable to abortion or premature delivery were caused by bacterial placentitis [1,2]. The impact of these losses on the equine industry is emotional and financial. As a result, recent work has been directed at understanding the pathophysiology of the disease and formulating effective means for diagnosis and treatment. This article reviews these efforts.

Pathophysiology

Placentitis in mares is most commonly caused by bacteria ascending through the vagina [2–4]. The pathogens implicated in equine placentitis include *Streptococcus equi* subspecies *zooepidemicus*, *Escherichia coli*, *Klebsiella pneumoniae*, and *Pseudomonas aeruginosa* [5]. Although bacterial infection initiates disease, work in human beings and nonhuman primates has shown that the ensuing disease process is a result of inflammation. Bacteria ascend from the vagina [6], infect maternal and fetal gestational tissues near the cervix, and establish an inflammatory focus. Infection of gestational tissues activates decidual macrophages, resulting in production of proinflammatory cytokines (interleukin [IL]-1β, IL-6, IL-8, and tumor necrosis factor-α [TNFα]) as well as arachidonic acid metabolites by decidual and chorion cells [7,8]. These inflammatory processes result in prostaglandin production (PGE_2 and $PGF_{2\alpha}$) and stimulation of myometrial contractility [9,10].

Workers from the University of Florida [11–16] established a model of equine placentitis that has provided useful information regarding the

---

A portion of this work was supported by the State of Florida Parimutuel Wagering Trust and the Grayson Jockey Club Research Foundation.

E-mail address: macphersonm@mail.vetmed.ufl.edu

pathophysiology of placental disease in mares. In several coordinated studies, placentitis was induced in 16 pony mares using an intracervical inoculum of *S equi* subsp *zooepidemicus* between 280 and 295 days of gestation [13,14,17]. Four mares served as uninfected controls. Fourteen of the 16 infected mares delivered dead or nonviable foals. Two foals born prematurely (days 311 and 313 of gestation) experienced accelerated maturation and lived with minimal neonatal care. The duration and intensity of uterine contractions were higher in infected mares [13].Concentrations of PGE_2 and $PGF_{2\alpha}$ in allantoic fluid from mares with placentitis were elevated; however, allantoic concentrations of cytokines (IL-1, IL-6, and TNFα) were not different between infected and control mares [11]. Concentrations of IL-6 and IL-8 were elevated in the placentas of infected mares. All infected mares exhibited a necrotizing, suppurative, acute placentitis localized in the area of the cervical star [16]. Common placental findings included bacteria on the chorionic surface, allantoic inflammation, and inflammation on the umbilical cord surface. Bacteria were isolated in fetal lungs from seven fetuses [16]. The authors proposed that fetal infection occurred by passage of bacteria through fetal membranes and into the amniotic fluid. The fetus inhaled or swallowed the fluid. Interestingly, not all fetuses became infected from inoculated mares. These important data showed that infection and inflammation likely play a role in placentitis-induced preterm delivery, similar to other species.

As mentioned, some foals experience accelerated fetal maturation in the face of chronic placentitis [17,18]. These foals are delivered prematurely but are mature enough to survive in the extrauterine environment. In human beings, it is thought that indirect stimulation of the fetal hypothalamic-pituitary-adrenal axis by proinflammatory cytokines is responsible for precocious fetal maturation [8,19]. If this phenomenon is also true for equine fetuses, delaying premature labor long enough to allow accelerated fetal maturation to occur may improve foal survival rates. To achieve this goal, it is necessary to diagnose and treat the disease effectively and promptly.

Diagnosis of placentitis

Diagnosis of equine placentitis often occurs well after establishment of disease. The most common signs of placentitis in mares are premature udder development (± streaming of milk) and vulvar discharge. Development of these clinical signs prompts further examination using ultrasound techniques and endocrinologic assays to diagnose and monitor progression of placentitis in mares. Endocrine evaluation of the late pregnant mare is reviewed in a separate article in this issue.

Ultrasonographic monitoring of mares with placentitis

Ultrasound is an excellent tool for monitoring fetal and placental changes in mares affected by placentitis. Transabdominal and transrectal evaluations can provide meaningful and somewhat different information. Neither tool is fail-proof. Mares often develop subclinical cases of placentitis without overt symptoms. Routine serial ultrasonographic evaluations are not commonly used in late-gestation mares; therefore, diagnosis in subclinically affected mares can be missed. Subclinical disease may also result in subtle ultrasonographic changes that are not easily distinguished from normal findings. In spite of these hurdles, ultrasound remains one of the best tools available for diagnosing equine placental infections.

Transrectal ultrasonography

Transrectal ultrasonography of the caudal allantochorion in late-gestation mares provides an excellent image of the placenta close to the cervical star [20]. Because this area is most frequently affected in ascending placentitis, it is an ideal area to monitor for disease. Under normal circumstances, the uterus and the placenta in this region are indistinguishable from one another. Therefore, the combined unit of the uterus and chorioallantois (ie, combined thickness of the uterus and placenta [CTUP]) is measured. A 5-MHz linear transducer should be positioned 1 to 2 inches cranial to the cervical-placental junction and then moved laterally until a major uterine vessel (possibly the middle branch of the uterine artery) is visible at the ventral aspect of the uterine body [20]. The area between the uterine vessel and the allantoic fluid is measured (Fig. 1). When possible, at least three measurements are taken and averaged. Measurements for the CTUP are obtained from the ventral aspect of the uterine body, because the dorsal aspect of the uteroplacental unit may be edematous, even in normal pregnant

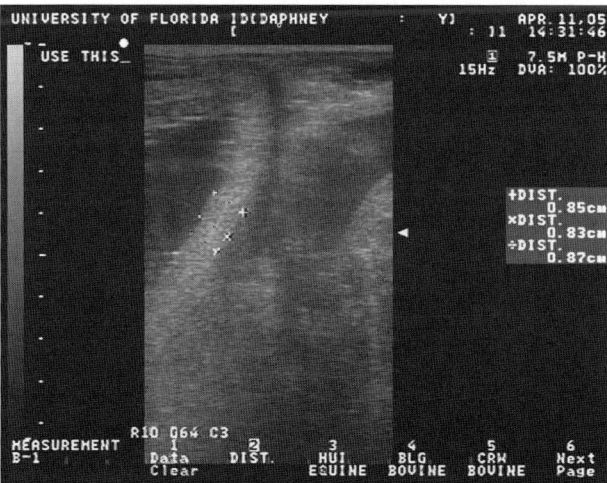

Fig. 1. CTUP measured using transrectal ultrasound on day 304 of gestation in a normal pregnant mare. The average measure from this mare was 8.5 mm. The normal reference value for this stage of gestation is a CTUP measurement less than 10 mm [21].

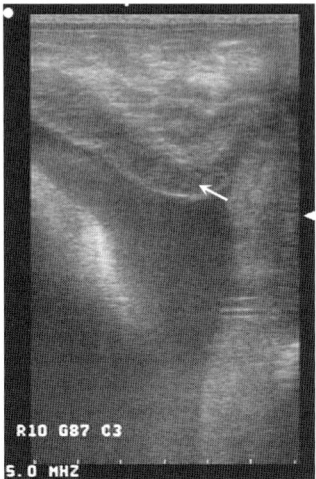

Fig. 2. Edema in the dorsal aspect of the uteroplacental unit (*arrow*) detected using transrectal ultrasonography. This finding is often normal in near-term mares. This image was obtained on day 323 of gestation, and a healthy foal was delivered 5 days later.

mares, in the last month of gestation (Fig. 2). Also, care should be taken to ensure that the amniotic membrane is not adjacent to the allantochorion, because this may result in a false increased CTUP. Normal values for the CTUP have been established [20]. Increases in the CTUP greater than 8 mm between days 271 and 300, greater than 10 mm between days 301 and 330, and greater than 12 mm after day 330 have been associated with placental failure and pending abortion (Fig. 3) [21]. Transrectal ultrasonographic examination is useful for identifying other abnormal conditions,

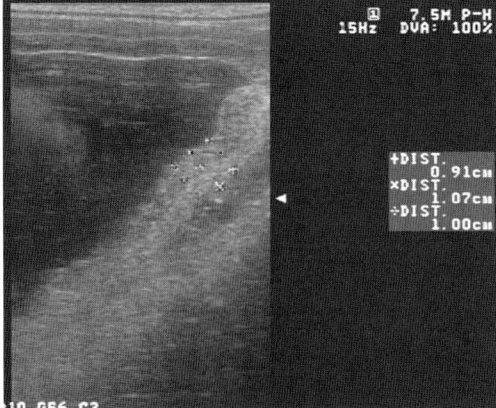

Fig. 3. Thickening of the CTUP detected using transrectal ultrasound. The average measure from this mare was 10 mm at 293 days of gestation. The normal reference value for this stage of gestation is a CTUP measurement less than 8.0 mm [21].

such as accumulation of purulent material between the uterus and placenta (Fig. 4). Measurements in these cases are meaningless, because one is no longer measuring the combined unit. Additionally, purulent fluid accumulation in the cervical star region would be pathognomonic for an ascending placental infection. Amniotic thickening would also be a strong indicator of inflammation and placental disease (Fig. 5).

Transabdominal ultrasonography

Ultrasonographic examinations of the placenta in mares that are considered at risk for abortion during late gestation can be performed by a transabdominal approach [22–24]. Using a 3.5- or 5-MHz sector scanner, four quadrants of the placenta should be examined: right cranial, right caudal, left cranial, and left caudal. Using this technique, mares with normal pregnancies should have a minimal CTUP of 7.1 ± 1.6 mm and a maximal CTUP of 11.5 ± 2.4 mm [22]. Pregnancies with an increased CTUP have been associated with the delivery of abnormal foals [22]. Using transabdominal ultrasonography, the caudal portion of the allantochorion (cervical star area) cannot be imaged, which prevents the clinician from diagnosing ascending placentitis in its early stages. Placental thickening and partial separation of the allantochorion from the endometrium can be detected using transabdominal ultrasonography in mares with placentitis originating from a hematogenous infection, however. In addition, mares infected with *Nocardia* spp bacteria often have placental separation and purulent material at the base of the gravid horn and the junction of the uterine body (Fig. 6) [2]. The transabdominal approach is the most accurate means for diagnosing nocardial placentitis.

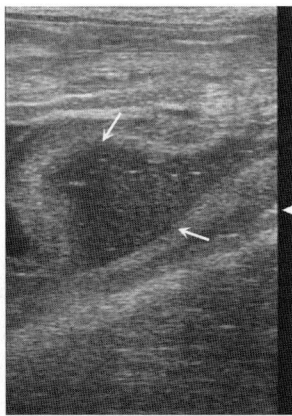

Fig. 4. This transrectal ultrasound image depicts separation of the chorioallantois from the endometrium in the area of the cervical star (*arrows*). Note the accumulation of purulent material between the chorioallantois and endometrium.

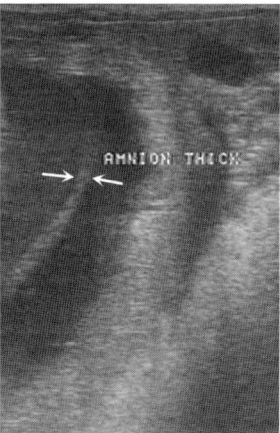

Fig. 5. Thickening of the amnion (*arrows*) was noted with transrectal ultrasonography in a mare with placentitis.

In addition to diagnosing placental disease, transabdominal ultrasonography is useful for monitoring fetal health. Fetal heart rate measures can easily be achieved using this technique. The average fetal heart rate in a fetus greater than 300 days of gestation is 75 ± 7 beats per minute (bpm) [22]. The fetal heart rate slows by approximately 10 bpm at greater than 330 days of gestation. Fetal heart rates vary with activity level, which should be considered when examining a mare. Consistently low or high fetal heart rates are associated with fetal stress. Foals experiencing fetal distress often become bradycardic initially and then become tachycardic in the terminal phase of life [25,26]. Serial examinations should be performed to verify fetal well-being or distress. Once-daily transabdominal ultrasonographic assessments are commonly performed in mares "at risk." Fetuses experiencing distress are often evaluated several times a day. This is particularly true when determining if fetal distress is significant enough to prompt intervention, such as

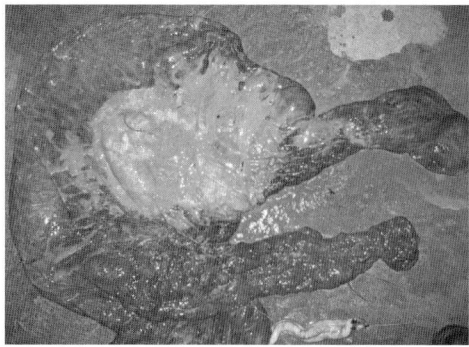

Fig. 6. This placenta was affected by nocardial placentitis. Note the characteristic mucoid exudate located at the base of the pregnant uterine horn.

induction of parturition. Induced parturition would typically be reserved for noninfectious causes of pregnancy compromise, such as hydrallantois, hydramnios, or rupture of the prepubic tendon. It would be less likely that a mare experiencing placentitis would undergo induced parturition unless the fetal or maternal compromise was significant enough to be life threatening.

Treatment of equine placentitis

Treatment strategies for mares with ascending placentitis are currently ill defined. Many treatment regimens have been extrapolated from other species, such as human beings. Treatment efforts are directed at several factors, including combating infection, reducing inflammation, and controlling myometrial activity.

Antimicrobial and anti-inflammatory therapy

Most placental infections are caused by opportunistic bacteria migrating into the uterus from the caudal reproductive tract. Therefore, broad-spectrum antibiotic therapy is an essential first step in treating placentitis. Antibiotic efficacy for reducing the incidence of preterm labor in nonhuman primates, when used alone, has been limited [27–29]. Anti-inflammatory and immunomodulatory therapies have been shown to suppress inflammatory components of preterm labor in experimental models [30,31]. Recent work in nonhuman primates [32] showed that antibiotic therapy (ampicillin) combined with dexamethasone (immunomodulator) and indomethacin (cyclooxygenase inhibitor) was more effective in suppressing bacterial infection, amniotic fluid cytokines, prostaglandins, and uterine contractions than antibiotic therapy alone. Studies in these species indicate that combined therapy is necessary to stem the bacterial infection as well as to suppress the subsequent inflammatory and uterine responses.

Treatment approaches for equine placentitis have been largely anecdotal. Early studies evaluated the ability of commonly used antibiotics to penetrate the placenta in normal pregnant mares [33,34]. Sertich and Vaala [33] administered intravenous potassium penicillin G (22,000 IU/kg every 6 hours) and intravenous gentamicin sulfate (2.2 mg/kg every 6 hours) alone and in combination or oral trimethoprim sulfadiazine (5 mg/kg every 12 hours) to 11 normal late pregnant mares. Samples were obtained from allantoic and amniotic fluid, when possible, and serum. Penicillin and gentamicin were detected in the mares' serum at normal concentrations but not in amniotic fluid or foal serum. Penicillin was detected in the allantoic fluid of 1 mare. Trimethoprim sulfadiazine was recovered from amniotic (n = 2) and allantoic (n = 4) fluid and was detectable in neonatal serum of two foals. The authors concluded that trimethoprim sulfadiazine penetrated fetal membranes sufficiently to combat bacteria that were sensitive to the drug.

Santschi and Papich [34] monitored the pharmacokinetics of gentamicin in late pregnancy and early lactation. Seven mares were treated with one dose of gentamicin sulfate (6.6 mg/kg administered intravenously) before parturition and again after parturition, and pharmacokinetic analysis was performed on serum samples. The authors also studied the pharmacokinetics of gentamicin sulfate in a subpopulation of foaling mares (n = 3). Parturition was induced in three mares using oxytocin within 60 minutes of gentamicin administration. Amniotic fluid was collected from one mare. Serum samples were collected from foals after delivery. Gentamicin was detected in all the mare serum samples at expected concentrations. Gentamicin was not detected in foal serum or in the amniotic fluid sample. The authors concluded that lack of gentamicin in foal serum or amniotic fluid indicated that gentamicin did not readily pass the equine placenta or that the time between drug administration and sample collection may have been too short for sufficient drug distribution.

Recently, workers from the University of Florida [35] used in vivo microdialysis to collect highly purified samples from allantoic fluid and blood of pregnant pony mares treated with commonly used drugs. In the first study, five reproductively normal mares (269–271 days of gestation) had microdialysis probes placed in the allantoic cavity and jugular vein. Mares were treated intravenously with potassium penicillin G (22,000 IU/kg every 6 hours), gentamicin (6.6 mg/kg every 24 hours), and flunixin meglumine (1 mg/kg every 12 hours). Allantoic fluid and blood were collected for 24 hours. Both antibiotics were present in allantoic fluid, albeit at lower concentrations than present in serum. Concentrations of penicillin in allantoic fluid achieved the minimum inhibitory concentration (MIC) against *S equi* subsp *zooepidemicus*. Gentamicin concentrations in allantoic fluid were adequate to be effective against *E coli* or *K pneumoniae*. Flunixin meglumine was not detected in allantoic fluid. The authors speculated that the protein-bound drug was unable to penetrate the microdialysis membrane pores; therefore, the drug was undetectable using this system.

The same regimen was tested in two mares with experimentally induced placentitis. Mares were inoculated with *S equi* subsp *zooepidemicus* directly into the cervix 10 days after the initial microdialysis experiment. Drugs were administered to mares beginning 4 days after inoculation. Penicillin and gentamicin were detected in allantoic fluid of the two infected mares after drug administration. The pharmacokinetics and efficacy of the drugs for treating placentitis could not be determined because of the limited number of mares and short treatment time.

Also using microdialysis, workers [36] studied the pharmacokinetics of trimethoprim sulfamethoxazole and pentoxifylline in allantoic fluid of 10 pregnant pony mares from 277 to 300 days of gestation. The drugs were chosen because of oral bioavailability and good uterine penetration. Pentoxifylline was evaluated because it seems to downregulate proinflammatory cytokines [37,38]. Five mares were inoculated intracervically with *S equi* subsp *zooepidemicus* 5 days before drug administration and measurement of allantoic drug concentrations by microdialysis. Five mares underwent microdialysis but were not inoculated (controls). All mares were treated with trimethoprim sulfamethoxazole (30 mg/kg twice daily) and pentoxifylline (8.5 mg/kg twice daily) orally for 14 days. Trimethoprim sulfamethoxazole and pentoxifylline penetrated fetal membranes and were detected in allantoic fluid of infected and control mares. Differences in allantoic drug concentrations were not detected between groups. Peak drug concentrations in allantoic fluid were delayed when compared with serum drug concentrations in control and infected mares. All control noninfected mares delivered live foals at term. Four of the five infected mares aborted. One mare aborted on day 13 of drug therapy, three mares aborted after termination of drug therapy (10, 17, and 19 days after the last day of treatment), and one mare carried a normal foal to term (40 days after cessation of drug therapy). These data suggested that trimethoprim sulfamethoxazole and pentoxifylline might delay preterm delivery in mares with placentitis but that treatment time was not sufficient to improve neonatal outcome consistently.

Workers at the University of Florida (Jennifer Graczyk, personal communication, 2005) are currently investigating the effects of long-term treatment with trimethoprim sulfamethoxazole and pentoxifylline on pregnancy outcome in mares with experimentally induced placentitis. Eleven mares were inoculated intracervically with *S equi* subsp *zooepidemicus*. Six mares were treated with the drug regimen described previously from the onset of clinical signs until delivery or abortion. Five mares served as infected untreated controls. Five of 6 treated mares aborted up to 27 days (mean = 15 days) after bacterial inoculation. One mare delivered a healthy live foal. Four of 5 control mares aborted up to 10 days (mean = 4 days) after bacterial inoculation. One mare delivered a healthy live foal. The treatment regimen did not improve fetal viability in this model, but treated mares ($P = .06$) tended to carry pregnancies longer than untreated mares after inoculation. Furthermore, fetal and placental tissues were analyzed for presence of trimethoprim sulfamethoxazole and pentoxifylline. Drugs were detected in all fetal and placental tissues analyzed.

Data from these important drug studies verify that commonly used drugs (penicillin, gentamicin, trimethoprim sulfamethoxazole, and pentoxifylline) penetrate fetal membranes in normal mares and mares with placentitis. Although the efficacy of these particular drug combinations for preventing preterm labor is not clear from this experimental model, the data are encouraging. Additional drugs, such as progestins or steroids, may be instrumental in completing an effective therapeutic regimen.

Progestins

Progestin therapy is currently being implemented in human beings to halt preterm labor. A recent study [39] showed a beneficial effect when women with a documented history of spontaneous preterm delivery were treated with progesterone. The incidence of recurring spontaneous preterm delivery was significantly lower in women treated with 17α-hydroxyprogesterone than in untreated women (36.3% versus 54.9%, respectively). Presumably, the anti-prostaglandin effect of progestins would contribute to reduced myometrial activity by interfering with upregulation of prostaglandin and oxytocin receptors [40]. Without receptor formation, gap junction formation would be inhibited and uterine contractility prevented.

Treatment with progestins has long been advocated to promote uterine quiescence in mares with high-risk pregnancies. Daels and coworkers [41] tested the effects of progesterone and altrenogest, a synthetic progestin, on pregnancy maintenance in mares treated with the prostaglandin analogue cloprostenol. Sixteen mares with pregnancies ranging from 93 to 153 days of gestation were included in the study. Cloprostenol (250 μg) was administered to all mares intramuscularly for 5 consecutive days. Progesterone (300 mg once daily) was administered intramuscularly to 8 mares, and altrenogest (44 mg once daily) was administered orally to 8 mares. Cloprostenol-treated control mares were extrapolated from a previous study. Five (63%) of 8 mares in the progesterone-treated group maintained pregnancies after cloprostenol treatment, whereas 3 mares aborted during treatment. All 8 mares (100%) treated with altrenogest maintained pregnancies. None of the control mares (0%) maintained pregnancies after cloprostenol treatment. Administration of exogenous progestins to mares treated with cloprostenol was associated with an endogenous decrease in prostaglandin metabolite concentrations. This important study demonstrated that progestin supplementation was able to prevent prostaglandin-induced abortion in most cases.

Tocolytics

The goal of tocolytic therapy is to prevent or disrupt uterine contractions and premature labor. A variety of agents have been used in women with preterm labor, including magnesium sulfate, β-sympathomimetic agents (eg, ritodrine, terbutaline), prostaglandin synthesis inhibitors (eg, indomethacin, sulindac, ibuprofen, aspirin), calcium channel blockers (nifedipine), and oxytocin antagonists (atosiban) [28]. Tocolytic agents have not been shown to prolong pregnancy significantly or to improve neonatal outcome when used alone. Historically, tocolytics prolong pregnancy for up to 48 hours; during that time, glucocorticoids can be administered to the mother in an effort to expedite fetal maturation. Side effects from tocolytic agents can be significant [42].

Clenbuterol, a β-sympathomimetic agent, has been used as a tocolytic agent in clinical equine practice. The effects of clenbuterol administration on uterine tone and maternal and fetal heart rates were examined by Card and Wood [43]. Clenbuterol was administered intravenously (300 μg) to four pregnant mares throughout gestation until parturition. The final dose was administered when the mares were thought to be close to parturition as indicated by concentration of calcium and magnesium (120 ppm) measured using water-hardness test strips. Fetal heart rate, maternal heart rate, and uterine tone (measured by palpation) were recorded after drug administration. Mares and fetuses experienced transient tachycardia after drug administration at all time points. Resting uterine tone changed significantly after clenbuterol administration to mares early in gestation. Uterine relaxation after clenbuterol administration was less profound later in gestation when uterine tone was decreasing naturally. Uterine relaxation occurred within 3 minutes of drug administration and persisted for up to 120 minutes. The authors concluded that clenbuterol was effective in causing uterine relaxation throughout gestation and that the side effects were minimal and transient.

A more recent study [44] reported the effects of clenbuterol when administered to 29 mares late in gestation. Beginning on day 320 of gestation, mammary secretion electrolyte changes were monitored using a calcium strip test. Treatment started when calcium levels reached a maximum level of 13 mmol (four squares reacted on the strip test). Mares were treated with varying doses of clenbuterol administered intravenously: 0.6 mg (n = 6), 1 mg (n = 5), and 1.5 mg (n = 4). Fifteen control mares were treated with saline. All mares were treated once daily at the same time until parturition. No differences were detected between groups for length of gestation, number of treatments, or time to foaling after the last dose was administered. Treatment dose did not affect outcomes. Mares in the low-dose treatment groups (0.6 mg and 1 mg) showed no side effects, whereas mares treated with 1.5 mg showed transient signs of abdominal distress and sweating. All foals were clinically normal, except one foal from the treatment group that died after demonstrating dystocia. The authors concluded that clenbuterol was not effective in preventing the onset of myometrial contractions in normal foaling mares at term. Treated mares in this study actually foaled earlier in the evening than untreated mares. The authors speculated that the relaxant effects of clenbuterol may have promoted cervical relaxation and subsequent parturition. Based on side effects detected when clenbuterol is administered to pregnant mares [43–44] and lack of effect for delaying normal parturition, the authors suggest that this agent has limited usefulness in horses. Furthermore, these agents have not been prescribed for horses in the same manner that has proven most useful for human beings (ie, tocolytics plus glucocorticoids over a 48-hour period for fetal maturation). The success of these drugs may be more apparent if they can be combined with an agent that promotes fetal maturation before delivery.

Combined therapy for equine placentitis in a clinical setting

Work from a large-scale clinical trial examined the efficacy of multipronged long-term therapy for treating equine placentitis [45]. Investigators examined records of 477 mares over 6 years. Fifteen mares were diagnosed with placentitis. Criteria for treatment included increased thickness of the uteroplacental unit using transrectal ultrasound, placental separation or vulvar discharge, and udder development. The average gestational age at diagnosis was 8.6 months. Mares were treated with a combination of systemic antibiotics (trimethoprim sulfamethiazole, ceftiofur or penicillin, and gentamicin), pentoxifylline, altrenogest, and nonsteroidal anti-inflammatory agents. Mares were treated until abortion or delivery of a foal. Twelve (84%) of 15 treated mares carried their foals to term, and 11 (73%) of 15 mares delivered live foals. Birth weights of surviving foals from mares treated for placentitis were similar to those of foals from nonaffected mares. Data from these studies suggest that long-term antibiotic and anti-inflammatory treatment may have a positive impact on pregnancy outcome in mares with placentitis.

Summary

Effective diagnosis and treatment for equine placentitis remain elusive. Mares "at risk" for placentitis (eg, multiparous, poor perineal conformation, previous history of placentitis) may benefit from prospective monitoring of ultrasonographic and endocrine parameters. The same parameters can be useful for monitoring resolution of disease after the onset of therapy. Combined therapies (antibiotics, anti-inflammatory agents, and progestins) show the most promise for interrupting preterm labor.

References

[1] Giles RC, Donahue JM, Hong CB, et al. Causes of abortion, stillbirth, and perinatal death in horses—3,527 cases (1986–1991). J Am Vet Med Assoc 1993;203(8):1170–5.
[2] Hong CB, Donahue JM, Giles RC, et al. Etiology and pathology of equine placentitis. J Vet Diagn Invest 1993;5(1):56–63.
[3] Platt H. Infection of the horse fetus. J Reprod Fertil Suppl 1975;23:605–10.
[4] Whitwell K. Equine infectious diseases V. 5th edition. Lexington (KY): University of Kentucky Press; 1988.
[5] Acland HM. Abortion. In: McKinnon AO, Voss JL, editors. Equine reproduction. Philadelphia: Lea & Febiger; 1993. p. 554–61.
[6] Romero R, Mazor M. Infection and preterm labor. Clin Obstet Gynecol 1988;31(3):553–84.
[7] Dudley DJ, Trautman MS. Infection, inflammation, and contractions—the role of cytokines in the pathophysiology of preterm labor. Semin Reprod Endocrinol 1994;12(4):263–72.
[8] Gravett MG, Hitti J, Hess DL, et al. Intrauterine infection and preterm delivery: evidence for activation of the fetal hypothalamic-pituitary-adrenal axis. Am J Obstet Gynecol 2000; 182(6):1404–10.
[9] Dudley DJ. Pre-term labor: an intra-uterine inflammatory response syndrome? J Reprod Immunol 1997;36(1–2):93–109.
[10] Pollard JK, Mitchell MD. Intrauterine infection and the effects of inflammatory mediators on prostaglandin production by myometrial cells from pregnant women. Am J Obstet Gynecol 1996;174(2):682–6.

[11] Leblanc MM, Giguere S, Brauer K, et al. Premature delivery in ascending placentitis is associated with increased expression of placental cytokines and allantoic fluid prostaglandins E-2 and F-2 alpha. Theriogenology 2002;58(2–4):841–4.
[12] Hendry JM, Lester GD, Hansen PJ, et al. Patterns of uterine myoelectrical activity in reproductively normal mares in late gestation and in mares with experimentally induced ascending placentitis. Theriogenology 2002;58(2–4):853–5.
[13] McGlothlin JA, Lester GD, Hansen PJ, et al. Alteration in uterine contractility in mares with experimentally induced placentitis. Reproduction 2004;127(1):57–66.
[14] Kelleman AA, Luznar SL, Lester GD, et al. Evaluation of transrectal ultrasonographic combined thickness of the uterus and placenta (CTUP) in a model of induced ascending placentitis in late gestation in the pony mare. Theriogenology 2002;58(2–4):845–8.
[15] O'Donnell LJ, Sheerin BR, Hendry JM, et al. 24-Hour secretion patterns of plasma oestradiol 17 beta in pony mares in late gestation. Reprod Domest Anim 2003;38(3):233–5.
[16] Mays MBC, Leblanc MM, Paccamonti D. Route of fetal infection in a model of ascending placentitis. Theriogenology 2002;58(2–4):791–2.
[17] Stawicki RJ, Ruebel H, Hansen PJ, et al. Endocrinological findings in an experimental model of ascending placentitis in the mare. Theriogenology 2002;58(2–4):849–52.
[18] Silver M, Fowden AL, Knox J, et al. Relationship between circulating tri-iodothyronine and cortisol in the perinatal-period in the foal. J Reprod Fertil 1991;5:619–26.
[19] Besedovsky HO, delRey A. Immune-neuro-endocrine interactions: facts and hypotheses. Endocr Rev 1996;17(1):64–102.
[20] Renaudin CD, Troedsson MHT, Gillis CL, et al. Ultrasonographic evaluation of the equine placenta by transrectal and transabdominal approach in the normal pregnant mare. Theriogenology 1997;47(2):559–73.
[21] Renaudin CD, Liu IKM, Troedsson MHT, et al. Transrectal ultrasonographic diagnosis of ascending placentitis in the mare: a report of two cases. Equine Vet Educ 1999;11(2):69–74.
[22] Reef VB, Vaala WE, Worth LT, et al. Ultrasonographic assessment of fetal well-being during late gestation: development of an equine biophysical profile. Equine Vet J 1996;28(3):200–8.
[23] Adams-Brendemuehl C, Pipers FS. Antepartum evaluation of the equine fetus. J Reprod Fertil Suppl 1987;35:565–73.
[24] Vaala WE, Sertich PL. Management strategies for mares at risk for periparturient complications. Vet Clin North Am Equine Pract 1994;10(1):237–65.
[25] Pipers FS, Adamsbrendemuehl CS. Techniques and applications of trans-abdominal ultrasonography in the pregnant mare. J Am Vet Med Assoc 1984;185(7):766–71.
[26] Pipers FS, Zent W, Holder R, Asbury A. Ultrasonography as an adjunct to pregnancy assessments in the mare. J Am Vet Med Assoc 1984;184(3):328–34.
[27] Ramsey PS, Rouse DJ. Therapies administered to mothers at risk for preterm birth and neurodevelopmental outcome in their infants. Clin Perinatol 2002;29(4):725–43.
[28] Lamont RF. Can antibiotics prevent preterm birth—the pro and con debate. BJOG 2005;112:67–73.
[29] Lamont RF. Infection in the prediction and antibiotics in the prevention of spontaneous preterm labour and preterm birth. BJOG 2003;110:71–5.
[30] Sadowsky DW, Haluska GJ, Gravett MG, et al. Indomethacin blocks interleukin 1beta-induced myometrial contractions in pregnant rhesus monkeys. Am J Obstet Gynecol 2000;183(1):173–80.
[31] Sadowsky DW, Novy MJ, Witkin SS, et al. Dexamethasone or interleukin-10 blocks interleukin-1 beta-induced uterine contractions in pregnant rhesus monkeys. Am J Obstet Gynecol 2003;188(1):252–63.
[32] Gravett M, Sadowsky D, Witkin S, et al. Immunomodulators plus antibiotics to prevent preterm delivery in experimental intra-amniotic infection (IAI) [abstract]. Am J Obstet Gynecol 2003;189(6):S56.
[33] Sertich PL, Vaala WE. Concentrations of antibiotics in mares, foals and fetal fluids after antibiotic administration in late pregnancy. Proc Am Assoc Equine Pract 1992;38:727–36.

[34] Santschi EM, Papich MG. Pharmacokinetics of gentamicin in mares in late pregnancy and early lactation. J Vet Pharmacol Ther 2000;23(6):359–63.
[35] Murchie TA, Macpherson ML, Leblanc MM, et al. A microdialysis model to detect drugs in the allantoic fluid of pregnant pony mares. Proc Am Assoc Equine Pract 2003;49:118–9.
[36] Rebello SA, Macpherson ML, Murchie TA, et al. The detection of placental drug transfer in equine allantoic fluid [abstract]. Theriogenology 2005;64(3):776–7.
[37] Lauterbach R, Pawlik D, Zembala M, et al. Pentoxifylline in and prevention and treatment of chronic lung disease. Acta Paediatr 2004;93:20–2.
[38] Lauterbach R, Zembala M. Pentoxifylline reduces plasma tumour necrosis factor-alpha concentration in premature infants with sepsis. Eur J Pediatr 1996;155(5):404–9.
[39] Meis PJ, Klebanoff M, Thom E, et al. Prevention of recurrent preterm delivery by 17 alpha-hydroxyprogesterone caproate. N Engl J Med 2003;348(24):2379–85.
[40] Garfield RE, Kannan MS, Daniel ME. Gap junction formation in the myometrium: control by estrogens, progesterone and prostaglandins. Am J Physiol 1980;238:C81–9.
[41] Daels PF, Besognet B, Hansen B, et al. Effect of progesterone on prostaglandin F-2 alpha secretion and outcome of pregnancy during cloprostenol-induced abortion in mares. Am J Vet Res 1996;57(9):1331–7.
[42] Goldenberg RL. The management of preterm labor. Obstet Gynecol 2002;100(5):1020–37.
[43] Card CE, Wood MR. Effects of acute administration of clenbuterol on uterine tone and equine fetal and maternal heart rates. Biol Reprod Monogr 1995;1:7–11.
[44] Palmer E, Chavette-Palmer P, Duchamp G, et al. Lack of effect of clenbuterol for delaying parturition in late pregnant mares. Theriogenology 2002;58(2–4):797–9.
[45] Troedsson MHT, Zert WW. Clinical evaluation of the equine placenta as a method to successfully identify and treat mares with placentitis. Proceedings Workshop on the Equine Placenta. SR 2004-1. 2004. p. 66–7.

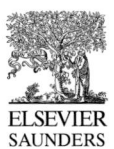

Laparoscopic Cryptorchidectomy and Ovariectomy in Horses

Dean Hendrickson, DVM, MS

Department of Clinical Sciences, James L. Voss Veterinary Teaching Hospital, Colorado State University, 300 West Drake Road, Fort Collins, CO 80523-1678, USA

Laparoscopic surgery has become commonplace in the field of equine urogenital surgery. The surgical procedures that are most commonly performed include cryptorchidectomy and ovariectomy. No doubt in time, other procedures, such as oviductal insemination, oviductal ligation, and other reproductive procedures, should become routine. As with most surgical procedures, the limiting factors in developing new surgical techniques are limited to the patient size and demeanor, the skills of the surgeon, and the available equipment. There are more companies that offer laparoscopic equipment now than there were 10 years ago. Some of the companies offer equipment that is specifically designed for equine laparoscopy, such as Surgical Direct (DeLand, Florida) and Karl Storz Veterinary Endoscopy (Goleta, California). Other companies provide equipment designed for human use that can be adapted for equine laparoscopy in some cases. Some of the greatest benefits of laparoscopic surgery in the horse include better visualization of the important structures; tension-free amputation of the testes or ovaries, which generally leads to less postoperative pain; and the ability to evaluate the transected stump carefully to make sure there is no hemorrhage. This article is limited to the use of laparoscopy for cryptorchidectomy and ovariectomy.

Presurgical preparation

Laparoscopic surgery is based on the concept of triangulation. The telescope and the instruments enter the abdomen from different angles, allowing the surgeon to access the structure of interest. To perform the surgical technique, an operating space must be created in the peritoneal cavity. This is

---

E-mail address: Dean.Hendrickson@colostate.edu

accomplished by withholding food from the animal for 24 or more hours and by insufflating the peritoneal space with carbon dioxide (CO_2). Standing surgery generally does not require food withholding for as long as does surgery with the patient in dorsal recumbency. The other benefit of longer food withholding or feeding low-bulk diets for cases undergoing general anesthesia is that when the horse is tipped into the Trendelenburg position (head down and tail elevated), less weight is placed on the diaphragm. This is especially true in the case of a dorsally recumbent ovariectomy, where the horse needs to be aggressively tipped. Water should be given free choice until the time of surgery. It is generally recommended that nonsteroidal anti-inflammatory drugs be given before surgery. The author typically uses phenylbutazone at a dose of 4.4 mg/kg administered orally before surgery and 2.2 mg/kg administered orally twice daily for 3 to 5 days after surgery. It would be reasonable to use flunixin meglumine in place of the phenylbutazone at a dose of 1.1 mg/kg before surgery and at a dose of 0.5 mg/kg twice daily after surgery. The biggest determinant is generally the ease of dosing with oral phenylbutazone. The use of antibiotics is based solely on the surgeon's preference. The author does not routinely use antibiotics before surgery; however, when indicated, a single dose of procaine penicillin G (20,000 IU/kg) administered intramuscularly is generally adequate. The need for blood work is based on the type of sedation and anesthesia planned. For standing procedures, an assessment of packed cell volume (PCV) and total protein (TP) levels is generally acceptable, whereas for general anesthesia and dorsal or lateral recumbency, a complete blood cell count (CBC) and presurgical panel are desired. Other specifics are dealt with in the following sections for individual techniques.

Laparoscopic cryptorchidectomy

Laparoscopic cryptorchidectomy is one of the primary indications for laparoscopic surgery. Although cryptorchid castration can be performed using many different techniques, the laparoscope allows direct visualization of the testis location. This can be especially valuable in animals that have had prior surgical attempts performed to remove an abdominal testis or testes [1]. Unless the anatomy has been disrupted, the gubernaculum is almost always attached to the vaginal ring (Fig. 1). The two laparoscopic approaches for cryptorchidectomy are standing and dorsal recumbency. The main benefit of standing laparoscopic cryptorchidectomy is the absence of general anesthesia and its associated complications. Another benefit is that the testis is generally more easily identifiable. The most significant detraction to standing laparoscopic cryptorchidectomy is associated with unruly horses that do not stand in the stocks for surgery. Consequently, for horses that do not seem likely to stay in the stocks, it is best to plan on general anesthesia and dorsally recumbent surgery.

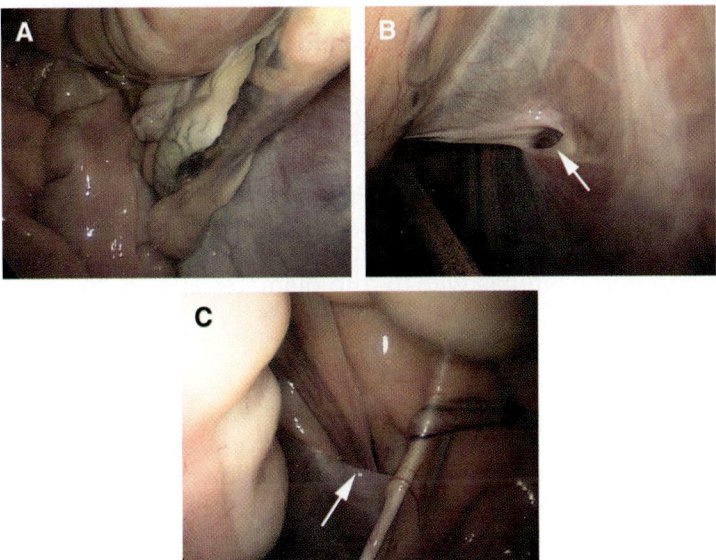

Fig. 1. Intra-abdominal view of a standing left flank laparoscopic cryptorchidectomy. (*A*) Left abdominally retained testis in the normal position. (*B*) Left vaginal ring (*arrow*) with the attached gubernaculum. (*C*) Right vaginal ring (*arrow*) viewed with a laparoscope under the descending colon.

Standing laparoscopic cryptorchidectomy

Surgical technique

The required instrumentation for the surgical technique [2,3] is listed in Box 1. The horses are sedated with intravenous xylazine (0.3 mg/kg) and placed in stocks for surgery. At this point, the caudal tail head area is clipped and prepared for a caudal epidural with detomidine (40 µg/kg brought to a total volume of 10 mL with 0.9% sodium chloride [NaCl]), or the neck area over the jugular vein is prepared for a catheter for intravenous infusion of detomidine (20 mg in polyionic replacement fluids [1 L]) given to effect. The appropriate flank(s) are clipped and aseptically prepared for surgery. For left-sided cryptorchids, the left flank is prepared; for right-sided cryptorchids, the right flank is prepared; and for bilateral cryptorchids or for horses with an uncertain castration history, both flanks are prepared (Fig. 2). Instrument portals are as previously described, with the middle portal at the level of the ventral aspect of the tuber coxae midway between the last rib and the tuber coxae and one portal 10 cm dorsal and 5 cm rostral and another portal 10 cm ventral. The portal sites are infiltrated directly with 2% lidocaine (10–15 mL) or mepivacain (Fig. 3). The animals are draped with a water-impervious paper drape to allow access to the appropriate flank(s). Insufflation is achieved using an 8-mm diameter mare urinary catheter (Fig. 4A) or a 10-mm diameter or 20-cm long laparoscopic cannula

Box 1. Instruments needed for standing laparoscopic cryptorchidectomy

30° telescope (author prefers length of 57 cm)
Videocamera and monitor
300-W xenon light source and large-diameter fiberoptic cable
Insufflator and CO_2 tank
Insufflation cannula and insufflation tubing
Three to four cannulas with 10-mm diameter and 15- to 20-cm length
Laparoscopic injection needle
Atraumatic grasping forceps: 10-mm diameter and 45-cm length
1 to 2 acute claw grasping forceps: 10-mm diameter and 45-cm length
Scissors: 10-mm diameter and 45-cm length
Pedicle ligation instruments
One to four ligating loops using size 1 Maxon with a knot pusher and knot protector or Ligasure device (Tyco Health Care/Kendall, Mansfield, Massachusetts)
Standard surgical pack

with a blunt obturator (see Fig. 4B) in the middle portal site. If the laparoscopic cannula is used, the telescope can be introduced before insufflation to confirm entry into the peritoneal cavity. Either cannula is placed by directing the cannula toward the opposite stifle. The insufflation tubing is attached to the insufflator and the cannula to confirm negative pressure within the peritoneal cavity. When using the mare urinary catheter, the

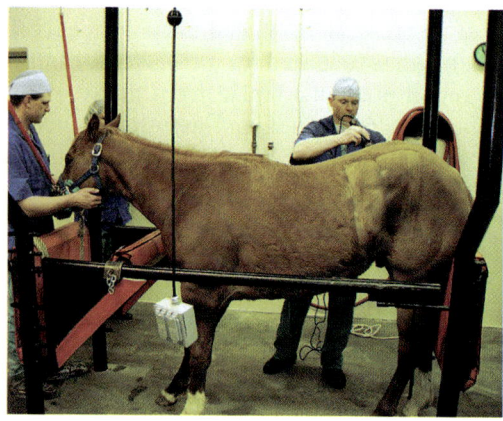

Fig. 2. Photograph of a horse in stocks after epidural sedation in preparation of both flanks for surgery.

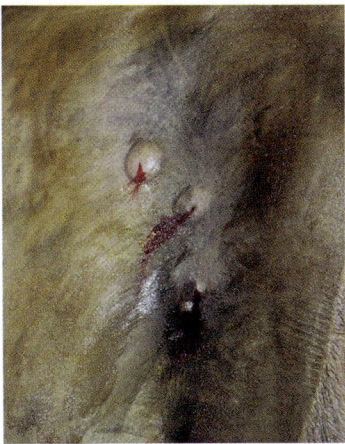

Fig. 3. Photograph of the left flank of the horse in Fig. 2 shows local infiltration of lidocaine in the portal sites.

intra-abdominal pressure is taken to 12 to 15 mm Hg, and a 10-mm diameter or 20-cm long cannula with a blunt obturator is then placed through the dorsal portal site. As soon as a laparoscopic cannula is in place, the laparoscope with an attached videocamera is placed through the cannula and an

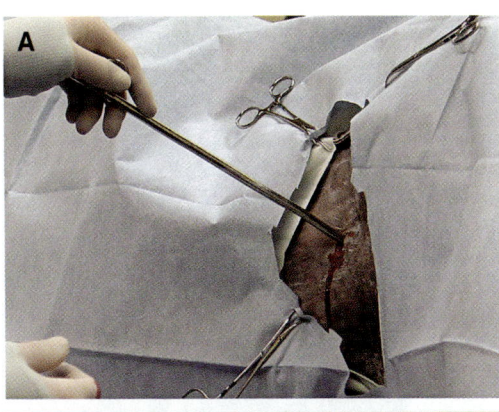

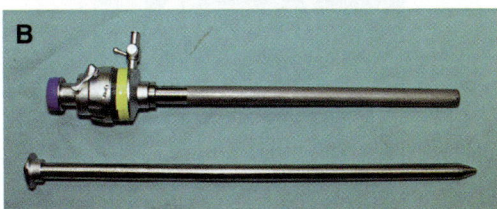

Fig. 4. Photograph of insufflation trochars. (*A*) Eight-millimeter diameter mare urinary catheter in the middle portal of the left flank. (*B*) Ten-millimeter diameter 20-cm length cannula with a blunt trochar.

exploratory procedure is performed. For bilateral cryptorchids, a fourth cannula can be placed in the left flank to allow amputation of both testes from the left side (Fig. 5).

After the abdomen has been explored and both inguinal rings have been identified (a long grasper can be used to elevate the descending colon to view the contralateral inguinal ring; see Fig. 1C), the testis or testes or respective mesorchia are identified and injected with 2% lidocaine (10–20 mL) to provide analgesia (Fig. 6). After waiting for 10 minutes, the ipsilateral testis in cases with a single retained testis or the contralateral testis in cases of bilaterally retained testes is grasped for ligation and amputation. There are two primary methods that the author uses to ligate the mesorchium. The first method involves the use of an encircling ligature using size 1 polyglyconate (Maxon, Kendall/TycoHealthcare, Mansfield, Massachusetts) with a 4S modified Roeder knot [4,5] to ligate the mesorchium, followed by amputation with tissue scissors (Fig. 7). The second technique involves the use of a Ligasure vessel sealing device (TycoHealth Care/Kendall, Mansfield, Massachusetts) with 10-mm Atlas surgical shears (TycoHealth Care/Kendall), where sequential application of the shears, followed by application of the cutting blade, ligates and divides the mesorchium at the same time. The loop technique requires less equipment but more expertise than does the Ligasure device. Another technique that has been described involves the use of bipolar electrosurgery in much the same manner as the Ligasure device [6]. In cases of bilateral cryptorchids, if possible, the contralateral testis is ligated and amputated first, followed by the ipsilateral testis. This requires the use of a third instrument cannula to hold onto the contralateral testis while the ipsilateral testis is ligated and amputated. In some instances, the

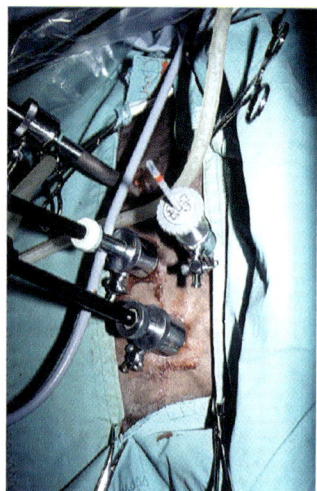

Fig. 5. Photograph of left flank with four portals for removing bilateral cryptorchid testes from one flank.

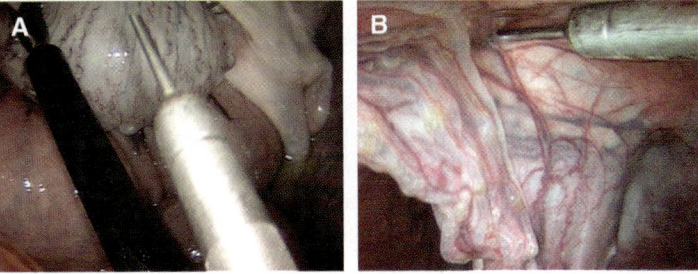

Fig. 6. Photograph shows intra-abdominal injection of lidocaine in the testis (*A*) or mesorchium (*B*) before surgery.

distance to the contralateral testis is too great for the instrument length or the length of the gubernaculum, and a portal must be established in both flanks for surgery. After amputation of the testis or testes, the most ventral cannula portal is extended by sharp dissection through the skin and external abdominal oblique muscle and by blunt dissection through the internal abdominal oblique and transverses muscles, and the testis or testes are removed. Once the testis or testes have been removed from the peritoneal space, all cannulas are opened to desufflate the peritoneal cavity. In the extended incision, the external abdominal oblique muscle is closed using size 0 polyglyconate (Maxon, Kendall/TycoHealthcare, Mansfield, Massachusetts) in a simple continuous pattern, followed by size 2-0 nylon in a simple continuous

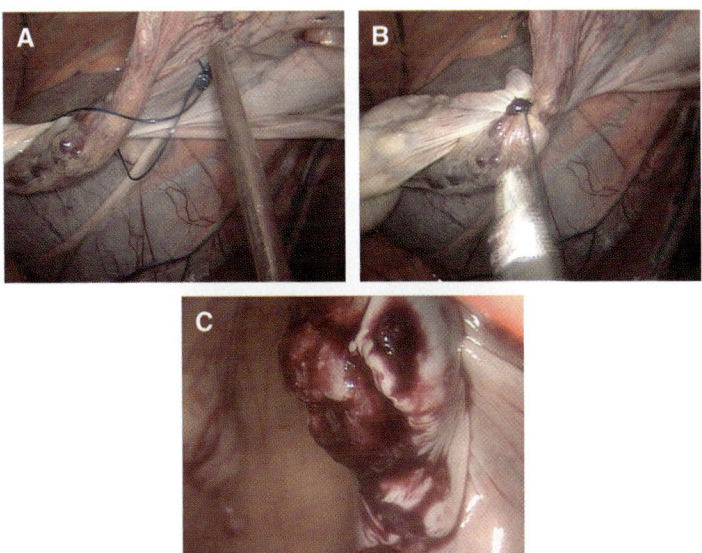

Fig. 7. Photographs show ligation of the mesorchium. (*A*) 4S modified Roeder knot with size 1 Maxon encircling the mesorchium. (*B*) Tightened knot just before suture transection. (*C*) Stump of the mesorchium after amputation of the testis.

pattern. The other portals are closed using size 2-0 nylon in a cruciate pattern (Fig. 8). If there is a descended testis, it is removed via standing castration or standard castration using a short-acting anesthetic regimen.

After surgery, the horses are allowed to eat as soon as they have fully recovered from the sedation. Phenylbutazone is continued at a dose of 2.2 mg/kg administered orally two times daily for 3 to 5 days. No further antibiotics are given, and the animals begin light exercise the day after surgery, with full exercise in 5 to 7 days.

Dorsally recumbent laparoscopic cryptorchidectomy

Surgical technique

The surgical technique [1,7] requires specific instrumentation (Box 2). The horses are sedated, and the neck over the jugular vein is clipped and aseptically prepared for catheter placement. Anesthetic induction and maintenance are performed as desired. It is important to have an anesthetic machine that is capable of positive-pressure ventilation to ensure adequate oxygenation when the horse is tipped into the Trendelenburg position. Once the horse is anesthetized and placed in dorsal recumbency, the ventral abdomen from the xiphoid rostrally, the pelvis caudally, and folds of the flanks laterally is aseptically prepared for surgery. The ventral abdomen is draped with a water-impermeable drape that allows access to the umbilicus and both parainguinal regions.

A 1-cm incision is made through the skin and linea alba just rostral to the umbilicus. A long teat cannula (Fig. 9), an 8-mm diameter mare urinary catheter, or a 10-mm diameter and 20-cm long laparoscopic cannula with a blunt obturator can be used to enter the peritoneal space for insufflation. If the laparoscopic cannula is used, the telescope can be introduced before

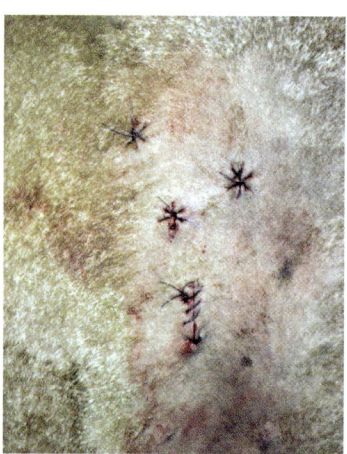

Fig. 8. Photograph of the left flank after a standing laparoscopic bilateral cryptorchidectomy.

Box 2. Instruments needed for dorsally recumbent laparoscopic cryptorchidectomy

30° telescope (30- or 57-cm length, author prefers 57-cm length)
Videocamera and monitor
300-W xenon light source and large-diameter fiberoptic cable
Insufflator and CO_2 tank
Insufflation cannula and insufflation tubing
Three to four cannulas with 10-mm diameter or 15- to 20-cm length cannulas
Laparoscopic injection needle
Atraumatic grasping forceps
One to two acute claw grasping forceps
Scissors
Ligation instruments
One to four ligating loops using size 1 Maxon with a knot pusher and knot protector or Ligasure device
Standard surgical pack
Surgical table that tilts at least 20°
Ability to provide positive-pressure ventilation

insufflation to confirm entry into the peritoneal cavity. In most cases, there is not negative pressure in the peritoneal space when the animal is positioned in dorsal recumbency. The insufflation cannula or laparoscopic cannula is attached to the insufflator with insufflation tubing, and the peritoneal space is insufflated to a pressure of 15 mm Hg. The abdomen is explored while the horse is tilted into the Trendelenburg position. The horse is only tilted far enough to be able to see the abdominally retained testis or testes (Fig. 10). The testis or testes are generally located laterally to the bladder,

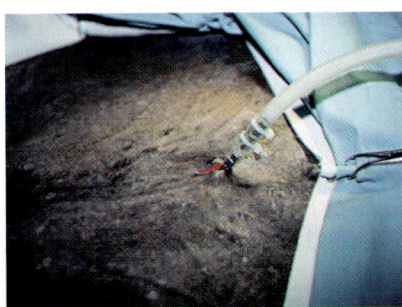

Fig. 9. Photograph of insufflation of a dorsally recumbent horse. Note that a teat cannula has been placed through an incision at the umbilicus.

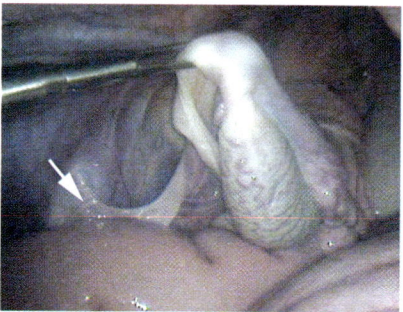

Fig. 10. Photograph shows an abdominally retained left testis in a horse in dorsal recumbency. The arrow denotes the left vaginal ring with gubernacular attachment.

with the gubernaculum attached to the vaginal ring, unless previous surgical attempts have disrupted the architecture. After the abdominal exploration, two additional portals are created approximately 15 cm on each side of the midline and 10 cm rostral to the external inguinal ring. To create these portals, a 1-cm skin incision is made in the skin and external rectus sheath. A 10-mm diameter 10- to 20-cm long cannula with a blunt obturator is advanced under direct vision into the peritoneal space. Once the testis or testes are identified, they are grasped with an atraumatic grasper to make sure the entire complex is located within the abdomen. The testis or testes are ligated and amputated as described for the standing laparoscopic cryptorchidectomy. In cases of bilaterally retained testes, a third instrument portal is helpful to maintain possession of the first amputated testis. After the testis or testes have been amputated, one of the parainguinal incisions is enlarged to remove the testis or testes from the peritoneal space. Once the testis or testes have been removed from the peritoneal space, all cannulas are opened to desufflate the peritoneal cavity. As the abdomen is desufflated, the horse is tipped back into a normal position to reduce the weight load on the thoracic cavity. The external rectus sheath of the enlarged portal is closed with size 0 polyglyconate (Maxon, Kendall/TycoHealthcare, Mansfield, MA) in a simple continuous pattern, and the external rectus sheath of the standard portals is closed with size 0 polyglyconate (Maxon, Kendall/TycoHealthcare, Mansfield, MA) in a simple interrupted pattern. The skin of the enlarged portal is closed with size 2-0 polyglyconate glycomer 631 (Biosyn, Kendall/TycoHealthcare, Mansfield, MA) using a simple continuous pattern or intradermal pattern, and the skin over the standard portals is closed using size 2-0 glycomer 631 (Biosyn, Kendall/TycoHealthcare, Mansfield, MA) using a cruciate or an intradermal pattern. If there is a descended testis, it is removed via standard castration. The horse is allowed to recover from anesthesia.

After surgery, the horses are allowed to eat as soon as they have fully recovered from the anesthesia. Phenylbutazone is continued at a dose of

2.2 mg/kg administered orally two times daily for 3 to 5 days. No further antibiotics are given, and the animals begin light exercise the day after surgery, with full exercise in 7 to 10 days.

Laparoscopic ovariectomy

Laparoscopic ovariectomy has become a much more common procedure in the past 5 years. In most cases of laparoscopic ovariectomy, the indication is for mares with behavioral problems associated with estrus. Although there may be some debate on the likelihood of improving aberrant behavior after ovariectomy, unpublished data from the author would indicate a good possibility of positive behavioral change after ovariectomy in the mare. The laparoscopic procedure can be performed in a standing, laterally recumbent, or dorsally recumbent position. The benefits of standing laparoscopic ovariectomy are identical to those of standing laparoscopic cryptorchidectomy. The limiting factors associated with standing laparoscopic ovariectomy are mares that do not stay in the stocks during surgery and mares with large granulosa thecal cell tumors (ovaries larger than 15–18 cm). When performing laterally recumbent ovariectomies, it is important to realize that only the ipsilateral ovary is approachable. The most limiting factor when performing a dorsally recumbent laparoscopic ovariectomy is a surgery table that can tilt at least 30°. When performing recumbent laparoscopic ovariectomies, it is useful to put the mares on a pelleted ration 4 to 5 days before holding off feed to reduce the bulk in the colon. One study has suggested that it is feasible to leave the ovaries of young horses free in the abdomen after ligation and transection with no untoward effects [8].

Standing laparoscopic ovariectomy

Surgical technique

The required instrumentation for the surgical technique [9–11] is listed in Box 3. The surgical technique is similar to that of horses undergoing standing laparoscopic cryptorchidectomy. The horses are sedated intravenously with xylazine (0.3 mg/kg) and placed in stocks for surgery. At this point, the caudal tail head area is clipped and prepared for a caudal epidural with detomidine (40 µg/kg brought to a total volume of 10 mL with 0.9% NaCl), or the neck area over the jugular vein is prepared using a catheter for intravenous infusion of detomidine (20 mg in polyionic replacement fluids [1 L]) given to effect. The appropriate flank(s) are clipped and aseptically prepared for surgery. For mares with small to moderately sized (less than 15- to 20-cm long) granulosa thecal cell tumors that are presented for ovariectomy, only the affected side is surgically prepared, whereas for bilateral ovariectomy, both flanks are prepared. Instrument portals are as previously described, with the middle portal at the level of the ventral aspect of the tuber coxae midway between the last rib and the tuber coxae and one

> **Box 3. Instruments needed for standing laparoscopic ovariectomy**
>
> 30° telescope (author prefers 57-cm length)
> Videocamera and monitor
> 300-W xenon light source and large-diameter fiberoptic cable
> Insufflator and CO_2 tank
> Insufflation cannula and insufflation tubing
> Three to six cannulas with 10-mm diameter and 15- to 20-cm length
> Laparoscopic injection needle
> Atraumatic grasping forceps, 10-mm diameter, 45-cm length
> Two to three acute claw grasping forceps, 10-mm diameter, 45-cm length
> Scissors, 10-mm diameter, 45-cm length
> Ligating instruments
> Two to four ligating loops using size 1 Maxon with a knot pusher and knot protector or Ligasure device
> Standard surgical pack

portal 10 cm dorsal and 5 cm rostral and another portal 10 cm ventral. The portal sites are infiltrated directly with 2% lidocaine (10–15 mL) or mepivicaine. The animals are draped with a water-impervious paper drape to allow access to the appropriate flank(s). Insufflation is achieved using an 8-mm diameter mare urinary catheter or a 10-mm diameter or 20-cm long laparoscopic cannula with a blunt obturator in the middle portal site (see previous section on standing laparoscopic cryptorchidectomy). If the laparoscopic cannula is used, the telescope can be introduced before insufflation to confirm entry into the peritoneal cavity. Either cannula is placed by directing the cannula toward the opposite stifle. The insufflation tubing is attached to the insufflator and the cannula to confirm negative pressure within the peritoneal cavity. When using the mare urinary catheter, the intra-abdominal pressure is taken to 12 to 15 mm Hg, and a 10-mm diameter or 20-cm long cannula with a blunt obturator is then placed through the dorsal portal site. As soon as a laparoscopic cannula is in place, the laparoscope with an attached videocamera is placed through the cannula and an exploratory procedure is performed (Fig. 11). Unlike standing laparoscopic cryptorchidectomy, it is generally not possible to visualize the contralateral ovary because of the mesocolon and the location of the ovary.

After the abdomen has been explored and the ipsilateral ovary has been identified, the ovary is grasped and the mesovarium is identified and injected with 2% lidocaine (10–20 mL) to provide analgesia [12]. After waiting for 10 minutes, the ipsilateral ovary is grasped for ligation and amputation. There

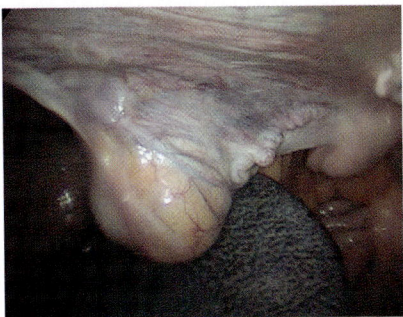

Fig. 11. Photograph of the left ovary, oviduct, and ovarian horn from the left flank in a standing laparoscopy.

are two primary methods that the author uses to ligate the mesovarium. The first method involves two encircling ligatures using size 1 polyglyconate (Maxon, Kendall/TycoHealthcare, Mansfield, MA) with a 4S modified Roeder knot [4,5] to ligate the mesovarium. The caudal pole of the ovary is sharply dissected to provide a more distinct pedicle for ligation. It is important to dissect the mesovarium approximately midway between the ovary and the uterine horn and to dissect in a straight line toward the dorsal body wall (Fig. 12A) After two loops are applied, the mesovarium is transected with tissue scissors (see Fig. 12B). It is helpful to rotate the ovary into the loop to speed the process. The second technique involves the use of a Ligasure vessel sealing device with 10-mm Atlas surgical shears, where sequential application of the shears, followed by application of the cutting blade, ligates and divides the mesovarium at the same time (Fig. 13) [13]. The loop technique requires less equipment but more expertise than does the technique with the Ligasure device. After amputation of the first ovary, the security of the grasper is ensured and a similar technique is performed on the other side of the horse. Other techniques that have been described for ligation and amputation of the ovary include bipolar electrosurgery [14]

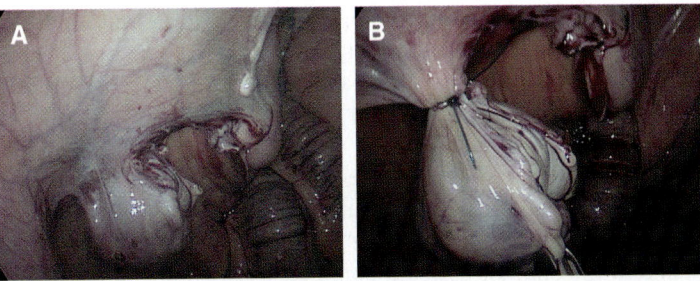

Fig. 12. Photographs show dissection (*A*) and ligation (*B*) of an ovary using a pretied knot using size 1 Maxon with a 4S modified Roeder knot.

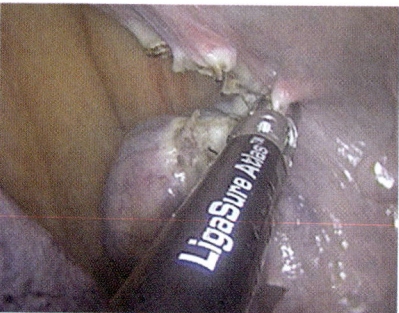

Fig. 13. Photograph shows amputation of an ovary using a Ligasure Atlas wand.

and ultrasonic cutting or coagulating shears [15,16]. In most cases, the left side is operated on first, followed by surgery on the right side when bilateral ovariectomy is planned. After amputation of the desired ovaries, the most ventral cannula portal (generally on the left side for bilateral ovariectomy) is extended by sharp dissection through the skin and external abdominal oblique muscle and by blunt dissection through the internal abdominal oblique and transverses muscles, and the ovaries are removed. It is important to make the incision large enough to remove the ovaries without difficulty, because ovaries that have been dropped in the abdomen can be difficult to find. In cases of bilateral ovariectomy, the right ovary is passed under the small colon to the left side of the abdomen for removal from the same enlarged incision. Once the amputated ovaries have been removed from the peritoneal space, all cannulas are opened to desufflate the peritoneal cavity. In the extended incision, the external abdominal oblique muscle is closed using size 0 polyglyconate (Maxon, Kendall/TycoHealthcare, Mansfield, MA) in a simple continuous pattern, followed by size 2-0 nylon in a simple continuous pattern. The other portals are closed using size 2-0 nylon in a cruciate pattern. The standing laparoscopic approach can be used successfully to remove moderately sized granulosa thecal cell tumors. The main limiting factor is the size of the ovary. Ovaries up to 15 cm can generally be successfully removed using hand-tied ligating loops; however, it is much more technically demanding than when removing a normal-sized ovary. The author has successfully removed an ovary that was 18 cm long using the Ligasure device. It is much easier to remove an enlarged ovary with the Ligasure device than it is with ligating loops.

After surgery, the horses are allowed to eat as soon as they have fully recovered from the sedation. Phenylbutazone is continued at a dose of 2.2 mg/kg administered orally two times daily for 3 to 5 days. No further antibiotics are given, and the animals are stall-confined with hand walking for 2 weeks and then begin an increasing exercise program. Most mares are back in full work in 2 to 4 weeks.

Laterally recumbent laparoscopic ovariectomy

Surgical technique

The required instrumentation is listed in Box 4. The surgical technique is similar to that of horses undergoing standing laparoscopic ovariectomy. The horses are sedated and anesthetized as desired. When mares are placed in lateral recumbency, only the ipsilateral ovary is approachable. Consequently, this approach is generally reserved for mares with moderately sized granulosa thecal cell tumors. The "up" flank is clipped and aseptically prepared for surgery. Instrument portals are as previously described, with the middle portal at the level of the ventral aspect of the tuber coxae midway between the last rib and the tuber coxae and one portal 10 cm dorsal and 5 cm rostral and another portal 10 cm ventral [11]. The portal sites can be infiltrated directly with 2% lidocaine (10–15 mL) or mepivicaine. The animals are draped with a water-impervious paper drape to allow access to the flank. Insufflation is achieved using an 8-mm diameter mare urinary catheter or a 10-mm diameter or 20-cm long laparoscopic cannula with a blunt obturator in the middle portal site (see previous section on standing laparoscopic cryptorchidectomy). If the laparoscopic cannula is used, the telescope can be introduced before insufflation to confirm entry into the peritoneal cavity. Either cannula is placed by directing the cannula toward the opposite stifle. When using the mare urinary catheter, the intra-abdominal pressure is taken to 12 to 15 mm Hg, and a 10-mm diameter or 20-cm long cannula

---

Box 4. Instruments needed for laterally recumbent laparoscopic ovariectomy

30° telescope (author prefers 57-cm length)
Videocamera and monitor
300-W xenon light source and large-diameter fiberoptic cable
Insufflator and CO_2 tank
Insufflation cannula and insufflation tubing
Three to four cannulas with 10-mm diameter and 15- to 20-cm length
Laparoscopic injection needle
Atraumatic grasping forceps, 10-mm diameter, 45-cm length
One to two acute claw grasping forceps, 10-mm diameter, 45-cm length
Scissors, 10-mm diameter, 45-cm length
Ligating instruments
Two ligating loops using size 1 Maxon with a knot pusher and knot protector or Ligasure device
Standard surgical pack
Ability to perform positive-pressure ventilation

with a blunt obturator is then placed through the dorsal portal site. As soon as a laparoscopic cannula is in place, the laparoscope with an attached videocamera is placed through the cannula and an exploratory procedure is performed (Fig. 14A). It is not possible to visualize the contralateral ovary.

After the abdomen has been explored and the ipsilateral ovary has been identified, the ovary is grasped and the mesovarium is identified and injected with 2% lidocaine (10–20 mL) to provide analgesia [12]. After waiting for 10 minutes, the ipsilateral ovary is grasped for ligation and amputation. The techniques for ligation and amputation are the same as for a standing flank laparoscopic ovariectomy. Because the most common reason for performing a laterally recumbent ovariectomy is to remove a granulosa thecal cell tumor, it is useful to have a Ligasure device available. It is possible to use an encircling ligature to ligate ovaries up to 15 cm long (see Fig. 14B, C). After amputation of the ovary, the most ventral cannula portal is extended by sharp dissection through the skin and external abdominal oblique muscle and by blunt dissection through the internal abdominal oblique and transverses muscles, and the ovary is removed. It is important to make the incision large enough to remove the ovary without difficulty, because ovaries that have been dropped in the abdomen can be difficult to find. Once the amputated ovaries have been removed from the peritoneal space, all cannulas are opened to desufflate the peritoneal cavity. In the extended incision, the external abdominal oblique muscle is closed using size 0 polyglyconate (Maxon, Kendall/TycoHealthcare, Mansfield, MA) in a simple continuous

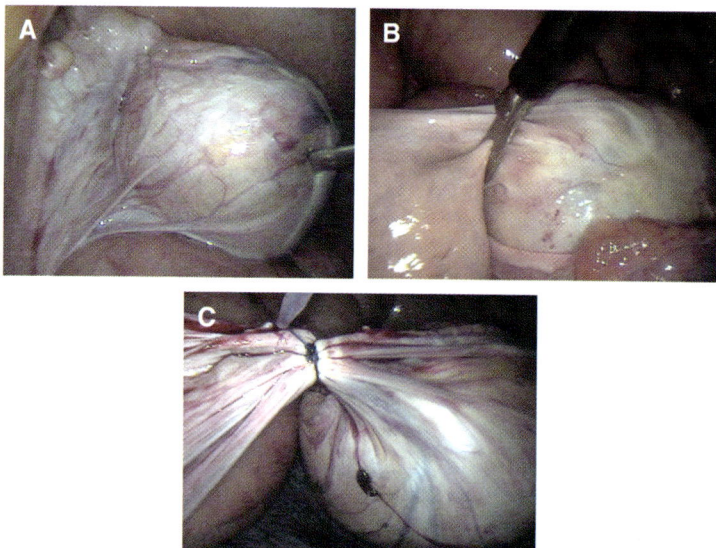

Fig. 14. Photographs of a left laterally recumbent laparoscopic ovariectomy. (*A*) Normal location of the ovary. (*B*) Dissection of the caudal pole of the ovary. (*C*) Ligation of the ovary with a pretied knot using size 1 Maxon with a 4S modified Roeder knot.

pattern, followed by size 2-0 nylon in a simple continuous pattern. The other portals are closed using size 2-0 nylon in a cruciate pattern.

After surgery, the horses are allowed to eat as soon as they have fully recovered from the anesthesia. Phenylbutazone is continued at a dose of 2.2 mg/kg administered orally two times daily 3 to 5 days. No further antibiotics are given, and the animals are stall-confined with hand walking for 2 weeks and then begin an increasing exercise program. Most mares are back in full work in 2 to 4 weeks.

Dorsally recumbent ovariectomy

Surgical technique

The required instrumentation for the surgical technique [17] is listed in Box 5. The surgical technique is similar to that of horses undergoing dorsally recumbent laparoscopic cryptorchidectomy. The biggest difference is that the mare generally has to be tipped farther into the Trendelenburg position than do stallions for cryptorchidectomy. The main reason for this is that the abdominally retained testes are generally located near the bladder, whereas the ovaries are more dorsal and rostral. Consequently, this approach is generally reserved in the author's practice for horses that are not tractable to having standing laparoscopic ovariectomy. The horses are sedated, and the neck over the jugular vein is clipped and aseptically

---

Box 5. Instruments needed for dorsally recumbent laparoscopic ovariectomy

30° telescope (author prefers 57-cm length)
Videocamera and monitor
300-W xenon light source and large-diameter fiberoptic cable
Insufflator and CO_2 tank
Insufflation cannula and insufflation tubing
Three to four cannulas with 10-mm diameter and 15- to 20-cm length cannulas
Laparoscopic injection needle
Atraumatic grasping forceps, 10-mm diameter, 45-cm length
1 to 2 acute claw grasping forceps, 10-mm diameter, 45-cm length
Scissors, 10-mm diameter, 45-cm length
Ligating instruments
Two ligating loops using size 1 Maxon with a knot pusher and knot protector or Ligasure device
Standard surgical pack
Surgical table that tilts at least 30°
Ability to perform positive-pressure ventilation

prepared for catheter placement. Anesthetic induction and maintenance are performed as desired. It is important to have an anesthetic machine that is capable of positive-pressure ventilation to ensure adequate oxygenation when the horse is tipped into the Trendelenburg position. Once the horse is anesthetized and placed in dorsal recumbency, the ventral abdomen from the xiphoid rostrally, the pelvis caudally, and folds of the flanks laterally is aseptically prepared for surgery. The ventral abdomen is draped with a water-impermeable drape that allows access to the umbilicus and both parainguinal regions.

A 1-cm incision is made through the skin and linea alba just rostral to the umbilicus. A long teat cannula, an 8-mm diameter mare urinary catheter, or a 10-mm diameter or 20-cm long laparoscopic cannula with a blunt obturator can be used to enter the peritoneal space for insufflation. If the laparoscopic cannula is used, the telescope can be introduced before insufflation to confirm entry into the peritoneal cavity. In most cases, there is no negative pressure in the peritoneal space when the animal is in dorsal recumbency. The insufflation cannula or laparoscopic cannula is attached to the insufflator with insufflation tubing, and the peritoneal space is insufflated to a pressure of 15 mm Hg. The abdomen is explored while the horse is tilted into the Trendelenburg position (head down, tail elevated). The horse is generally tilted to at least 30°, or until the large colon has moved far enough rostrally to visualize the uterine body dorsal to the bladder (Fig. 15). After the abdominal exploration, two additional portals approximately 15 cm on each side of the midline and 10 cm rostral to the external inguinal ring are created. To create these portals, a 1-cm skin incision is made in the skin and external rectus sheath. A 10-mm diameter 10- to 20-cm long cannula with a blunt obturator is advanced under direct vision into the peritoneal space. A third instrument portal is generally helpful to secure the first ovary after ligation and amputation. This cannula is used similar to and at the same

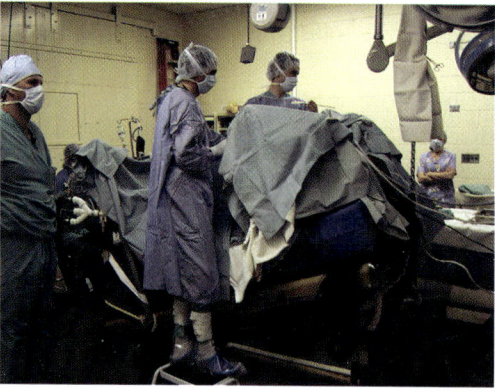

Fig. 15. Photograph of the overall surgery room with a mare in dorsal recumbency and the Trendelenburg position for laparoscopic ovariectomy.

level as got the other two instrument portals but on midline. Atraumatic grasping forceps are used to move any overlying bowel to gain access to the ovaries. Once the ovaries are identified, they are grasped with a traumatic grasper to ligate and amputate (Fig. 16). The ovaries are ligated and amputated as described for the standing or laterally recumbent laparoscopic ovariectomy. After the ovaries have been amputated, one of the parainguinal incisions is enlarged to remove the ovaries from the peritoneal space. Once the ovaries have been removed from the peritoneal space, all cannulas are opened to desufflate the peritoneal cavity. As the abdomen is desufflated, the horse is tipped back into a normal position to reduce the weight load on the thoracic cavity. The external rectus sheath of the enlarged portal is closed with size 0 polyglyconate (Maxon, Kendall/TycoHealthcare, Mansfield, MA) in a simple continuous pattern, and the external rectus sheath of the standard portals is closed with size 0 polyglyconate (Maxon, Kendall/TycoHealthcare, Mansfield, MA) in a simple interrupted pattern. The skin of the enlarged portal is closed with size 2-0 glycomer 631 (Biosyn, Kendall/TycoHealthcare, Mansfield, MA) using a simple continuous pattern or intradermal pattern, and the skin over the standard portals is closed using size 2-0 glycomer 631 (Biosyn, Kendall/TycoHealthcare, Mansfield, MA) with a cruciate or intradermal pattern. The horse is allowed to recover from anesthesia.

After surgery, the horses are allowed to eat as soon as they have fully recovered from the anesthesia. Phenylbutazone is continued at a dose of 2.2 mg/kg administered orally two times daily for 3 to 5 days. No further antibiotics are given, and the animals are stall-confined with hand walking for 2 weeks and then begin an increasing exercise program. Most mares are back in full work in 2 to 4 weeks.

Complications

Complications associated with laparoscopic surgery have generally been minimal [18,19]. The most common complication has been subcutaneous

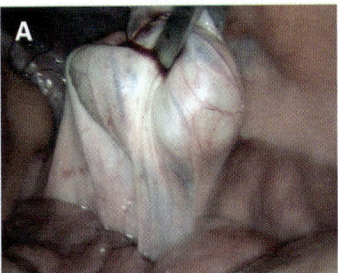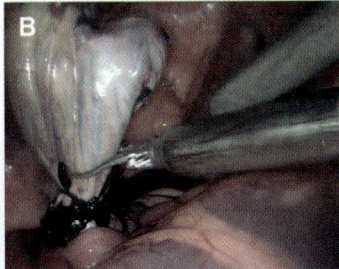

Fig. 16. Intra-abdominal photographs of the mare in Fig. 15. (*A*) Right ovary in the normal position. (*B*) Ovary after ligation with two pretied knots using size 1 Maxon with a 4S modified Roeder knot.

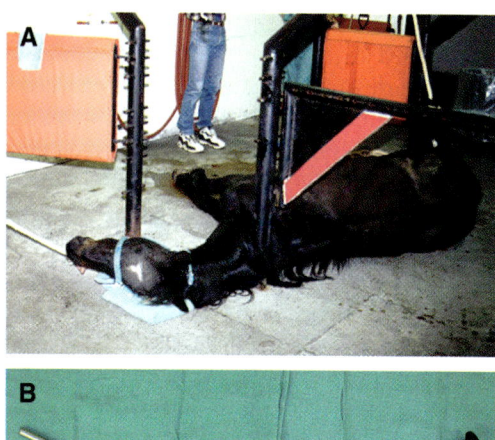
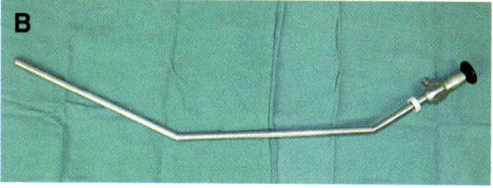

Fig. 17. Photographs of a horse in lateral recumbency after too high a dose of detomidine hydrochloride (*A*) and the laparoscope after the horse fell on it (*B*).

emphysema at the incision sites. Other minor complications include excessive bleeding at an incision site, retroperitoneal insufflation, and slippage of ligatures [20]. More severe complications have included bowel perforation, recumbency secondary to epidural detomidine [21], and recumbency secondary to surgical manipulation (Fig. 17). If care is taken during insufflation (eg, catheter placement) using a blunt cannula, the chances of bowel perforation are dramatically reduced. Careful administration of sedative drugs can minimize recumbency during surgery, as can infiltration of the mesovarium or mesorchium with local anesthetic.

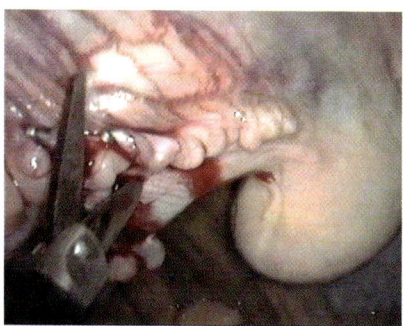

Fig. 18. Intra-abdominal photograph showing clip placement and cutting of oviduct for oviductal ligation.

Other uses

Other uses for laparoscopy for reproductive purposes have included treating horses with continued bleeding after castration [22], assessment of the uterus after foaling for tears, and diagnosis of uterine or ovarian abnormalities [23]. Oviductal ligation for gamete intrafallopian transfer (GIFT)–recipient mares has been described (Fig. 18) [24], and oviductal insemination is being explored.

References

[1] Wilson DG, Hendrickson DA, Cooley AJ, et al. Laparoscopic methods for castration of equids. J Am Vet Med Assoc 1996;209:112–4.
[2] Hendrickson DA, Wilson DG. Laparoscopic cryptorchid castration in standing horses. Vet Surg 1997;26:335–9.
[3] Trumble TN, Hendrickson DA. Standing male urogenital endoscopic surgery. Vet Clin North Am Equine Pract 2000;16(2):269–84.
[4] Shettko DL, Frisbie DD, Hendrickson DA. A comparison of knot security of commonly used hand-tied laparoscopic slipknots. Vet Surg 2004;33:521–4.
[5] Carpenter EM, Hendrickson DA, James S, et al. A mechanical study of ligature security of commercially available pre-tied ligatures versus hand tied ligatures for use in equine laparoscopy. Vet Surg 2006;35:55–9.
[6] Hanrath M, Rodgerson DH. Laparoscopic cryptorchidectomy using electrosurgical instrumentation in standing horses. Vet Surg 2002;31:117–24.
[7] Wilson DG. Dorsally recumbent male equine urogenital endoscopic surgery. Vet Clin North Am Equine Pract 2000;16(2):285–300.
[8] Shoemaker RW, Read EK, Duke T, et al. In situ coagulation and transection of the ovarian pedicle: an alternative to laparoscopic ovariectomy in juvenile horses. Can J Vet Res 2004;68: 27–32.
[9] Hanson CA, Galuppo LD. Bilateral laparoscopic ovariectomy in standing mares: 22 cases. Vet Surg 1999;28:106–12.
[10] Hendrickson DA. Minimally invasive surgery of the reproductive system in large animals. In: Freeman L, editor. Veterinary endosurgery. St. Louis (MO): Mosby; 1999. p. 217–25.
[11] Dechant JE, Hendrickson DA. Standing female urogenital endoscopic surgery. Vet Clin North Am Equine Pract 2000;16(2):301–16.
[12] Farstvedt E, Hendrickson DA. Intraoperative pain responses following intraovarian versus mesovarian injection of lidocaine in mares undergoing laparoscopic ovariectomy. J Am Vet Med Assoc 2005;227:593–6.
[13] Hand R, Rakestraw P, Taylor T. Evaluation of a vessel-sealing device for use in laparoscopic ovariectomy in mares. Vet Surg 2002;31:240–4.
[14] Rodgerson DH, Belknap JK, Wilson DA. Laparoscopic ovariectomy using sequential electrocoagulation and sharp transection of the equine mesovarium. Vet Surg 2001;30:572–9.
[15] Dusterdieck KF, Pleasant RS, Lanz OI, et al. Evaluation of the harmonic scalpel for laparoscopic bilateral ovariectomy in standing horses. Vet Surg 2003;32:242–50.
[16] Alldredge JG, Hendrickson DA. Use of high-power ultrasonic shears for laparoscopic ovariectomy in mares. J Am Vet Med Assoc 2004;225:1578–80.
[17] Ragle CA. Dorsally recumbent urinary endoscopic surgery. Vet Clin North Am Equine Pract 2000;16(2):343–50.
[18] Shettko DL. Complications in laparoscopic surgery. Vet Clin North Am Equine Pract 2000; 16(2):377–83.
[19] Desmaizieres LM, Martinot S, Lepage OM, et al. Complications associated with cannula insertion techniques used for laparoscopy in standing horses. Vet Surg 2003;32:501–6.

[20] Rodgerson DH, Hanson RR. Ligature slippage during standing laparoscopic ovariectomy in a mare. Can Vet J 2000;41:395–7.
[21] Wittern C, Hendrickson DA, Trumble TN, et al. Complications associated with administration of detomidine into the caudal epidural space in a horse. J Am Vet Med Assoc 1998;213: 516–8.
[22] Trumble TN, Ingle-Fehr J, Hendrickson DA. Laparoscopic intra-abdominal ligation of the testicular artery following castration in a horse. J Am Vet Med Assoc 2000;216:1596–8.
[23] Radcliffe RM, Hendrickson DA, Richardson GL, et al. Standing laparoscopic-guided uterine biopsy in a Southern White Rhinoceros (Ceratotherium Simum Simum). J Zoo Wildl Med 2000;31:201–7.
[24] McCue PM, Hendrickson DA, Hess MB. Fertility of mares after unilateral laparoscopic tubal ligation. Vet Surg 2000;29:543–5.

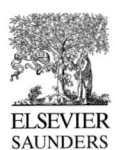

Granulosa Cell Tumors of the Equine Ovary

Patrick M. McCue, DVM, PhD[a],*,
Janet F. Roser, PhD[b], Coralie J. Munro, BS[c],
Irwin K.M. Liu, DVM, PhD[c], Bill L. Lasley, PhD[c]

[a]*Department of Clinical Sciences, College of Veterinary Medicine and Biomedical Science, Colorado State University, Fort Collins, CO 80523, USA*
[b]*Department of Animal Science, University of California-Davis, Davis, CA 95616, USA*
[c]*Department of Population Health and Reproduction, University of California-Davis, Davis, CA 95616, USA*

Tumors may develop from any tissue type located within the equine ovary. Histologic classification of an ovarian tumor is usually based on the World Health Organization (WHO) system, which includes three basic types: tumors of the surface germinal epithelium, tumors of sex cord–stromal tissue, and tumors of germ cell origin [1,2]. In addition, tumors of mesenchymal tissue (ie, fibromas, hemangiomas) may develop within the ovary, and secondary tumors that originate in another location (ie, lymphosarcoma, melanoma) may metastasize to the ovary. The presence of more than one tumor type in the same mare has also been reported [3].

The goal of this review is to describe the clinical parameters, diagnostic techniques, pathophysiology, potential complications, differential diagnoses, and treatment options for mares with ovarian granulosa cell tumors (GCTs).

Granulosa cell tumors

The GCT is a sex cord–stromal tumor and is by far the most common tumor of the equine ovary [4–9]. GCTs account for more than 85% of equine reproductive tract tumors [10] and approximately 2.5% of all neoplasms in horses [11]. Some sex cord–stromal tumors are composed primarily of granulosa cells and are termed *granulosa cell tumors*, whereas

---

* Corresponding author.
E-mail address: pmccue@colostate.edu (P.M. McCue).

others contain granulosa and theca cells and are consequently termed *granulosa–theca cell tumors* (GTCTs) [12]. The general term *granulosa cell tumor* is used throughout this review unless otherwise noted.

On gross examination, GCTs are typically polycystic (Fig. 1) with some areas of solid tissue [13]. Focal areas of necrosis and hemorrhage are common. Histologically, the cysts seem to be a disorganized attempt at follicle formation, with multiple layers of granulosa-type cells within the follicular structures and a supporting stroma that may contain theca-type cells [14]. Sex cord–stromal tumors in all species have the potential to be hormonally active.

Clinical parameters

There is no breed predilection for the formation of GCTs in mares. In the largest retrospective study reviewing clinical parameters in multiple cases of mares with GCTs, the average age of affected mares was reported to be 10.6 years and ranged from 2 to 20 years of age [8]. Juvenile GCTs have been reported in a newborn Thoroughbred filly [15], a 7-day old Thoroughbred filly [16], and a 3-month-old Arabian filly [17]. In adult horses, GCTs have been detected in maiden [8,18,19], barren [4,18], pregnant [4,8], and foaling [8,18,20,21] mares.

Most GCTs are benign [12,13,22], although malignant tumors have been reported [8,23]. GCTs are usually unilateral, and the contralateral ovary is almost always small and inactive [7,8,24–27]. Reports of mares with bilateral tumors have been published, however [28,29]. A few cases have been described in which mares continued to cycle despite the presence of a GCT [30–32]. It is likely that these situations represent tumors in early stages of development and that suppression of follicular growth would have occurred given sufficient time.

Affected mares may exhibit one of three behavioral abnormalities: prolonged anestrus, continuous or intermittent estrus (nymphomania behavior), or aggressive stallion-like behavior (Fig. 2) [4,5,7,8,18,19,27,33]. The

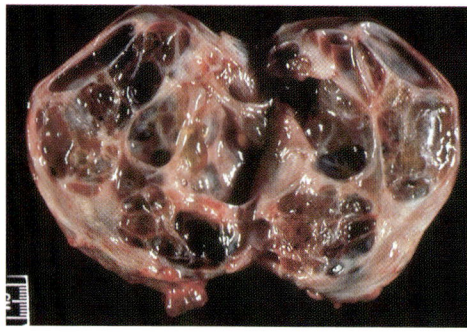

Fig. 1. Photograph of a GCT containing multiple cysts. (*From* McCue PM. Neoplasia of the female reproductive tract. Vet Clin North Am Equine Pract 1998;14(3):509; with permission.)

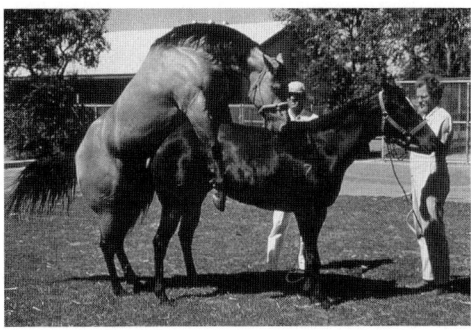

Fig. 2. Photograph of a mare with a GTCT mounting a mare in estrus. (*Courtesy of* John P. Hughes, DVM, Davis, CA.)

type of behavior expressed is dependent on the tumor cell type and the predominant steroid hormone produced. Meagher and coworkers [8] reported that 20 (31.7%) of 63 mares with GCTs exhibited anestrus behavior, whereas 14 (22.2%) of 63 and 29 (46.0%) of 63 showed continuous estrus or stallion-like behavior, respectively.

Mares with androgen-producing GCTs may also develop a crested neck, increased muscle mass, and an enlarged clitoris [5,8,34,35]. Less frequent clinical signs associated with the presence of a GCT include lameness [8], colic [35–37], and weight loss [35].

Diagnostic techniques

The classic clinical presentation of a mare with a GCT is a unilaterally enlarged ovary and a small inactive contralateral ovary. The ultrasonographic appearance of the affected ovary, behavioral changes, and endocrine parameters may be of assistance in confirming the diagnosis. Other techniques, such as laparoscopy, biopsy, or aspiration of an ovarian mass, have occasionally been used for diagnostic purposes [38–41] but are not routinely used in clinical practice. The definitive diagnosis is made by histopathologic examination.

Palpation and ultrasonography

The detection of a unilaterally enlarged ovary in the presence of a small inactive contralateral ovary during the physiologic breeding season is suggestive of a GCT. GCTs can present in all shapes and sizes. Most affected ovaries range from 10 to 20 cm in diameter [8]. A small GCT may be difficult to detect and may not have an effect on the opposite ovary if detected early in the course of the disease. Large tumors are much more obvious and are typically associated with suppression of follicular development in the contralateral ovary. One of the largest GCTs recorded was a 59.1-kg mass that weighed approximately 350 kg, which was removed from a 9-year-old Quarter Horse mare [35].

It has been reported that the ovulation fossa is usually obliterated by the presence of a GCT and that the absence of an ovulation fossa may be a means to differentiate this tumor from other ovarian abnormalities [42]. Nevertheless, a case has been described in which a mare had a slightly enlarged ovary with a histologically verified GCT on one pole that, on surgical removal, had a well-defined ovulation fossa present [43]. It was hypothesized that the tumor was in the early stages of development and that the ovulation fossa had not yet been eliminated by tumor expansion. The effect on the ovulation fossa may not be unique to the GCT, because development of other tumors has been reported to abolish the presence of the ovulation fossa [38].

Ultrasound examination may be valuable in diagnosing the presence of a GCT, but the appearance of the affected ovary can be quite variable [30,44]. GCTs can appear as a multicystic ("honeycombed") mass (Fig. 3), as a solid ovarian mass, or as a single large fluid-filled cyst (Fig. 4). The affected ovary often has a thick capsule or tunica albuginea surrounding a multicystic core [41]. The opposite ovary usually has little or no follicular activity noted on ultrasound [30].

Endocrinology

Endocrine assays may be valuable in the diagnosis or confirmation of a presumptive clinical diagnosis of GCT. Unfortunately, there are often

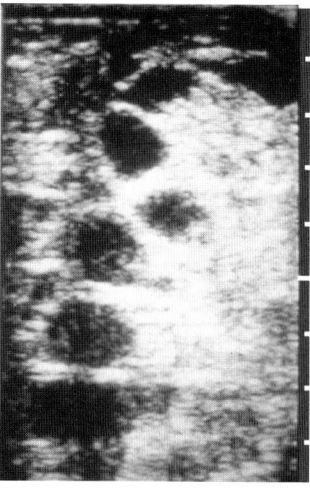

Fig. 3. Ultrasound photograph of a GCT shows multiple cystic areas. (*From* McCue PM. Neoplasia of the female reproductive tract. Vet Clin North Am Equine Pract 1998;14(3):508; with permission.)

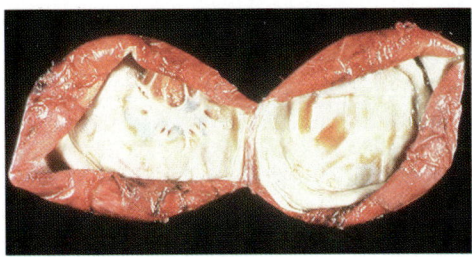

Fig. 4. Photograph of a GCT consisting of one large cyst. (*From* McCue PM. Neoplasia of the female reproductive tract. Vet Clin North Am Equine Pract 1998;14(3):509; with permission.)

substantial differences in assay components (ie, antibodies, standards) and techniques between endocrine laboratories. As a consequence, the range of normal values may be quite different between laboratories and a direct comparison of results may be impossible. Diagnostic laboratories should have a normal range of values established for each hormone, however. Test results for a given mare can be compared against the normal range established for that laboratory. For this review, comparisons are made relative to the normal ranges of hormone values (Table 1) established by the Endocrinology Laboratory, University of California, Davis.[1]

Testosterone

Testosterone concentrations have been reported to be elevated above the normal range of cycling mares in 40% to 50% of mares with GCTs [20,27], and measurement of testosterone levels has been used historically as a diagnostic marker for the presence of an ovarian tumor. Testosterone concentrations in normal cycling mares range from 20 to 45 pg/mL [45]. McCue [46] noted that testosterone levels in mares with histologically confirmed GCTs ranged from 24.9 to 420 pg/mL (average: 101.4 ± 19.5 pg/mL) and were elevated in 14 (66.7%) of 21 affected mares (Table 2). In contrast, Bailey and colleagues [47] noted that there was no statistical difference in detectable testosterone levels in mares with a GCT (304 ± 107 pg/mL) and control mares (146 ± 32 pg/mL). Furthermore, it was noted that testosterone levels in an Arabian mare collected at 12-hour intervals for 21 days fluctuated widely, ranging from undetectable (21 of 41 samples) to 268 pg/mL. It was suggested that evaluation of testosterone levels in a single sample may not accurately estimate the rate of testosterone secretion.

Mares with anestrus or persistent estrus behavior usually have normal testosterone concentrations [7,8,19,27,48]. Mares with GCTs expressing

---

[1] Endocrinology Laboratory, Department of Population Health and Reproduction, Tupper Hall, Room 1114, School of Veterinary Medicine, University of California, Davis, Davis, CA 95616.

Table 1
Normal values for inhibin, testosterone, estradiol, and progesterone in cycling mares

Hormone	Normal range
Inhibin	0.1–0.7 ng/mL
Testosterone	20–45 pg/mL
Estradiol	20–45 pg/mL
Progesterone (estrus)	<1.0 ng/mL
Progesterone (diestrus)	>1.0 ng/mL

aggressive male behavior often have testosterone concentrations greater than 100 pg/mL [27,29,30]. Elevated testosterone concentrations have been associated with the presence of a large number of theca (ie, a GTCT) within the interstitial tissue of the tumor [12,13,27]. Plasma testosterone concentrations decline to basal levels within 12 to 24 hours after surgical removal of the tumor [7,27].

Estradiol

Concentrations of estradiol in mares with GCTs are variable and not always clearly related to the predominant behavior expressed [27,48,49].

Table 2
Inhibin, testosterone, follicle-stimulating hormone, and luteinizing hormone concentrations in 21 mares with histologically confirmed granulosa cell tumors

Mare no.	Inhibin (ng/mL)	Testosterone (pg/mL)	FSH (ng/mL)	LH (ng/mL)
1	1.77	144.9	1.04	50.33
2	2.13	127.8	1.67	5.61
3	1.88	78	1.17	30.72
4	1.29	420	2.65	141.45
5	2.18	53	1.09	18.9
6	1.09	41.1	2.64	63.51
7	1.39	54.6	1.66	2.4
8	0.52	34.4	16.16	31.88
9	1.57	189.9	1.12	5.57
10	1.78	38.5	1.48	14.46
11	3.00	97	0.98	1.93
12	1.95	35.1	1.16	1.62
13	1.93	24.9	0.8	2.07
14	2.19	186.3	1.97	8.6
15	3.00	98.5	1.17	0.48
16	1.03	44.1	4.46	3.51
17	1.67	203	4.55	28.37
18	0.80	56.8	1.97	63.71
19	0.58	100.9	10.19	59.9
20	3.00	54.1	1.1	2.76
21	1.32	45.6	10.95	90.93

Abbreviations: FSH, follicle stimulating hormone; LH, luteinizing hormone.
Data from McCue PM. Pathophysiology of follicular development [PhD dissertation]. Davis (CA); University of California, Davis; 1993. p. 148–75.

Aromatization of testosterone to estradiol in mares with GCTs may be reduced, because mares with extremely high testosterone concentrations do not necessarily have concomitantly high estradiol concentrations [27]. Watson and Thomson [50] noted that granulosa cells from mares with GCTs exhibited little staining for the enzyme aromatase cytochrome P-450 as compared with granulosa cells from normal follicles. The authors concluded that GCT tissue has a limited capacity to aromatize androgens to estrogens.

Plasma estradiol levels in mares with a GCT are not usually elevated above the normal range of cycling mares (20–45 pg/mL), even in mares expressing continuous estrus. It is hypothesized that the behavioral estrus of affected mares is driven by the low levels of estradiol that are present. As a consequence, measurement of estradiol levels is generally of limited value in the diagnosis of GCTs in the mare.

Progesterone

Progesterone concentrations are almost invariably low (<1.0 ng/mL) in mares with GCTs, consistent with the absence of active luteal tissue [27]. Because most mares with GCTs are acyclic, the detection of elevated progesterone (>1.0 ng/mL) suggests that a GCT is not present. GCTs have been reported in several mares in which ovulation was detected, however, and the presence of active luteal tissue was verified by elevations in plasma progesterone levels [31,51]. Therefore, caution must be taken before attempting to exclude the diagnosis of GCT based solely on progesterone values.

Inhibin

Inhibin is a glycoprotein hormone produced in female animals by granulosa cells of the ovary [52]. Inhibin, activin, and follistatin are classified as members of the transforming growth factor-β (TGFβ) superfamily [53]. Inhibin is composed of two subunits: an α subunit and one of two β subunits ($β_A$ or $β_B$), yielding inhibin A (α-$β_A$) or inhibin B (α-$β_B$). Immunohistochemically, the inhibin α subunit and inhibin α-$β_A$ and α-$β_B$ subunits have been localized in the granulosa and theca interna cells of large follicles in the mare [54]. The primary physiologic role of inhibin is the specific suppression of follicle-stimulating hormone (FSH) secretion from the anterior pituitary [55]. Inhibin plays an active role in the regulation of follicular development and in limiting the number of ovulations in horses through the negative feedback effect on FSH [56].

The pattern of inhibin secretion throughout the equine estrous cycle has been defined [54,57,58]. Inhibin levels increase with follicular development during estrus, achieve peak concentrations on or near the day of ovulation, and reach a nadir during the middle of diestrus. Concentrations of inhibin are positively correlated with concentrations of estradiol [57,58]. Concentrations of FSH are inversely correlated with levels of inhibin and estradiol during the equine estrous cycle [54,57,58]. Roser and colleagues [58] reported that the range of inhibin concentrations in normal cycling mares was 0.1 to 0.7 ng/mL. Inhibin is undetectable in the plasma of ovariectomized mares and geldings [58]. The radioimmunoassay (RIA) described by Roser and colleagues [58] used an inhibin antiserum raised in rabbits against 31-kd bovine inhibin and was validated for the horse. The antibody does not exhibit cross-reaction with bovine α- or β-subunits but does show significant cross-reaction with a pro-α-subunit [59]. The antibody recognizes the free α- subunit, proαC, and the inhibin dimer. The presence and relative amount of free α- subunit in the horse has not been established [58].

Inhibin has been described as a diagnostic marker for the presence of GCTs in women [60] and Sertoli cell tumors in dogs [61]. Equine GCTs were reported to express mRNA for inhibin [62]. This led to the hypothesis that measurement of circulating inhibin concentrations may be of clinical use in the diagnosis of equine GCTs [46,63]. In the original study, concentrations of inhibin in 21 mares with GCTs ranged from 0.5 to 3.0 ng/mL and averaged 1.7 ± 0.2 ng/mL (see Table 2) [46]. Inhibin concentrations in mares with GCTs were elevated above values established for normal cycling mares (0.1–0.7 ng/mL) in 19 (90.5%) of 21 cases. Inhibin concentrations declined to undetectable levels within 24 hours after surgical removal of the affected ovary. Concentrations of inhibin and testosterone were not correlated in mares with GCTs ($r = -0.02$; $P > .05$). In an expanded study, concentrations of inhibin were reported to be elevated in 34 (87%) of 39 mares with histologically confirmed GCTs [63].

Other studies have since confirmed the presence of elevated inhibin concentrations in mares with GCTs [47,64,65]. Christman and coworkers [64] reported that concentrations of the inhibin dimer ($\alpha\beta_A$-inhibin) were elevated in 3 of 6 mares with GCTs. The assay used was a two-site immunoradiometric assay (IRMA) that incorporated antibodies against the α-subunit and the A-form of the β-subunit (β_A). A subsequent study [47] compared the measurement of dimeric $\alpha\beta_A$-inhibin using an IRMA with measurement of the inhibin α-subunit, described as a combination of monomeric (free) inhibin α-subunit and dimeric $\alpha\beta_A$-inhibin, in 22 mares with GCTs and 31 normal cycling mares. The α-inhibin RIA used an antiserum against the N-terminal 25 amino acids of the ovine inhibin αC-subunit. A strong positive correlation ($r = 0.91$) was noted between concentrations of α-inhibin and tumor diameter. It was concluded that measurement of α-inhibin using an RIA was a more reliable indicator of the presence of a GCT than measurement of the $\alpha\beta_A$-inhibin dimer using an IRMA.

Watson and colleagues [65] evaluated concentrations of inhibin in 6 mares with GCTs and from 14 normally cycling mares. It was reported that concentrations of plasma inhibin isoforms containing pro- and -αC immunoreactivity were increased in all 6 mares compared with those of normal mares in estrus, diestrus, or anestrus. Concentrations of inhibin A were elevated in 4 of the 6 mares. Testosterone concentrations were elevated in 4 of the 6 mares with GCTs.

Inhibin is a more accurate indicator of the presence of a GCT than testosterone [47,63,65]. When inhibin and testosterone measurements were used together diagnostically, 95.2% of equine GCTs were detected [63]. Currently, the only clinical endocrinology laboratory performing inhibin assays in equine samples is the Clinical Endocrinology Laboratory at the University of California, Davis. The recommended tumor panel is a combination of inhibin, testosterone, and progesterone.

Follicle-stimulating hormone

The mean concentration of FSH in the 21 mares with GCTs was 3.3 ± 4.1 ng/mL (see Table 2). Three of the mares had high FSH levels (10.2, 11.0, and 16.2 ng/mL, respectively), and 2 of these 3 mares had low inhibin concentrations (<0.7 ng/mL). If the values from those 3 mares are excluded as statistical outliers, the mean FSH concentration in the remaining 18 mares was 1.8 ± 0.3 ng/mL, which was significantly ($P < .01$) lower than the mean concentration of FSH in normal cycling mares during estrus (4.0 ± 0.6 ng/mL) or diestrus (5.6 ± 0.8 ng/mL) (Table 3). Concentrations of FSH in mares with GCTs were inversely correlated with inhibin concentration ($r = -0.63$, $P < .01$) but not testosterone ($r = -0.1$, $P > .05$).

The pituitary function of 5 mares with GCTs and 6 normal mares in seasonal anestrus (January), estrus (day 3 of estrus), and diestrus (day 7 after ovulation) was assessed after administration of a single 50-μg intravenous bolus of gonadotropin-releasing hormone (GnRH) [46]. The objective was to compare the gonadotropin response to an exogenous GnRH challenge in mares with GCTs versus normal mares. Plasma samples were collected at 20-minute intervals before and after GnRH treatment. Administration of GnRH resulted in significantly higher ($P < .05$) secretion of FSH (Fig. 5) and luteinizing hormone (LH; not shown) in normal mares in diestrus and seasonal anestrus versus normal mares in estrus or mares with GCTs.

Table 3
Average concentrations of inhibin, testosterone, follicle-stimulating hormone, and luteinizing hormone in mares with granulosa cell tumors and normal mares in estrus and diestrus

	Mares with GCTs	Normal Estrus	Mares Diestrus
No. Mares (n)	21	8	8
Inhibin (ng/mL)	1.7 ± 0.2^a	0.5 ± 0.1^b	0.2 ± 0.1^c
Testosterone (pg/mL)	101.4 ± 19.5^a	29.4 ± 6.2^b	18.8 ± 1.5^b
FSH (ng/mL)^d	1.8 ± 0.3^a	4.0 ± 0.6^b	5.6 ± 0.8^b
LH (ng/mL)	29.9 ± 7.9^a	15.1 ± 3.3^a	2.9 ± 0.4^b

Values presented are the mean ± SEM.

Abbreviations: FSH, follicle-stimulating hormone; GCT, granulosa cell tumor; LH, luteinizing hormone.

[a,b,c] Values within each row with different superscripts are significantly different ($P < .05$).

[d] Mean FSH concentration for mares with GCTs excludes three mares as outliers.

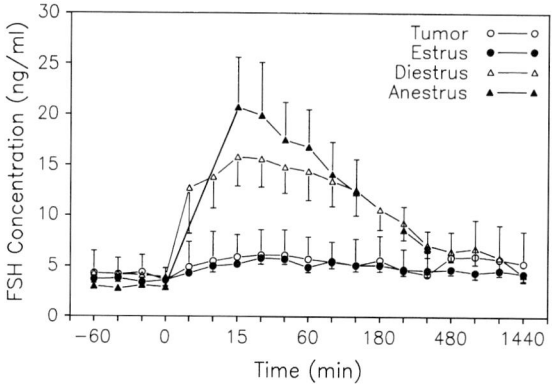

Fig. 5. FSH response to a 50-μg intravenous injection of native GnRH in five mares with GCTs and 6 normal mares in estrus, diestrus, or seasonal anestrus (Time 0 is time of injection).

Bailey and coworkers [47] noted a tendency toward a negative correlation ($r = -0.41$, $P = .08$) between concentrations of FSH and $\alpha\beta_A$-inhibin but not between FSH and α-inhibin.

Luteinizing hormone

McCue [46] noted that concentrations of LH in mares with tumors were highly variable and that the mean concentration (29.9 ± 7.9 ng/mL) was not significantly different ($P > .05$) than in normal mares in estrus (15.1 ± 3.3 ng/mL). This is similar to the variability of LH levels in mares with GCTs reported previously [7]. A positive correlation ($r = 0.46$, $P = .05$) was noted between LH and testosterone in mares with a GCT [47].

Pathophysiology

The GCT is the only ovarian abnormality in the mare associated with inactivity of the contralateral ovary. The physiologic basis for dysfunction of the contralateral ovary is presumed to be mediated through suppression of pituitary FSH secretion attributable to the production of inhibin and possibly other hormones from the affected ovary [63]. Reduction of FSH levels causes suppression of the function of an otherwise healthy contralateral ovary.

The FSH suppression hypothesis is supported by the facts that (1) concentrations of inhibin are inversely correlated with concentrations of FSH during the estrous cycle of normal mares [57,58] and mares with GCTs [46,47], (2) administration of inhibin in the form of steroid-free follicular fluid to cycling mares results in suppression of FSH secretion and follicular development [57,66], and (3) inactivation of inhibin biologic activity through active immunization has been demonstrated to increase FSH levels and results in enhanced follicular development and superovulation [67,68].

Secretion of ovarian steroids by the tumor may also affect the development of follicles in the contralateral ovary. Administration of testosterone or estradiol to normal intact or ovariectomized mares results in a decrease in FSH secretion [69,70]. Although not all mares with ovarian GCTs have increased concentrations of testosterone or estradiol, continuous secretion of steroids by the affected ovary, even at concentrations within the normal range, may result in inhibition of FSH secretion.

Potential complications

Medical complications attributable to or associated with the presence of a GCT are uncommon. Although most equine granulosa cells are benign, metastasis has been reported [8,23,71,72]. Patrick and colleagues [72] noted that only 2 of 112 reported cases of GCTs had metastasized. Metastasis is generally confined to the abdominal cavity, although extension to thoracic and sublumbar lymph nodes and emboli within the vasculature of the lungs has been noted [23].

Large GCTs may cause colic or other gastrointestinal problems [8,21,35]. Van der Zaag and coworkers [73] reported that a postpartum Arabian mare developed colic secondary to a 31.5-kg GCT. Intermittent colic was also noted in a mare with an extremely large GCT [35]. Wilson and colleagues [37] described a case in which a GCT caused rupture of the small colon in a 10-year-old Quarter Horse mare. The rupture was secondary to impaction caused by occlusion of the small colon between the enlarged left ovary and its suspensory ligament.

Rupture of juvenile- and adult-form GCTs with subsequent intra-abdominal hemorrhage has been reported [15,36,74]. In one case, tumor rupture was diagnosed in a neonatal foal [15]. It was hypothesized that the rupture occurred during foaling. Affected animals are typically presented with abdominal pain, distention, and anemia [15,36]. Hemoperitoneum is confirmed by transabdominal ultrasonography and abdominocentesis [74]. Alexander and coworkers [74] reported on the successful surgical treatment of two mares with ruptured ovarian GCTs. There are no documented cases of metastasis after rupture of a GCT in mares.

Adhesions of unruptured GCTs to adjacent abdominal structures, including the abdominal wall, bladder, uterus, spleen, omentum, and intestinal tract, have been described [41]. Rupture of the tumor or adhesion of the tumor to adjacent structures may follow localized ischemia and necrosis of the tunica albuginea induced by pressure of rapid neoplastic growth within the encapsulated ovary [41].

Torsion of the ovary containing a GTCT has been described in a 3-month-old Arabian filly [17] and a 12-year-old Morgan mare [75]. The filly had a 3-day history of abdominal distention and colic. Necropsy revealed a 360° torsion of the affected ovary, which measured 32 cm × 27 cm × 27 cm. The mare had a 45-day history of stallion-like behavior, and initial examination revealed an enlarged multicystic left ovary and a small inactive right ovary. Serum levels of testosterone and inhibin were elevated above normal values. A complete blood cell count (CBC) evaluation revealed mild anemia, and abdominocentesis indicated that recent intra-abdominal hemorrhage had occurred. The mare became acutely painful, and surgical exploration of the abdomen confirmed a 720° torsion of the enlarged ovary. The ovary was removed, and the mare recovered. Gross and histologic evaluation of the ovary revealed extensive necrosis and hemorrhage.

Hypertrophic osteopathy (HO) associated with the presence of an ovarian GCT with metastasis to the abdominal cavity was noted in a pregnant 8-year-old Quarter Horse mare [71]. Similar syndromes have been reported in a 4-year-old Arab-cross mare with an ovarian dysgerminoma with metastasis to the abdominal lymph nodes [76] and an 8-year-old Arabian mare with metastases throughout the abdomen [77]. Although the pathogenesis of HO is unclear, it has been associated with neoplasia or inflammatory conditions of the thoracic or abdominal cavity [71].

Hensen and colleagues [78] reported the association between a GTCT and histiolymphocytic lymphoma in a 9-year-old Arabian mare. The mare exhibited signs of stallion-like behavior around other mares and had multiple subcutaneous masses on the trunk and limbs. A generalized regression of the subcutaneous tumors occurred within a month after surgical removal of the GTCT. It was hypothesized that steroid hormones produced by the GTCT may have influenced the growth and development of the lymphoma.

Secondary diabetes mellitus was noted in a 10-year-old American Saddle Horse with bilateral GCTs. The horse had markedly elevated serum and urine glucose levels and abnormal results of a glucose tolerance test [28]. The cause of the diabetes condition was not determined, but exposure to gonadal steroids or other hormones produced by the tumor was suggested as a possibility.

Differential diagnosis

The differential diagnosis may be based on ovarian enlargement or behavioral changes. The differential diagnosis for ovarian enlargement in the mare includes tumors, such as a GCT, teratoma, serous cystadenoma, or dysgerminoma as well as a persistent anovulatory follicle, multiple corpora lutea of pregnancy, and other causes. The differential diagnosis for stallion-like behavior includes GTCT, pregnancy, anabolic steroid administration, and developmental abnormalities (eg, male pseudohermaphroditism). The primary differential diagnosis for persistent estrus is the vernal transition period.

Teratomas presumably arise from pluripotent germ or stem cells within the ovary that undergo somatic differentiation into two or more germinal cell layers (ie, ectoderm, mesoderm, endoderm) [14]. Teratomas may contain a variety of tissue types, including hair, skin, sebaceous glands, adipose tissue, nerve tissue, cartilage, bone, active bone marrow, teeth, muscle, respiratory epithelium, and other tissues [4,38,79,80]. Ultrasound examination may reveal the presence of cystic and solid hyperechoic structures within the affected ovary.

Teratomas are considered to be the second most common ovarian tumors of mares; however, in reality, they are rare [3,40,80]. The frequency of diagnosis of an ovarian teratoma relative to a GCT in horses has been noted to be 1:18 [3]. In the horse, teratomas are usually unilateral, slow growing, and benign. Metastasis is extremely uncommon but has been reported [81]. The tumor is not hormonally active, the opposite ovary is unaffected, and mares with a teratoma may continue to cycle [38,80,81]. Affected mares may be presented for colic, or the enlarged ovary may be diagnosed during routine examination [81]. Diagnosis is usually based on the presence of a unilaterally enlarged ovary with ultrasonographically echogenic and cystic areas and a normal contralateral ovary. Teratomas have been diagnosed in mares along with a GCT [3].

The serous cystadenoma is the primary ovarian epithelial tumor of the mare and is reported to be the third most common ovarian tumor [80]. Cystadenomas arise from the surface germinal epithelium, which is only located within the ovulation fossa or the rete ovarii in the mare [13,16]. The serous cystadenoma derives its name from the fluid-filled cystic or polycystic nature of the tumor.

Cystadenomas are rare benign unilateral tumors that do not metastasize and do not affect the development of the contralateral ovary [82]. In general, cystadenomas are not considered to be hormonally active, although several individual cases in which affected mares had elevated serum testosterone levels have been reported [7,83]. In one case, plasma testosterone concentrations declined from 0.15 to 0.09 ng/mL after surgical removal of the tumor [83].

Mares with cystadenomas may continue to cycle and may become pregnant [83,84]. The cystic spaces are lined by a single layer of flattened cuboidal epithelium, which may be ciliated [16]. Cystadenomas have been reported to resemble germinal inclusion cysts (fossa cysts) at the macroscopic level [16]. It has been suggested that cystadenomas may arise indirectly from fossa cysts [83].

Dysgerminomas are another type of germ cell tumor and are considered to be the ovarian equivalent of the testicular seminoma of stallions [85]. The tumor is thought to arise from follicular oocytes, primordial or immature germ cells, or testicular rudiments or their homologues within the ovary [13]. Dysgerminomas differ from teratomas in that they do not exhibit somatic differentiation [12]. Ovarian dysgerminomas are extremely rare, are unilateral, and do not produce steroid hormones. Dysgerminomas in the mare are composed of broad sheets, cords, or nests of large uniform cells separated by connective tissue septae [14,85]. Equine dysgerminomas have a high tendency for metastasis [76,85,86]. In addition, in at least two cases, the presence of a dysgerminoma was associated with the development of HO [76,77].

Other causes of ovarian enlargement include tumors, such as melanomas, epitheliomas, hemangiomas, adenocarcinomas, arrhenoblastomas, and hemoblastomas [87–89].

The ovaries of mares may enlarge greatly during pregnancy because of the formation of secondary corpora lutea [90,91]. Secondary corpora lutea begin to form at approximately day 40 of gestation and are associated temporally with the onset of equine chorionic gonadotropin (eCG) production. Regression of secondary corpora lutea begins between days 160 and 180 of gestation. Pregnant mares may exhibit aggressive or stallion-like behavior associated with increased androgen production during midgestation.

Treatment options

Surgical removal of the affected ovary is recommended. The tumor may continue to increase slowly in size and may eventually cause colic [30,35,73], weight loss [10], gastrointestinal obstruction, or other problems. Ovarian tumors can be surgically removed by a colpotomy approach [92] or through a flank, ventral midline, paramedian, or diagonal paramedian laparotomy approach [93]. In addition, standing flank and ventral abdominal laparoscopic techniques for removal of GCTs have been described [94,95]. Advantages of specific procedures, details of surgical techniques, and potential complications are provided elsewhere [93–95].

Testosterone and inhibin concentrations decline rapidly after surgical removal of the affected ovary [7,27,47,63]. The contralateral ovary returns to normal function in most mares after removal of the neoplastic ovary. In one report, 42 of 57 mares returned to estrus an average of 8.5 months after surgery (range: 2–16 months) and 30 of 39 eventually produced live foals [8]. Stabenfeldt and colleagues [27] noted that 8 of 10 mares resumed normal estrous cycles from the contralateral ovary the spring after surgical removal of the GCT-affected ovary. Two mares did not ovulate until 341 and 392 days, respectively, after surgery, and 1 additional mare still had not ovulated by 524 days after surgery.

Summary

The GCT is the most common ovarian tumor in mares. A clinical diagnosis can be made based on the presence of a unilaterally enlarged ovary and a small inactive contralateral ovary. Endocrine testing may be beneficial to confirm a diagnosis. Plasma inhibin and testosterone concentrations are elevated in approximately 90% and 50% to 60%, respectively, of mares with GCTs. Testosterone is elevated if the tumor has a significant thecal cell component, and affected mares exhibit stallion-like behavior. Hormones produced by the tumor result in suppression of pituitary FSH secretion and inactivity in the opposite ovary. Surgical removal of the tumor eliminates the adverse effect on pituitary function and results in resumption of follicular development and ovulation over time.

Acknowledgment

This article is dedicated to the memory of Dr. John P. Hughes and Dr. George H. Stabenfeldt, pioneers in the area of equine ovarian abnormalities.

References

[1] Chen VW, Ruiz B, Killeen JL, et al. Pathology and classification of ovarian tumors. Cancer 2003;97:2631–42.
[2] Kennedy PC, Cullen JM, Edwards JF, et al. Histological classification of the tumors of the genital system. In: Schulman FY, editor. World Health Organization, histological classification of tumors of domestic animals. Washington (DC): The Armed Forces Institute of Pathology; 1998. p. 24–8.
[3] Panciera RJ, Slusher SA, Hayes KE. Ovarian teratoma and granulosa cell tumor in two mares. Cornell Vet 1991;81:43–50.
[4] Bosu WTK, Smith CA. Ovarian abnormalities. In: McKinnon AO, Voss JL, editors. Equine reproduction. Philadelphia: Lea & Febiger; 1993. p. 397–407.
[5] Clark TL. Clinical management of equine ovarian neoplasms. J Reprod Fertil Suppl 1975; 23:331–4.
[6] Cordes DO. Equine granulosa tumours. Vet Rec 1969;85:186–8.
[7] Hughes JP, Kennedy PC, Stabenfeldt GH. Pathology of the ovary and ovarian disorders in the mare. In: Proceedings of the Ninth International Congress on Animal Reproduction and Artificial Insemination. Madrid, Spain; 1980. p. 203–22.
[8] Meagher DM, Wheat JD, Hughes JP, et al. Granulosa cell tumors in mares—a review of 78 cases. Proc Am Assoc Equine Pract 1977;23:133–43.
[9] Norris HJ, Taylor HB, Garner FM. Equine ovarian granulosa tumours. Vet Rec 1968;82: 419–20.
[10] McCue PM, Taylor HB, Garner FM. Neoplasia of the female reproductive tract. Vet Clin Equine 1998;14:505–15.
[11] Sundberg JP, Burnstein T, Page EH, et al. Neoplasms of equidae. J Am Vet Med Assoc 1977; 170:150–2.
[12] Jubb KVF, Kennedy PC, Palmer N. Pathology of domestic animals, vol. 3. 3rd edition. New York: Academic Press; 1985. p. 305–23.
[13] Nielsen SW, Kennedy PC. Tumors of the genital systems. In: Moulton JE, editor. Tumors in domestic animals. 3rd edition. Berkeley (CA): University of California Press; 1990. p. 479–517.
[14] MacLachlan NJ. Ovarian disorders in domestic animals. Environ Health Perspect 1987;73: 27–33.
[15] Green SL, Specht TE, Dowling SC, et al. Hemoperitoneum caused by rupture of a juvenile granulosa cell tumor in an equine neonate. J Am Vet Med Assoc 1988;193:1417–9.
[16] Buergelt CD. Ovarian tumors. In: Color atlas of reproductive pathology of domestic animals. St. Louis (MO): Mosby; 1997. p. 100–11.
[17] Hultgren BD, Zack PM, Pearson EG, et al. Juvenile granulosa cell tumor in an equine weanling. J Comp Pathol 1987;97:137–42.
[18] Baumann LE, Sillerud CL, Spolar-Kilroy CR. Equine granulosa cell tumors. A review of fifteen cases. Minn Vet 1985;25:52–4.

[19] Stickle RL, Erb RE, Fessler JF, et al. Equine granulosa cell tumors. J Am Vet Med Assoc 1975;167:148–51.
[20] Bergeron H, Crouch GM, Bowen JM. Granulosa theca cell tumor in a mare. Compend Contin Educ Pract Vet 1983;5(Suppl):S141–4.
[21] Schmidt GR, Cowles RR, Flynn DV. Granulosa cell tumor in a broodmare. J Am Vet Med Assoc 1976;169:635.
[22] McEntee K. Reproductive pathology of domestic animals. New York: Academic Press; 1990. p. 79–84.
[23] Gift LJ, Gaughan EM, Schoning P. Metastatic granulosa cell tumor in a mare. J Am Vet Med Assoc 1992;200:1525–6.
[24] Fessler JF, Brobst DF. Granulosa cell tumor. Cornell Vet 1972;62:110–23.
[25] Howard FA. Granulosa cell tumor of the equine ovary—a case report. J Am Vet Med Assoc 1949;114:134–5.
[26] Perino LJ, Didier PJ. Equine granulosa cell tumors. Equine Pract 1985;7:14–7.
[27] Stabenfeldt GH, Hughes JP, Kennedy PC, et al. Clinical findings, pathological changes and endocrinological secretory patterns in mares with ovarian tumours. J Reprod Fertil Suppl 1979;27:277–85.
[28] McCoy DJ. Diabetes mellitus associated with bilateral granulosa cell tumors. J Am Vet Med Assoc 1986;188:733–5.
[29] Turner TA, Manno M. Bilateral granulosa cell tumor in a mare. J Am Vet Med Assoc 1983; 182:713–4.
[30] Hinrichs K, Hunt PR. Ultrasound as an aid to diagnosis of granulosa cell tumour in the mare. Equine Vet J 1990;22:99–103.
[31] McCue PM, LeBlanc MM, Akita GY, et al. Granulosa cell tumors in two cycling mares. J Equine Vet Sci 1991;11:281–2.
[32] Nie GJ, Momont H. Ovarian mass in three mares with regular estrous cycles. J Am Vet Med Assoc 1992;201:1043–4.
[33] Swisher HP. A clinical case of granulosa-cell tumor in a Thoroughbred mare. Southwest Vet 1967;20:234–5.
[34] Finocchio EJ, Johnson JH. Granulosa cell tumor in a mare. Veterinary Medicine/Small Animal Clinician 1969;64:322–7.
[35] Nyack B, Johnson AD. A mammoth granulosa cell tumor in a mare. Veterinary Medicine/Small Animal Clinician 1983;78:218–23.
[36] Gatewood DM, Douglass JP, Cox JH, et al. Intra-abdominal hemorrhage associated with a granulosa-thecal cell neoplasm in a mare. J Am Vet Med Assoc 1990;196:1827–8.
[37] Wilson DA, Foreman JH, Boero MJ, et al. Small colon rupture attributable to a granulosa cell tumor in a mare. J Am Vet Med Assoc 1989;194:681–2.
[38] Catone G, Marino G, Mancuso R, et al. Clinicopathological features of an equine ovarian teratoma. Reprod Domest Anim 2004;39:65–9.
[39] Fischer AT, Lloyd KC, Carlson GP, et al. Diagnostic laparoscopy in the horse. J Am Vet Med Assoc 1986;189:289–92.
[40] Pugh DG, Bowen JM, Gaughan EM. Equine ovarian tumors. Compend Contin Educ Pract Vet 1985;7(Suppl):S710–7.
[41] Rambags BP, Stout TA, Rijkenhuizen AB. Ovarian granulosa cell tumours adherent to other abdominal organs; surgical removal from 2 warmblood mares. Equine Vet J 2003; 35:627–32.
[42] Baker CB, Kenney RM. Systematic approach to the diagnosis of the infertile or subfertile mare. In: Morrow DA, editor. Current therapy in theriogenology. Philadelphia: WB Saunders; 1980. p. 721–36.
[43] Hinrichs K, Cochran SL, Schelling SH, et al. Granulosa-theca cell tumor associated with an ovulation fossa and normal ovarian stroma in a mare. J Am Vet Med Assoc 1992;200: 696–8.

[44] White RAS, Allen WR. Use of ultrasound echography for the differential diagnosis of a granulosa cell tumour in a mare. Equine Vet J 1985;17:401–2.
[45] McCue PM. Review of ovarian abnormalities in the mare. Proc Am Assoc Equine Pract 1998;45:125–33.
[46] McCue PM. Pathophysiology of follicular development [PhD dissertation]. Davis (CA): University of California, Davis; 1993. p. 148–75.
[47] Bailey MT, Troedsson MHT, Wheaton JE. Inhibin concentrations in mares with granulosa cell tumors. Theriogenology 2002;57:1885–95.
[48] Meinecke B, Gips H. Steroid hormone secretory patterns in mares with granulosa cell tumors. Zentralblatt fur Veterinarmedizen Reihe A 1987;34:545–60.
[49] Kenney RM, Ganjam VK. Selected pathological changes of the mare uterus and ovary. J Reprod Fertil Suppl 1975;23:335–9.
[50] Watson ED, Thomson SRM. Immunolocalization of aromatase P-450 in ovarian tissue from pregnant and nonpregnant mares and in ovarian tumours. J Reprod Fertil 1996;108: 239–44.
[51] Hinrichs K, Watson ED, Kenney RM. Granulosa cell tumor in a mare with a functional contralateral ovary. J Am Vet Med Assoc 1990;197:1037–8.
[52] Cuevas P, Ying SY, Ling N, et al. Immunohistochemical detection of inhibin in the gonad. Biochem Biophys Res Commun 1987;142:23–30.
[53] Phillips DJ. Activins, inhibins and follistatins in the large domestic species. Domest Anim Endocrinol 2005;28:1–16.
[54] Nagamine N, Nambo Y, Nagata S, et al. Inhibin secretion in the mare: localization of inhibin α, β_A, and β_B subunits in the ovary. Biol Reprod 1998;59:1392–8.
[55] de Kretser DM, Robertson DM. The isolation and physiology of inhibin and related proteins. Biol Reprod 1989;40:33–47.
[56] Ginther OJ. Selection of the dominant follicle in cattle and horses. Anim Reprod Sci 2000; 60–61:61–79.
[57] Bergfelt DR, Mann BG, Schwartz NB, et al. Circulating concentrations of immunoreactive inhibin and FSH during the estrous cycle of mares. J Equine Vet Sci 1991;11: 319–22.
[58] Roser JF, McCue PM, Hoye E. Inhibin activity in the mare and stallion. Domest Anim Endocrinol 1994;11:87–100.
[59] Robertson DM, Giacometti M, Foulds LM, et al. Isolation of inhibin α subunit precursor proteins from bovine follicular fluid. Endocrinology 1989;125:2141–9.
[60] Lappohn RE, Burger HG, Bouma J, et al. Inhibin as a marker for granulosa-cell tumors. N Engl J Med 1989;321:790–3.
[61] Grootenhuis AJ, van Sluijs FJ, Klaij IA, et al. Inhibin, gonadotropins and sex steroids in dogs with Sertoli cell tumours. J Endocrinol 1990;127:235–42.
[62] Piquette GN, Kenney RM, Sertich PL, et al. Equine granulosa-theca cell tumors express inhibin α- and β_A-subunit messenger ribonucleic acids and proteins. Biol Reprod 1990;43: 1050–7.
[63] McCue PM. Equine granulosa cell tumors. Proc Am Assoc Equine Pract 1992;38:587–93.
[64] Christman SA, Bailey MT, Wheaton JE, et al. Dimeric inhibin concentrations in mares with granulosa-theca cell tumors. Am J Vet Res 1999;60:1407–10.
[65] Watson ED, Heald M, Leask R, et al. Detection of high circulating concentrations of inhibin pro- and -αC immunoreactivity in mares with granulosa-theca cell tumours. Equine Vet J 2002;34:203–6.
[66] Evans MJ, Loy RG, Taylor TB, et al. Administration of steroid-free follicular fluid (FF) to cyclic mares; FSH response to exogenous GnRH [abstract]. J Anim Sci 1981;53:313.
[67] McCue PM, Carney NJ, Hughes JP, et al. Ovulation and embryo recovery rates following immunization of mares against an inhibin alpha-subunit fragment. Theriogenology 1992; 38:823–31.

[68] McKinnon AO, Brown RW, Pashen RL, et al. Increased ovulation rates in mares after immunization against recombinant bovine inhibin α-subunit. Equine Vet J 1992;24: 144–6.
[69] Thompson DL, Reville-Moroz SI, Derrick DJ, et al. Effects of testosterone, dihydrotestosterone and estradiol on gonadotropin release after gonadotropin releasing hormone administration in cyclic mares. Biol Reprod 1983;29:970–6.
[70] Thompson DL, Garza F, St. George RL, et al. Relationships among LH, FSH and prolactin secretion, storage and response to secretagogue and hypothalamic GnRH content in ovariectomized pony mares administered testosterone, dihydrotestosterone, estradiol, progesterone, dexamethasone or follicular fluid. Domest Anim Endocrinol 1991;8:189–99.
[71] Lavoie JP, Carlson GP, George L. Hypertrophic osteopathy in three horses and a pony. J Am Vet Med Assoc 1992;201:1900–4.
[72] Patrick DJ, Kiupel M, Gerber V, et al. Malignant granulosa-theca cell tumor in a two-year-old Miniature Horse. J Vet Diagn Invest 2003;15:60–3.
[73] Van der Zaag EJ, Rijkenhuizen ABM, Kalsbeek HC, et al. A mare with colic caused by an ovarian tumour. Vet Q 1996;18:60–2.
[74] Alexander GR, Tweedie MA, Lescun TB, et al. Haemoperitoneum secondary to granulosa cell tumour in two mares. Aust Vet J 2004;82:481–4.
[75] Sedrish SA, McClure JR, Pinto C, et al. Ovarian torsion associated with granulosa-theca cell tumor in a mare. J Am Vet Med Assoc 1997;211:1152–4.
[76] McLennan MW, Kelly WR. Hypertropic osteopathy and dysgerminoma in a mare. Aust Vet J 1977;53:144–6.
[77] Meuten DJ, Rendano V. Hypertrophic osteopathy and dysgerminoma in a mare. J Equine Med Surg 1978;2:445–50.
[78] Henson KL, Alleman AR, Cutler TJ, et al. Regression of subcutaneous lymphoma following removal of an ovarian granulosa theca cell tumor in a horse. J Am Vet Med Assoc 1998;212: 1419–22.
[79] Hovell GJR, Hignett SL. Equine ovarian granulosa tumours. Vet Rec 1968;83:607.
[80] Lefebvre R, Theoret C, Dore M, et al. Ovarian teratoma and endometritis in a mare. Can Vet J 2005;46:1029–33.
[81] Frazer GS, Threlfall WR. Differential diagnosis of enlarged ovary in the mare. Proc Am Assoc Equine Pract 1986;32:21–8.
[82] Held J-P, Buergelt C, Colahan P. Serous cystadenoma in a mare. J Am Vet Med Assoc 1982; 181:496–8.
[83] Hinrichs K, Frazer GS, deGannes RVG, et al. Serous cystadenoma in a normally cyclic mare with high plasma testosterone values. J Am Vet Med Assoc 1989;194:381–2.
[84] Bridges ER, Lowder MQ, Gorham SL, et al. Serous cystadenoma in a pregnant mare. Equine Pract 1994;16:15–7.
[85] Chandra AMS, Woodward JC, Merritt AM. Dysgerminoma in an Arabian filly. Vet Pathol 1998;35:308–11.
[86] Gehlen H, Haist V, Baumgartner W, et al. Malignant dysgerminoma in an 18-year-old Warmblood mare. 2006;26:23–6.
[87] Liu IKM. Ovarian tumors. In: Robinson NE, editor. Current therapy in equine medicine. Philadelphia: WB Saunders; 1983. p. 408–9.
[88] Lock TF, Macy DW. Equine ovarian lymphosarcoma. J Am Vet Med Assoc 1979;175:72–3.
[89] Van Camp SD, Mahler J, Roberts MC, et al. Primary ovarian adenocarcinoma associated with teratomatous elements in a mare. J Am Vet Med Assoc 1989;194:1728–30.
[90] Ginther OJ. Characteristics of the ovulatory season. In: Reproductive biology of the mare. Basic and applied aspects. 2nd edition. Cross Plains (WI): Equiservices; 1992. p. 173–232.
[91] Colbern GT, Reagan WJ. Ovariectomy by colpotomy in mares. Compend Contin Educ Pract Vet 1987;9:1035–9.
[92] Neely DP. Reproductive endocrinology and fertility in the mare. In: Equine reproduction. Nutley (NJ): Hoffman-LaRoche; 1983. p. 12–22.

[93] Embertson RM. Ovaries and uterus. In: Auer JA, Stick JA, editors. Equine surgery. St. Louis (MO): WB Saunders Elsevier; 2006. p. 855–64.
[94] Palmer SE. Laparoscopic removal of granulosa cell tumors in the standing horse. In: Fischer AT, editor. Equine diagnostic and surgical laparoscopy. Philadelphia: WB Saunders; 2002. p. 205–10.
[95] Ragle CA. Ventral abdominal approach for laparoscopic removal of granulosa cell tumors. In: Fischer AT, editor. Equine diagnostic and surgical laparoscopy. Philadelphia: WB Saunders; 2002. p. 197–204.

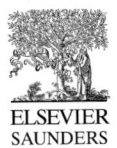

Superovulation in Mares

Edward L. Squires, PhD

*Animal Reproduction and Biotechnology Laboratory, ARBL Building,
Foothills Campus Colorado State University Fort Collins, CO 80523–1683, USA*

With the recent breed restriction changes that allow unrestricted foal registrations from a mare in a given year, the desire to obtain multiple embryos in a given breeding season has increased dramatically. This has created a renewed interest in superovulation. Recently, a commercial product has been made available (equine follicle-stimulating hormone [eFSH]) for superovulating mares. This has provided the practitioner with a hormonal product that is readily available for enhancing multiple ovulations. Additional benefits of stimulating multiple follicles include an increased number of follicles available for oocyte collection, availability of extra embryos for embryo freezing, enhancement of fertility in subfertile mares, and advancement of the first ovulation of the year. Superovulation was recently reviewed by McCue [1]. This article provides a short historical background, but most of it centers on the use of eFSH for stimulation of follicular development and ovulation in mares.

Historical background

There are two major reasons why superovulation has not become a common technique used in equine reproduction. The mare's ovary is considered to be "inside out," with the cortex in the interior of the ovary and the medulla toward the periphery. In addition, the surface germinal epithelium only lines a small portion of the ovary at the area of the ovulation fossa. This is the only area in which the follicle is capable of rupturing. Thus, the number of follicles that ovulate may be limited by the space available at the ovulation fossa. This anatomic constraint may limit the number of ovulations in the mare compared with other species, such as the cow. The other reason has been the unavailability of a hormonal product that would reliably induce multiple ovulations.

E-mail address: esquires@colostate.edu

Much of the early work done on superovulation in mares has centered on using porcine FSH or crude equine pituitary extract (EPE) that was primarily FSH. Douglas and colleagues [2] induced multiple ovulations in seasonally anovulatory mares using EPE. Further studies in this same laboratory stimulated multiple ovulations in mares during the physiologic breeding season [3]. Numerous other investigators used EPE to induce superovulation in cycling mares [4–8].

Squires and coworkers [4] reported 3.8 ovulations in response to EPE administration and an average of 2 embryos per mare flushed. This was in comparison to 1.2 ovulations and 0.65 embryo recovered per flush in untreated control mares. Squires and colleagues [9] summarized all the studies conducted on EPE at Colorado State University. Of 170 mares administered EPE during early diestrus and 130 untreated control mares, the ovulation rate and embryo recovery rate were 3.2 and 1.96 versus 1.2 and 0.65, respectively.

Porcine FSH and equine chorionic gonadotropin (eCG) are of limited value for superovulation in mares [1]. Administration of porcine FSH at a dose of 150 mg twice daily for several days resulted in only 1.7 ovulations per mare. Others also reported a poor response to porcine FSH [10,11]. It has been suggested that porcine FSH does not bind to the equine follicle with the same affinity as equine FSH. Extremely high doses of eCG have been used in an attempt to superovulate mares with a dismal response [12]. Although eCG is involved in follicular development and luteinization of follicles in pregnant mares, the level of eCG in the pregnant mare is approximately 100 IU/mL of blood. Clearly, EPE is much more effective in stimulating follicular development and superovulation than porcine FSH. This product has not been commercially available, however; thus, only a few client-owned mares have been administered EPE.

Other approaches to superovulating mares have included the use of gonadotropin-releasing hormone (GnRH). GnRH administration has been reported to induce ovulation and multiple follicles in seasonally anestrous mares. Ovulation rate in one study was related to the dose of GnRH administered [13]. The highest dose of GnRH (100 µg/h) resulted in 3.5 ovulations. In another study, anestrous mares receiving a GnRH agonist twice daily at a dose of 100, 200, or 400 µg exhibited multiple ovulation rates of 24%, 32%, and 37%, respectively [14]. Administration of GnRH to cycling mares was not effective in inducing multiple ovulations, however [15].

Immunization against the protein hormone inhibin has been shown to induce multiple ovulations in two studies [16]. Inhibin is a glycoprotein that suppresses the pituitary (and inhibits secretion of FSH). Thus, immunization against this hormone results in elevated levels of FSH. The ovulation rate in two studies with active immunization of mares against inhibin-α subunit resulted in 2.8 and 2.3 ovulations per mare [17]. Day 7 embryo recovery rates tended to be higher in immunized mares (1.6) than in control mares (0.7). A drawback to the use of active immunization of mares against inhibin is that multiple inoculations over several weeks are required. Adverse reactions, ranging from mild tissue swelling to abscessation, occasionally occurred at the immunization site, which makes this approach unacceptable for use in valuable mares.

Equine follicle-stimulating hormone

The remainder of this review centers on the use of a commercial product for superovulation of mares (eFSH; Bioniche Animal Health, Bogart, Georgia). This product was first made available in 2003, and several studies have been conducted evaluating the response of mares to eFSH. Niswender and colleagues [18] evaluated two doses of eFSH for superovulation of mares: 25 mg twice daily versus 12 mg twice daily (Table 1). The number of preovulatory follicles was greater in mares administered eFSH at a dose of 25 mg twice daily. For mares administered eFSH at a dose of 12 mg twice daily, half of the mares were given human chorionic gonadotropin (hCG) at the end of eFSH treatment and the other half were administered a GnRH agonist. The ovulation rate per mare was higher for mares administered hCG after eFSH treatment (3.3 and 3.4) versus those administered the GnRH agonist (1.8). Mares in all groups were inseminated with frozen semen. Pregnancy rates were determined 14 and 16 days after ovulation. Mares administered eFSH at a dose of 12 mg twice daily followed by hCG resulted in 1.8 embryonic vesicles per mare, which was higher than the pregnancy

Table 1
Ovulation and pregnancy rates for control and equine follicle-stimulating hormone–treated mares inseminated with frozen semen (experiment 1)

Parameters	Treatment groups			
	Control	eFSH-Des (25 mg)	eFSH-hCG (12 mg)	eFSH-Des (12 mg)
Mares (n)	29	10	5	5
Follicles (35 mm)	1.1 ± 0.1^c	6.7 ± 0.9^a	3.4 ± 0.7^b	3.8 ± 0.5^b
Ovulations per mare	1.1 ± 0.1^b	3.3 ± 0.9^a	3.4 ± 0.7^a	1.8 ± 0.7^b
Pregnancies per mare	0.6 ± 0.1^a	0.6 ± 0.3^a	1.8 ± 0.8^b	$0.8 \pm 0.5^{a,b}$
Pregnancy rate per ovulation	$54.5\%^a$	$18.2\%^b$	$52.9\%^a$	$44.4\%^{a,b}$

Abbreviations: Des, deslorelin; eFSH, equine follicle-stimulating hormone; hCG, human chorionic gonadotropin.

[a,b] Values within rows with different superscripts differ significantly ($P < .05$).

[c] Mares were injected twice daily beginning 5 or 6 days after ovulation and until most of the follicles reached 35 mm or greater, after which a gonadotropin-releasing hormone agonist (Des) or hCG was administered to induce ovulation.

Data from Niswender KD, Alvarenga MA, McCue PM, et al. Superovulation in cycling mares using equine follicle stimulating hormone (eFSH). J Equine Vet Sci 2003;23:497–500.

rate for mares in the control group (0.6) and for mares administered eFSH at a dose of 25 mg followed by GnRH agonist (0.6).

Based on this study, a 12-mg dose of eFSH given twice daily was used for a subsequent study conducted in Brazil. Sixteen cycling light-horse mares were used during the physiologic breeding season. On the first cycle, hCG at a dose of 2500 IU was administered to estrous mares after a 35-mm follicle was detected. Mares were subsequently inseminated with fresh semen from two stallions. An embryo collection procedure was performed 7 days after ovulation. On the day of embryo recovery, prostaglandin was administered to mares and eFSH treatment was initiated. Mares received eFSH at a dose of 12 mg twice daily until most of the follicles measured 35 mm in diameter; at that time, hCG was administered. Mares were inseminated, and embryo collection attempts were performed as described for the control cycle. Data from this study are presented in Table 2. Administration of eFSH resulted in a greater number of preovulatory follicles, ovulations per mare, and embryos per mare. The number of embryos per ovulation was similar between the two groups. Overall, 80% of mares in this study given eFSH had multiple ovulations.

A subsequent study conducted at Colorado State University evaluated the benefit of delaying hCG ("coasting the follicles") for 1.5 to 2 days after the end of eFSH treatment [19]. This project also evaluated the efficacy of single versus twice-daily injections of eFSH. A third objective of this trial was to determine if injecting eFSH combined with luteinizing hormone (LH) during the last 3.5 days of treatment would improve the ovulatory response. Administering eFSH at a dose of 12.5 mg twice daily with hCG administered 1.5 to 2 days after the last injection of eFSH (coast) resulted in

Table 2
Ovulation and embryo recovery rates for control and equine follicle-stimulating hormone–treated mares inseminated with fresh semen (experiment 2)

Parameters	Treatment groups	
	Control	eFSH-hCG (12 mg)[a]
Mares (n)	16	16
Follicles (35 mm)	1.0 ± 0.0^b	4.2 ± 0.5^c
Ovulations per mare	1.0 ± 0.0^b	3.6 ± 0.5^c
Embryos recovered per mare	0.5 ± 0.1^b	1.9 ± 0.3^c
Percentage of embryos recovered per ovulation	50.0%	52.8%

Mares in both groups were given hCG at a close of 2500 IU to induce ovulation.

Abbreviations: eFSH, equine follicle-stimulating hormone; hCG, human chorionic gonadotropin.

[a] Mares were treated with eFSH at a close of 12 mg twice daily starting on day 7 after ovulation.

[b, c] Means in rows with different superscripts differ ($P < .05$).

Data from Niswender KD, Alvarenga MA, McCue PM, et al. Superovulation in cycling mares using equine follicle stimulating hormone (eFSH). J Equine Vet Sci 2003;23:497–500.

the highest number of preovulatory follicles (n = 4.1; Table 3) and the greatest number of ovulations (n = 4.1). Furthermore, this treatment resulted in recovery of 2.6 embryos per cycle compared with 1.9 for all other groups. There was no advantage of adding LH to the eFSH preparation during the last part of the treatment period. Across all groups, the average number of days of treatment was 5.9, resulting in 3.4 ovulations and 2.0 embryos per cycle. Based on this study, the current recommended treatment for superovulation is eFSH at a dose of 12.5 mg given twice daily, followed by hCG 1.5 to 2 days after the end of eFSH treatment.

eFSH was also evaluated on a commercial Quarter Horse farm during the 2003 breeding season (J. Landers, personal communication, 2003). A total of 30 mares were treated with eFSH, and 74 additional mares served as untreated controls; eFSH treatment resulted in 3.1 ovulations and 1.5 embryos compared with 1.0 ovulation and 0.7 embryo in the untreated controls. The number of embryos recovered from each cycle of eFSH treatment was double that obtained from untreated controls.

Factors affecting the efficacy of equine follicle-stimulating hormone

Determining the correct time during the estrous cycle for initiation of treatment may be one of the more difficult aspects of superovulating mares. Mares have one or two follicular waves during the diestrous phase of the cycle [20]. Generally, 70% of mares have one follicular wave that begins in middle diestrus and culminates in one large dominant follicle that ovulates.

Table 3
Ovarian response (mean ± SEM) and embryo recovery of mares treated with equine follicle-stimulating hormone (cycles 1 and 2 combined)

Parameters	Treatment groups			
	12.5 mg[a]	12.5 mg[a] with coast[e]	eFSH 12.5 mg + LH[d]	25 mg[b] with coast[e]
Mares (n)	19	19	17	18
Days treated	5.9 ± 1.8	5.7 ± 1.5	5.9 ± 1.7	6.0 ± 2.5
Follicles ≥35 mm	2.8 ± 0.4[g]	4.1 ± 0.3[f]	3.0 ± 0.3[g]	2.5 ± 0.3[g]
Ovulations	3.3 ± 0.4[f, g]	4.1 ± 0.4[f]	3.5 ± 0.4[f, g]	2.8 ± 0.4[g]
Embryos per mare	1.9 ± 0.3	2.6 ± 0.3	1.9 ± 0.3	1.9 ± 0.3

Injections were from day 7 after ovulation until most of the follicles were 32 or 35 mm. Ovulations were induced by administration of hCG.

Abbreviations: eFSH, equine follicle-stimulating hormone; hCG, human chorionic gonadotropin; LH, luteinizing hormone.

[a] Two injections daily.
[b] Single injection daily.
[c] Human chorionic gonadotropin hCG was delayed 42 hours after the last eFSH treatment.
[d] Noncommercial preparation containing a 5:1 ratio of follicle-stimulating hormone to LH.
[e] hCG was delayed 54 hours after the last eFSH treatment.
[f, g] Values within rows with different superscripts differ significantly ($P < .05$).

Mares with two follicular waves during a diestrous phase make timing of initiation of eFSH treatment more difficult, however. If mares have two follicular waves, treatment may be initiated when some of the follicles from the first wave are becoming atretic and others from the second wave are in the growth phase. Studies have shown that during the follicular wave, a cohort of follicles begins to grow; this is termed the *growing phase* [21]. The beginning of deviation is characterized by the continual growth of a dominant follicle at a constant rate and a comparatively reduced rate of growth of subordinate follicles. The common growth phase extends from follicle emergence to the beginning of deviation. Once the largest follicle of a cohort obtains a size of approximately 23.5 mm, divergence occurs and the largest follicle continues to grow, whereas the other follicles become subordinate. Preferential growth of the largest follicle seems to be attributable to secretion of inhibin and estrogen from the dominant follicle, which suppresses FSH levels. Once FSH levels are suppressed, the smaller follicles become atretic and the dominant follicle continues to grow to the point of ovulation. In a normal cycle, an FSH peak occurs when the largest follicle is approximately 13 mm, and 3 to 4 days after the peak concentration of FSH, deviation occurs. If exogenous FSH is administered, such as during superovulation, deviation does not occur and several dominant follicles develop.

Day of initial treatment

There are several approaches to determine when to initiate eFSH treatment for superovulation. One approach would be to start treatment on a given day after ovulation. Dippert and coworkers [5] in our laboratory compared the response of mares when treatment was initiated on day 5 versus day 12 after ovulation. The number of ovulations was higher for mares given EPE treatment initially on day 5 versus those in which treatment was delayed until day 12. Thus, in most of the subsequent studies, treatment with EPE or eFSH was initiated 5 to 7 days after ovulation, around the time of the first follicular wave. Another approach is to examine mares with ultrasonography beginning approximately 5 days after ovulation; once the largest follicle becomes 23 to 25 mm in size, eFSH treatment can be initiated. With this approach, one only initiates treatment once follicles arrive at a certain size. Thus, the number of treatments needed to induce superovulation is less with this approach. A slight variation is examination of mares with ultrasonography on the day of embryo recovery (typically day 7 or 8). If the largest follicle is 25 mm or less, treatment can be initiated on the day of embryo recovery. If follicles are greater than 25 mm, perhaps eFSH treatment should not be initiated and that particular cycle should be skipped. Conversely, if the largest follicle is less than 23 to 25 mm, perhaps the mare should be re-examined and treatment only initiated once the diameter of the largest follicle obtains a size of 23 to 25 mm.

In cows, exogenous progesterone and estrogen are generally administered before the administration of FSH [22]. The administration of steroids induces follicular regression, and at the end of the steroid treatment, a new wave of follicular development is initiated. In women, GnRH agonist typically is given to suppress follicular development before initiation of FSH treatment [23]. At least two studies have been conducted in which a GnRH agonist has been administered in an attempt to suppress follicular development and allow initiation of a new follicular wave after the end of GnRH treatment [5,7]. Unfortunately, administration of GnRH agonist before EPE did not enhance the superovulatory response. In a similar fashion, progesterone and estradiol also have been administered before eFSH treatment [24,25]. Progesterone was given at a dose of 150 mg/d plus estradiol at a rate of 10 mg for 10 days, and eFSH treatment was initiated at the end of the progesterone-estradiol treatment. In our study [24], mares administered progesterone and estradiol before eFSH treatment resulted in 3.0 ovulations and 1.1 embryos per cycle versus 5.6 ovulations and 2.7 embryos per cycle in mares administered only eFSH. Neither study demonstrated an advantage of administering progesterone and estrogen before eFSH treatment. Further studies are needed to evaluate the potential use of progesterone and estradiol more carefully for initiation of new follicular waves in mares.

Repetitive equine follicle-stimulating hormone treatment during the breeding season

The question arises as to whether one can superovulate mares several times in a breeding season. Recently, a study was conducted in which mares were treated at least three times during the breeding season [26]. Half of the mares were treated on three consecutive cycles, although the other half of the mares were treated on an every-other-cycle basis. There was no difference in the number of ovulations in these two groups or in the number of embryos recovered. It was somewhat surprising that consecutive treatments did not adversely affect ovulation rate or embryo recovery. Mares that were administered eFSH on three consecutive cycles had an average of 4.1 ovulations and 1.8 embryos compared with 5.5 ovulations and 2.1 embryos for mares that were treated with eFSH on an every-other-cycle basis.

Viability of embryos from superovulated mares

Early studies by Woods and Ginther [6] suggested that embryos collected from superovulated mares were less viable than those from single-ovulating mares. Subsequent studies did not support this finding, however. Squires and colleagues [8] transferred embryos from single- and multiple-ovulating mares and reported similar pregnancy rates between the groups. Dippert and coworkers [27] recovered oviductal embryos from superovulated and single-ovulating mares and cultured the embryos for 10 days. They reported similar development in culture between embryos recovered from superovulated mares and single-ovulating mares. Recently, Hudson and colleagues [28] reported on the effects of cooling and vitrification of embryos from mares treated with eFSH on pregnancy rates after nonsurgical transfer. Embryos were collected from 38 eFSH-treated mares 6.5 days after ovulation or, if ovulations were asynchronous, 8 days after administration of hCG. On identification, each embryo was measured, graded, and rinsed in holding medium. Embryos were assigned to be vitrified immediately or placed in holding medium, packaged, and stored in a passive cooling device for 12 to 19 hours before vitrification. Embryos were stored in liquid nitrogen until nonsurgical transfer. After nonsurgical transfer, pregnancy was determined by ultrasonography 6 to 10 days after transfer. Pregnancy rates were similar for embryos in the two groups. For embryos cooled for 12 to 19 hours before vitrification, 13 of 20 embryos resulted in an embryonic vesicle versus 15 of 20 pregnancies from embryos vitrified immediately on collection. Overall, a pregnancy rate of 70% was obtained for these vitrified embryos. This percentage is nearly identical to that obtained with fresh embryos from single-ovulating mares. Thus, based on this study, pregnancy rates after nonsurgical transfer were not affected by superovulation or vitrification.

Potential problems after superovulation

One of the greatest problems with superovulating mares with eFSH is the tremendous variation in response. Most of the response is attributable to individual mare variation. This is not unlike what is obtained with superovulating cows, in which some cows respond favorably to FSH and are considered great embryo donors, whereas others are poor donors. The reason for the tremendous variation in response in cattle has not been determined nor has the cause of variation in the mare. In a study conducted last year in our laboratory [26], 30 mares were given eFSH on at least three cycles during the breeding season. The range in embryo recovery per cycle was 0.25 to 4.3 embryos.

It is our clinical impression that young normally cycling mares respond consistently to eFSH, whereas older mares have a much more variable response. Determining the appropriate dose of eFSH for a given donor is one of the major challenges. If the dose is too high, the ovaries become overstimulated and many of the follicles do not ovulate but become luteinized or develop an anovulatory follicle. Briant and coworkers [29] reported that if the dose of eFSH was too high, progesterone concentrations higher than 1 ng/mL were detected in treated mares before ovulation. This premature progesterone concentration was attributable to elevated LH, which resulted in premature ovulation or luteinization of follicles. They suggested that the reason for the high variability in response to eFSH was attributable to the individual sensitivity of the mare to the level of eFSH injected.

Squires and colleagues [26] reported on factors affecting the response to eFSH. This study combined data from the 2004 and 2005 breeding seasons. In 2005, donors were divided into good and poor donors based on embryo recovery. Good donors averaged at least 1.5 embryos per flush, and poor donors averaged less than 1.5 embryos per flush. There was a significant negative correlation between the total number of follicles on the day of initial eFSH treatment and the number of days of eFSH treatment. Significant positive correlations were also obtained for the number of follicles at the onset of treatment and the number of 35-mm follicles and number of ovulations. Those mares with 25-mm follicles at the onset of eFSH treatment were treated fewer days compared with mares with follicles less than 25 mm at the onset of treatment (4.6 versus 5.8 days). There was a significant positive correlation between the number of preovulatory follicles and the number of ovulations. Correlations between the number of ovulations and the number of embryos were significant. The number of follicles from 11 to 15 mm and from 16 to 20 mm at the onset of eFSH treatment was greater in mares considered good donors versus those categorized as poor donors. Good donors also had a higher number of preovulatory follicles and higher ovulation numbers than poor donors. Unfortunately, the repeatability of embryo recovery from cycle 1 to cycle 2 was poor. Being able to identify donor mares that respond favorably to eFSH based on follicular development, ovulation, and embryo recovery would be a great advantage. This would allow the breeder to concentrate on mares that respond favorably to eFSH and eliminate mares that respond poorly. Based on this study, mares that had follicles 25 mm or greater at the onset of treatment required fewer days of eFSH treatment. The best criteria as to whether or not a mare would be considered a good or poor donor were the number of follicles 11 to 15 mm and 16 to 20 mm at the onset of treatment, the number of preovulatory follicles at the end of treatment, and the number of ovulations.

Another potential problem with the use of eFSH is the failure of some mares to ovulate preovulatory follicles. The reason for the development of anovulatory follicles has not been determined. Other potential problems include overstimulation of the ovary and poor embryo recovery per ovulation. Finally, approximately 25% of the flushes that are conducted on superovulated mares result in no embryos. This is also similar to the 25% to 30% of the embryo flushes in cattle that result in no fertilized embryos. Obviously, further studies are needed to determine why poor embryo recovery per ovulation occurs and why some embryo recovery attempts result in no embryos being collected. It is likely that it may take years before the protocol for superovulation in mares is perfected.

Protocols for using equine follicle-stimulating hormone

Unlike the case in cattle, there are some situations in which mare owners desire to enhance embryo recovery but do not want more than one or two embryos on a given embryo flush. Their desire is to breed the mare to a given stallion for one cycle, recover embryos, and then switch to another stallion.

Recently, Logan and colleagues [30] published a study on how to use eFSH efficiently to enhance embryo recovery. Results of three studies using eFSH to superovulate mares for embryo recovery conducted over the past 2 years were reviewed. Practical considerations that improved the efficiency of using eFSH included (1) initiation of eFSH treatment only after mares obtained follicles that are 22 to 25 mm in diameter, (2) delaying administration of hCG for 1.5 to 2 days after the end of eFSH treatment, (3) decreasing the dose of eFSH from the standard 12.5 mg twice daily to perhaps 6 to 9 mg twice daily so that too many ovulations and embryos are not obtained, and (4) potentially treating mares for only 3 days during the time of follicular deviation. All these practices can minimize the number of days that mares are treated with eFSH and can reduce the total amount of eFSH needed for superovulation.

Based on the studies conducted, two protocols are recommended for the use of eFSH.

Protocol for maximizing embryo recovery
Step 1
  Ultrasound the mare beginning 5 to 7 days after ovulation (day 0 = day of ovulation).
Step 2
  Once mares have several follicles 22 to 25 mm, begin eFSH treatment.
Step 3
  Administer eFSH intramuscularly twice daily at a dose of 12.5 mg (1 mL).
Step 4
  Administer prostaglandin $F_{2\alpha}$ ($PGF_{2\alpha}$) on day 2 of treatment.
Step 5
  Once most of the follicles are 32 to 35 mm, stop eFSH. Generally, mares require 4 to 5 days of treatment.
Step 6
  Administer hCG 30 to 36 hours after the last eFSH treatment.
Step 7
  If mares are older or unresponsive to hCG, administer an implant or injectable deslorelin.
Step 8
  Inseminate according to standard procedure.
Step 9
  Flush mares for embryo recoveries 7 to 8 days after most of the ovulations for transfer of fresh embryos or 6.5 days after ovulation for the recovery of small embryos for cryopreservation.

Protocol for enhanced embryo recovery

Step 1
Ultrasound the mare beginning 5 to 7 days after ovulation (day 0 = day of ovulation).

Step 2
Once mares have several follicles 22 to 25 mm, begin eFSH treatment.

Step 3
Give eFSH intramuscularly twice daily at a dose of 6.25 mg (0.5 mL).

Step 4
Administer $PGF_{2\alpha}$ on day 2 of treatment.

Step 5
Once most of the follicles are 32 to 35 mm, stop eFSH. Generally, mares require 4 to 5 days of treatment.

Step 6
Administer hCG 30 to 36 hours after the last eFSH treatment.

Step 7
If mares are older or unresponsive to hCG, administer an implant or injectable deslorelin.

Step 8
Inseminate according to standard procedure.

Step 9
Flush mares for embryo recoveries 7 to 8 days after most of the ovulations for transfer of fresh embryos or 6.5 days after ovulation for the recovery of small embryos for cryopreservation.

References

[1] McCue PM. Superovulation. Vet Clin North America Equine Pract 1996;12:1–11.
[2] Douglas RH, Nuti L, Ginther OJ. Induction of ovulation and multiple ovulation in seasonally-anovulatory mares with equine pituitary fractions. Theriogenology 1974;2:133–42.
[3] Lappin DR, Ginther OJ. Induction of ovulation and multiple ovulations in seasonally anovulatory and ovulatory mares with an equine pituitary extract. J Anim Sci 1977;44:834–42.
[4] Squires EL, Garcia RH, Ginther OJ, et al. Comparison of equine pituitary extract and follicle stimulating hormone for superovulating mares. Theriogenology 1986;26:661–70.
[5] Dippert KD, Hofferer S, Palmer E, et al. Initiation of superovulation in mares 5 or 12 days after ovulation using equine pituitary extract with or without GnRH analog. Theriogenology 1992;38:695–710.
[6] Woods GL, Ginther OJ. Recent studies relating to the collection of multiple embryos in mares. Theriogenology 1983;19:101–8.
[7] Scoggin CF, Meira C, McCue PM, et al. Strategies to improve the ovarian response to equine pituitary extract in cycling mares. Theriogenology 2002;58:151–64.
[8] Squires EL, McKinnon AO, Carnevale EM, et al. Reproductive characteristics of spontaneous single and double ovulating mares and superovulating mares. J Reprod Fertil 1987;35:399–403.
[9] Squires EL, Carnevale EM, McCue PM, et al. Embryo technologies in the horse. Theriogenology 2003;59:151–70.
[10] Irvine CHG. Endocrinology of the estrous cycle of the mare: applications to embryo transfer. Theriogenology 1981;15:85–104.

[11] Fortune JE, Kimmich TL. Purified pig FSH increases the rate of double ovulation in mares. Equine Vet J 1993;15(Suppl):95–8.
[12] Allen WR. Embryo transfer in the horse. In: Adams CE, editor. Mammalian egg transfer. Boca Raton (FL): CRC Press; 1982. p. 135–54.
[13] Johnson AL, Becker SE. Use of gonadotropin-releasing hormone (GnRH) treatment to induce multiple ovulations in the anestrous mare. J Equine Vet Sci 1988;8:130–6.
[14] Ginther OJ, Bergfelt DR. Effect of GnRH treatment during the anovulatory season on multiple ovulation rate and on follicular development during the ensuing pregnancy in mares. J Reprod Fertil 1990;88:119–26.
[15] Squires EL, Rowley HR, Nett TM. Comparison of pulsatile vs constant release of GnRH for superovulation in mares [abstract]. Am Soc Anim Sci 1989;67(Suppl 1):391–2.
[16] McCue PM, Hughes JP, Lashley BL. Effect of ovulation rate of passive immunization rate of mares against inhibin. Equine Vet J 1993;15(Suppl):103–6.
[17] McKinnon AO, Brown RW, Pashen RL. Increased ovulation rate in mares after immunization against recombinant bovine inhibin α-subunit. Equine Vet J 1992;24:144–6.
[18] Niswender KD, Alvarenga MA, McCue PM, et al. Superovulation in cycling mares using equine follicle stimulating hormone (eFSH). J Equine Vet Sci 2003;23:497–500.
[19] Squires EL, Welch SA, Denniston DJ, et al. Evaluation of several eFSH treatments for superovulation in mares [abstract]. Theriogenology 2005;64:783.
[20] Ginther OJ. Major and minor follicular waves during the equine estrus cycle. J Equine Vet Sci 1993;13:18–25.
[21] Ginther OJ, Beg MA, Gastal MO, et al. Follicular dynamics and selection of mares. Anim Reprod 2004;1:45–63.
[22] Colazo MG, Martinez MF, Small JA, et al. Effect of estradiol valerate on ovarian follicular dynamics and superovulatory response in progestin-treated cattle. Theriogenology 2005;63:1454–68.
[23] Janssens RMJ, Vermeiden JP, Lambalk CB, et al. Gonadotropin-releasing hormone agonist dose-dependency of pituitary desensitization during controlled ovarian hyperstimulation in IVF. Hum Reprod 1998;13:2386–91.
[24] Logan N, McCue P, Alonso M, et al. The effect of administering progesterone and estradiol prior to eFSH on the superovulatory response of mares [abstract]. Reprod Fertil Dev 2006;18:290.
[25] Raz T, Green J, Corrigan M, et al. Folliculogenesis, embryo parameters, and post-transfer recipient pregnancy rate in eFSH treated donor mares [abstract]. In: Proceedings of the 2006 American Association of Equine Practitioners Annual Meeting, San Antonio, Texas.
[26] Squires EL, Logan N, Welch S, et al. Factors affecting the response to eFSH. Anim Reprod Sci 2006;94:408–10.
[27] Dippert KD, Jasko DJ, Seidel GE Jr, et al. Fertilization rates in superovulated and spontaneously ovulating mares. Theriogenology 1994;41:1411–23.
[28] Hudson J, McCue PM, Carnevale EM, et al. Effects of cooling and vitrification of embryos from mares treated with equine follicle stimulating hormone on pregnancy rates after nonsurgical transfer. J Equine Vet Sci 2006;26:51–4.
[29] Briant C, Toutain PL, Ottogalli M, et al. Kinetic studies and production rate of equine (e) FSH in ovariectomized pony mares. Applications to the determination of a dosage regimen for eFSH in a superovulation treatment. J Endocrinol 2004;182:43–54.
[30] Logan NL, McCue PM, Squires EL. How to use equine FSH efficiently to enhance embryo recovery [abstract]. In: Proceedings of the 2006 American Association of Equine Practitioners Annual Meeting, San Antonio, TX.

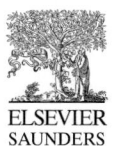

Vitrification of Equine Embryos
Elaine M. Carnevale, DVM, PhD

Animal Reproduction and Biotechnology Laboratory, College of Veterinary Medicine and Biomedical Sciences, Colorado State University, 3194 Rampart Road, Fort Collins, CO 80523, USA

Embryo transfer has been established as a valuable procedure to optimize productivity of the mare. Methods to cool (5°C) and store embryos for up to 24 hours have been developed to allow the shipment of embryos to distant farms or facilities for transfer. Although cooling embryos provides a limited duration of storage, embryo cryopreservation would allow storage for extended periods. The first foal was reported in 1982 [1] after an embryo was cryopreserved by conventional methods. Conventional cryopreservation involves the exposure of an embryo to increasing concentrations of permeating cryoprotectants, dehydrating the embryo while cooling at approximately 0.5°C per minute [2]. At approximately −6°C, the formation of ice crystals is induced and the temperature is further reduced. The embryo is eventually stored in liquid nitrogen at −196°C. The thawing process generally involves a series of steps, with embryos exposed to decreasing levels of cryoprotectants. Although successful, conventional cryopreservation is time-consuming, with the freezing process lasting approximately 1.5 hours, and embryos are usually frozen using specialized and often expensive equipment.

In contrast to conventional cryopreservation, vitrification is a rapid procedure that does not require special equipment. During vitrification, embryos are exposed to high concentrations of permeating cryoprotectants; ice crystals do not form [3], and a glass-like state is achieved. Vitrified embryos can be rapidly warmed within the straws and directly transferred from the straws into recipient uteri. Using this technique, the transfer procedure does not require special equipment and is rapid, resulting in a practical method for field conditions. This article reviews the procedures and

---

This research was supported by the Colorado Equine Racing Commission through the Research Council of the College of Veterinary Medicine and Biomedical Sciences at Colorado State University and the benefactors of the Preservation of Equine Genetics.
  E-mail address: emc@colostate.edu

limitations for vitrification of equine embryos. Emphasis is placed on the procedure currently being used for vitrification and warming of equine embryos in clinical environments.

Collection and evaluation of embryos

The success of cryopreservation is dependent on the size and stage of development of equine embryos. Cryopreservation, by conventional freezing or vitrification, is more successful when equine embryos are less than 300 μm in diameter [4–6], and embryos 250 μm or less in diameter are preferred. Embryos should be collected at the morula or early blastocyst stage of development. Embryo development after vitrification and warming of embryos 300 μm or less in diameter was not significantly different for morulae (9 [82%] of 11) and early blastocysts (19 [66%] of 29) [7].

The equine morula is approximately 160 μm in diameter and is surrounded by a thick zona pellucida (ZP) that is round or oval in shape. The embryo does not increase in diameter from the oocyte to the morula. Cells of the morula are dark and often do not extend to the inner edge of the ZP (Fig. 1). Morulae can be confused with unfertilized oocytes, which often remain within the oviduct but are inconsistently found within the mare's uterus. Within the ZP, contents of unfertilized oocytes can be dark, light, or mottled in appearance (Fig. 2). A partial or intact cell membrane and fragmentation may or may not be imaged (see Fig. 2; Fig. 3). Unfertilized oocytes are often flat when manipulated onto their side, and they may float to the surface of the medium and slowly sink.

A fluid-filled cavity, or blastocele, forms as the embryo develops into a blastocyst. The early blastocele can be difficult to image (see Fig. 3). The presence of a blastocele can usually be determined by the expansion

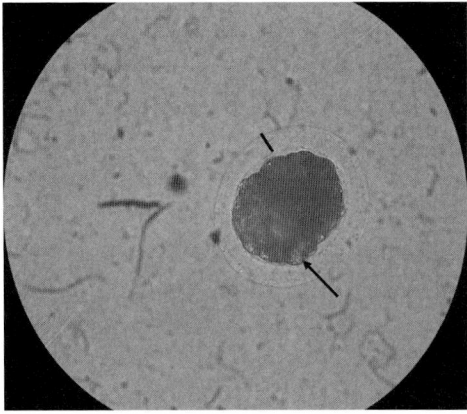

Fig. 1. The equine morula has a thick ZP (*line*) and compact mass of dark cells. The smooth borders of the cells are apparent (*arrow*), and the cell mass does not fill the ZP (*line*).

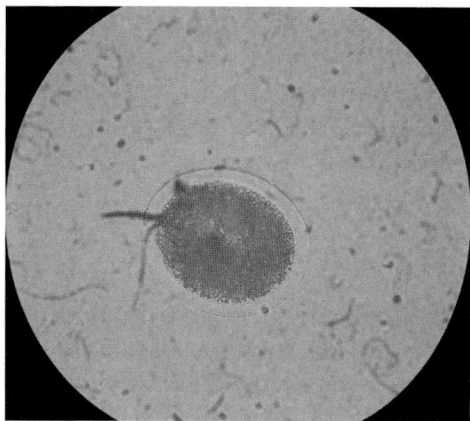

Fig. 2. The unfertilized oocyte is similar in size to the morula (see Fig. 1). The cell membrane is disrupted or absent (seen in this image), resulting in a poorly defined edge with inner contents that often fill the cavity within the ZP. This unfertilized oocyte has a grainy texture and was flat when manipulated onto its side.

of the cellular mass to fill the ZP. When imaging the embryo with a stereoscope, the cells lining the outside of the embryo are distinct, whereas the center cavity is blurred. As the embryo grows, two distinct cell types develop. Trophoblast cells line the outer surface of the embryo, and the inner cell mass is imaged as a thickened localized group of cells. In general, the trophoblast forms the placenta, and the inner cell mass develops into the embryo proper. At the early blastocyst stage, a glycoprotein layer forms between the ZP and trophoblast. This layer, or capsule, is acellular and

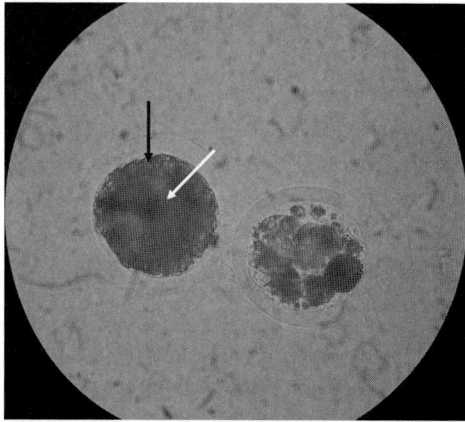

Fig. 3. The extremely early blastocyst (*left*) and unfertilized oocyte (*right*) are similar in size. The unfertilized oocyte is fragmented. When focusing on the extremely early blastocyst, a ring of cells (*black arrow*) may be apparent, with a less defined central area (*white arrow*) that develops into the blastocele.

reflective when imaged through a stereoscope. As the embryo develops into a blastocyst, the embryo becomes lighter in appearance with a distinct cellular pattern (Fig. 4). The ZP thins, and eventually disappears, as the capsule and inner cell mass become more distinct. The rapidly expanding blastocyst quickly grows to greater than 300 µm in diameter, usually by 7 days after ovulation.

Collection of small embryos

The equine embryo leaves the oviduct and enters the uterus at approximately 5.5 days after ovulation. Freeman and colleagues [8] determined the time of oviductal transport to be 5 days and from 10 to 22 hours. The morula is the earliest stage of embryo development to enter the uterus, with an average diameter of 168 µm [8]. By day 7, the embryo is often too large to cryopreserve with optimal success. Using once-daily examinations for the detection of ovulation, the mean diameters for embryos collected on days 6 and 7 were 208 and 406 µm, respectively [9]. Therefore, embryos to be vitrified would ideally be collected between 6 and 6.5 days after ovulation.

Different methods have been used to collect embryos at the optimal stage of development. Twice-daily examinations of the mare's reproductive tract can be used to determine the time of ovulation within approximately 12 hours, and embryo collections can be appropriately scheduled. Embryo collections can also be timed from ovulation induction. Ovulation occurs approximately 36 hours after the administration of human chorionic gonadotropin (hCG) and approximately 40 hours after administration of

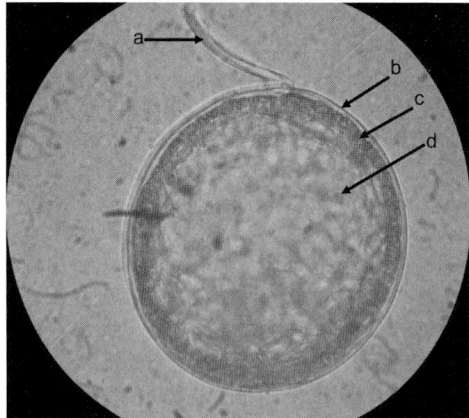

Fig. 4. This equine blastocyst has a ZP that has thinned and is separating from the embryo (a). The reflective layer over the surface of the blastocyst is the capsule (b). Under the capsule, the ring of trophoblast cells (c) can be imaged. The large blastocele (d) and defined capsule are indications that this embryo is too large for successful vitrification.

a gonadotropin-releasing hormone (GnRH) analogue (deslorelin). Eldridge and coworkers [6] administered hCG at a dose of 2000 IU when estrous mares had a follicle sized 35 mm or greater in diameter. Mares were inseminated, and their ovaries were examined daily by ultrasound. Ovulation was typically detected on the second day after administration of hCG, and embryo collection attempts were made approximately 8 days after administration of hCG or 6.5 days after the time of expected ovulation. In the study, embryos were collected after 78% of ovulations, and embryos ranged in diameter from 140 to 250 μm. Therefore, timing of embryo collections from administration of hCG resulted in high recovery rates of embryos at the preferred size for cryopreservation. Potential problems using this scheme would include mares that ovulate early or fail to ovulate in response to hCG. In addition, delayed embryo development could affect the optimal collection time. Embryo development could be delayed when embryos are collected from old mares, after insemination with frozen semen, or after postovulatory inseminations. In these cases, the timing of embryo collection may have to be altered.

Embryo vitrification

Procedures for vitrification of embryos

A successful and easy method for embryo vitrification has recently been described [6,10]. In contrast to other methods, the success of this procedure has been established [6,7], and it is currently being used for commercial purposes. Vitrification solutions (VSs) are commercially available or can be made using a base medium of modified phosphate-buffered saline (mPBS) without calcium and magnesium and supplemented with sodium pyruvate (0.3 mmol), glucose (3.3 mmol), and 20% fetal calf serum. Three VSs are required, with each solution containing various combinations of glycerol (Gly) and ethylene glycol (EG) as cryoprotectants (Table 1).

Before cryopreservation, embryos are collected, washed, and placed in a holding medium at a moderate room temperature. Commercial media are available for washing and holding embryos. Exposure of embryos to poor conditions before vitrification can reduce embryo viability; therefore, an appropriate holding medium that has been quality tested should be used. The embryos should remain in the holding medium for a minimal period, preferably less than 15 minutes, before vitrification.

During vitrification, embryos are sequentially exposed to three VSs: VS1 (Gly [1.4 M]), VS2 (Gly [1.4 M] plus EG [3.6 M]), and VS3 (Gly [3.4 M] plus EG [4.6 M]). A dilution solution (DS, galactose [0.5 M]) is also needed when loading straws. Before beginning the vitrification process, media are placed in drops within a Petri or four-well dish at room temperature (22°–24°C), allowing the organized movement of embryos through the various media and rapid loading of straws (Fig. 5). Straws have also been loaded using

Table 1
Preparation of dilution solution (10 mL) and vitrification solutions

Solution	Gly[a]	EG[b]	Gal[c]	mPBS[d]
VS1 (Gly [1.4 M])	1.0 mL	none		9.0 mL
VS2 (Gly [1.4 M] + EG [3.6 M])	1.0 mL	2.0 mL		7.0 mL
VS3 (Gly [3.4 M + EG [4.6 M])	2.4 mL	2.6 mL		5.0 mL
DS (galactose [0.5 m])			0.9 g	10.0 mL

Abbreviations: DS, dilution solution; EG, ethylene glycol; Gal, galactose; Gly, glycerol; mPBS, modified phosphate-buffered saline; VS, vitrification solution.

[a] Glycerol.
[b] Ethylene glycol.
[c] Galactose.
[d] Modified phosphate-buffered saline (without calcium and magnesium and supplemented with sodium pyruvate [0.3 mmol] glucose [3.3 mmol], and 20% fetal calf serum).

commercial media based on lengths of media columns within the straw (Bioniche Animal Health, Bogart, Georgia). After the vitrification process has started, the embryo must be moved at precise intervals into sequential media. Exposure of the embryo to a VS for an incorrect time can result in damage to the embryo.

To start the procedure, the embryo is removed from the holding medium and placed into VS1. Movements of the embryo should be with a small volume of medium (~1 μL), or the embryo should be gently moved within the solution to ensure that the embryo is exposed to the proper concentrations of cryoprotectants. The embryo remains in VS1 for 5 minutes. A timer can be used to ensure that the embryo is moved promptly into the next solution.

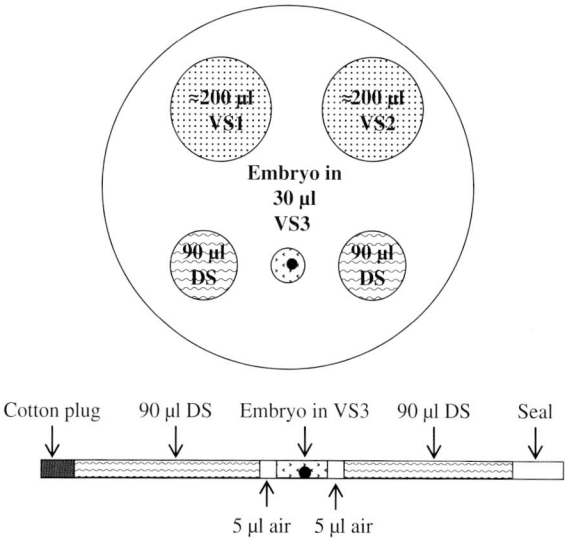

Fig. 5. Organization of VSs and DS in a Petri dish. Volumes of VS1 and VS2 can be approximated; however, precise volumes of DS and VS3 are required when loading the straw.

The embryo remains in VS2 for 5 minutes before placement into VS3. The interval of exposure of the embryo to VS3 is important. Too long of an exposure to VS3 can be toxic to the embryo. Therefore, the embryo is placed into a 30-μL drop of VS3, the volume to be pulled into the straw, to allow rapid loading of the straw. The embryo should remain in VS3 for less than 1 minute before exposure to liquid nitrogen vapor.

Straws (0.25 μL, nonirradiated, polyvinyl chloride) should be labeled before the beginning of vitrification. The straw can be labeled directly, or a straw adapter can be used to plug the end of the 0.25-μL straw and attach it to a 0.5-μL straw that is used for labeling. The 0.5-μL straw can be flattened and labeled before use, allowing easier labeling and handling of the straw for vitrification. The 0.25-μL straw is loaded for vitrification with DS (90 μL), air (5 μL), the embryo in VS3 (30 μL), air (5 μL), and DS (90 μL) (see Fig. 5). The DS should extend to the cotton plug of the straw to seal that end of the straw. The open end of the straw can be plugged with the straw adapter or double heat sealed.

Before beginning the vitrification process, liquid nitrogen should be placed in an insulated container. A cane, such as that used for storing frozen straws and containing a plastic goblet (10 or 13 mm in diameter), is held vertically in the liquid nitrogen, allowing the liquid nitrogen to surround the goblet but only permitting vapor within the goblet. Large forceps can be placed across the top of the container to grasp and hold the cane in position. The loaded straw is placed into the goblet containing liquid nitrogen vapor for 1 minute. The goblet and straw are then plunged into the liquid nitrogen. The straw can then be transferred into a holding tank.

Warming of embryos

To warm an embryo, the straw is removed from liquid nitrogen and held in air at room temperature for 10 seconds. The straw should be handled from an end, without touching the center of the straw containing media. The straw is then placed into water at 20°C to 22°C for 10 seconds. The straw is flicked, similar to a thermometer, to mix solutions (DS and VS3) and laid on a horizontal surface for 4 to 5 minutes. During this time, the embryo can be imaged under a stereoscope; the straw should be gently rotated, however, because the embryo sinks to the bottom. The straw should not be left on the lighted stage for any length of time. If the embryo is near an end of the straw, the straw can be held at an angle to allow the embryo to sink to a more desirable position.

Embryos are transferred into recipients 6 to 8 minutes after warming the straw. If the straw is heat sealed, the heat-sealed end can be cut. If a plastic adapter was used to seal the straw, this can be removed or the end of the straw can be cut to remove the adapter. The straw can then be loaded into a transfer rod (Agtech, Manhattan, Kansas; IMV, Maple Grove, Minnesota). The model of transfer rod depends on whether the straw was or was not cut ("deep chamber" rod for full-length straws and "shallow chamber" rod for cut straws). Embryo transfers can be performed according to the clinician's preferred method. Pregnancy rates after transfer of vitrified and thawed embryos were not different for transfer into recipients 5 or 6 days after ovulation [7], although most embryos were transferred on day 5. Recipients 4 to 6 days after ovulation would probably be acceptable for transfer.

Establishment of pregnancies from vitrified embryos

Vitrification of small embryos

Numerous methods have been used to evaluate embryos after vitrification and thawing, including cell staining and culture. Although useful, the results of these methods may not correlate with pregnancy rates after transfer into recipients. Therefore, only methods that have resulted in the establishment of pregnancies are emphasized in this review. In 1994, Hochi and colleagues [11] established the first pregnancies from vitrified and warmed embryos. The embryos were placed in 20% EG for 10 or 20 minutes before being placed into a VS (40% vol/vol EG, 18% wt/vol Ficoll, and sucrose [0.3 M] in mPBS). Embryos in VS (10 μL) were then loaded into a 0.25-μL straw, which also contained DS (150 μL) (sucrose [0.5 M] in mPBS). Within 2 minutes after exposing the embryos to VS, the straws were exposed to vapor 1 cm above liquid nitrogen before plunging. On warming, the embryos were placed in decreasing concentrations of sucrose before culture. Five embryos were selected for transfer into recipients 4 days after ovulation. Two embryos developed until the last examination on day 60.

Based on methods previously described for ovine embryos [12], a preliminary study was done in our laboratory [13]. Embryos were vitrified using solutions previously described (see Table 1); however, after warming, they were diluted by steps in vitro. Four of the six embryos 300 μm or less in diameter that were vitrified, warmed, and transferred into recipients resulted in embryonic vesicles, detected by ultrasound on day 16. Two pregnancies were allowed to develop until day 38; embryo development appeared normal during ultrasound examinations. In a subsequent study [6], the same basic procedures [13] were used, although modifications were made to allow for dilution of cryoprotectants within the straw and direct transfer into recipient uteri, resulting in the vitrification procedure previously described in detail. Embryo development rates to day 16 after transfer into recipient uteri were 45% (10 of 22 recipients) and 62% (16 of 26 recipients) for step dilutions in vitro and for direct transfer, respectively. The mean diameter of embryos used in the study was approximately 185 μm. Five pregnancies were allowed to develop to day 35, and ultrasound assessment of embryo development was normal.

Hudson and coworkers [7] recovered embryos 300 μm or less in diameter from mares superovulated with equine follicle-stimulating hormone (eFSH; Bioniche Animal Health). Embryos were vitrified (as described previously) at less than 1 hour after collection, or embryos were cooled (5°C–8°C) for 12 to 19 hours before vitrification. For cooling, the embryos were placed in medium (Vigro holding solution; AB Technology, Pullman, Washington) and packaged within a passive cooling container (Equitainer; Hamilton Thorne Biosciences, Beverly, Massachusetts). Pregnancy rates on day 16 were not significantly different when embryos were vitrified immediately or cooled before vitrification (15 [75%] of 20 embryos and 13 [65%] of 20 embryos, respectively). Results of the study confirm the success of vitrification procedures and suggest that embryos can be cooled for a period of time sufficient to transport them to another laboratory for vitrification.

Vitrification of large embryos

Embryo size is a major factor predicting the outcome of cryopreservation. In commercial programs, mares are often palpated daily for ovulation, with embryos collected 7 or 8 days after the detection of ovulation. Because mean embryo diameters are 406 and 1132 μm at days 7 and 8, respectively [9], embryos for cryopreservation are usually collected on day 6 to 6.5 so as to obtain embryos less than 300 μm in diameter. Occasionally, embryos larger than 300 μm in diameter are collected. Few studies have been conducted to evaluate the potential of vitrifying large embryos; however, success has been limited. Most research protocols for the vitrification of large embryos have only been tested in vitro, but transfers into recipients were done in a few studies. Caracciolo di Brienza and colleagues [13] vitrified embryos of different sizes. All (three of three) morulae and extremely early blastocysts developed into embryonic vesicles; in contrast, few blastocysts (one of three or none of three for blastocysts 300 μm or less in diameter and greater than 300 μm in diameter, respectively) developed after transfer. In the study by Eldridge-Panuska and coworkers [6], large embryos were vitrified similar to the method described by Caracciolo di Brienza and colleagues [13] (n = 10 with a mean diameter of 575 μm) or with the modification of a higher concentration of EG in VS3 (EG [6.6 M] plus Gly [1.4 M]; n = 10, with a mean diameter of 644 μm). None of the large embryos developed into embryonic vesicles.

Only in one study were pregnancies established after vitrification of large embryos. Campos-Chillon and coworkers [14] attempted three methods to vitrify large embryos, with one of the three methods resulting in success. In the study, 17 embryos between 300 and 750 μm in diameter were sequentially placed into EG [1.5 M] for 5 minutes; EG [3 M] for 10 minutes; EG [5 M] for 5 minutes; and EG [7 M], galactose [0.5 M], and 18% wt/vol Ficoll 70 for less than 1 minute. The base medium for VSs was mPBS. Straws (0.25 mL) were loaded with the embryos in 10 μL of the final VS and separate columns of DS. Straws were plunged vertically into liquid nitrogen, with the sealed end of the straw and the embryo submerged before the remaining portion of the straw. For warming, straws were held in air (24°C) for 10 seconds and then in water at 37°C for 10 seconds. Straws were shaken to mix contents; embryos were expelled and placed into solutions of galactose (0.3 and 0.15 M, respectively) for 3 minutes. Embryos were transferred into the recipient uteri 5 days after ovulation. The embryo development rate by approximately day 16 was 35% (6 of 17 recipients) overall. Although 6 (55%) of 11 embryos sized 300 to 400 μm in diameter resulted in embryo development, no embryos greater than 400 μm in diameter developed.

The cause of cryopreservation failure in large equine embryos is not known. The capsule that is present in larger embryos may impede the intracellular diffusion of cryoprotectants. In addition, the equine blastocyst is rapidly increasing in size with a large blastocele cavity and changing interactions between cells. Regardless of the cause, the reduced success with vitrification of embryos greater than 300 μm in diameter necessitates the collection of small embryos to optimize the success of the procedure at this time.

Summary

Vitrification can be used successfully to cryopreserve equine embryos. Embryos for vitrification should be collected from donor mares' uteri when they are 300 μm or less in diameter and at the morula of early blastocyst stage of development. During the vitrification procedure, embryos are moved through three media containing increasing concentrations of cryoprotectants (Gly and EG). A 0.25-μL straw is loaded with the embryo in a VS and a volume of DS to allow dilution of cryoprotectants in the straw after warming. No special equipment is required for vitrification; the straw containing the embryo is exposed to vapor for 1 minute before plunging it into liquid nitrogen. Warming of the straw requires no special equipment, and the embryo can be transferred directly from the straw into a recipient's uterus. Vitrification has been repeatedly successful when the procedure is used with small embryos and provides a method for the rapid cryopreservation of equine embryos.

References

[1] Yamamoto Y, Oguri N, Tsutsumi Y, et al. Experiments in the freezing and storage of equine embryos. J Reprod Fertil Suppl 1982;32:399–403.
[2] Seidel GE. Cryopreservation of equine embryos. Vet Clin North Am Equine Pract 1996;12: 85–99.
[3] Rall WF, Fahy GM. Ice-free cryopreservation of mouse embryos at −196°C by vitrification. Nature 1985;313:573–5.

[4] Slade NP, Takeda T, Squires EL, et al. A new procedure for the cryopreservation of equine embryos. Theriogenology 1985;24:45–57.
[5] Maclellan LJ, Carnevale EM, Coutinho da Silva MA, et al. Cryopreservation of small and large equine embryos pretreated with cytochalasin-B and/or trypsin. Theriogenology 2002; 58:717–20.
[6] Eldridge-Panuska WD, Caracciolo di Brienza V, Seidel GE Jr, et al. Establishment of pregnancies after serial dilution or direct transfer by vitrified equine embryos. Theriogenology 2005;63:1308–19.
[7] Hudson J, McCue PM, Carnevale EM, et al. The effects of cooling and vitrification of embryos from mares treated with equine follicle-stimulating hormone on pregnancy rates after nonsurgical transfer. J Equine Vet Sci 2006;26:51–4.
[8] Freeman DA, Weber JA, Geary RT, et al. Time of embryo transport through the mare oviduct. Theriogenology 1991;36:823–30.
[9] Squires EL, Cook VM, Voss JL. Collection and transfer of equine embryos. Bulletin no. 1. Fort Collins (CO): Animal Reproduction Laboratory; 1985.
[10] Carnevale EM, Eldridge-Panuska WD, Caracciolo di Brienza V. How to collect and vitrify equine embryos for direct transfer. In: Proceedings of the 50th Annual Convention of the American Association of Equine Practitioners. Denver (CO); 2004. p. 402–5.
[11] Hochi S, Fujimoto T, Braun J, et al. Pregnancies following transfer of equine embryos cryopreserved by vitrification. Theriogenology 1994;42:483–8.
[12] Naitana S, Loi P, Ledda S, et al. Effect of biopsy and vitrification on in vitro survival of ovine embryos at different stages of development. Theriogenology 1996;46:813–24.
[13] Caracciolo di Brienza V, Squires EL, Zicarelli L, et al. Establishment of pregnancies after vitrification of equine embryos [abstract]. Reprod Fertil Dev 2004;16:165.
[14] Campos-Chillon LF, Cox TJ, Seidel GE Jr, et al. Vitrification in vivo of large equine embryos after vitrification or culture [abstract]. Reprod Fertil Dev 2006;18:151.

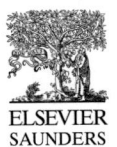

Collection, Evaluation, and Use of Oocytes in Equine Assisted Reproduction

Elaine M. Carnevale, DVM, PhD[a,*], Lisa J. Maclellan, PhD[b]

[a]*Animal Reproduction and Biotechnology Laboratory, College of Veterinary Medicine and Biomedical Sciences, Colorado State University, 3194 Rampart Road, Fort Collins, CO 80523, USA*
[b]*Seven Creeks Equine, PO Box 21, Euroa, Victoria, Australia 3666*

Assisted reproductive techniques have been developed to obtain pregnancies from subfertile mares and stallions and to salvage gametes after death. In recent years, these procedures have been used for clinical cases with repeated success. The basis for the success and future development of assisted reproductive techniques is our ability to collect and handle the equine oocyte successfully. This article focuses on important clinical aspects of oocyte collection and evaluation and briefly discusses the clinical use of assisted reproductive procedures in the horse.

Oocyte collection and culture

Oocytes can be removed from follicles at different stages of maturation or atresia. Immature oocytes can be collected from the follicles of live mares. The equine cumulus has a close and broad attachment to the follicular wall, however, with cumulus cell extensions into an underlying thecal pad [1]; this results in the surrounding cells firmly attaching the oocyte to the follicular wall. Consequently, collection rates from immature follicles are often less than 50%. When mares die or are euthanized for medical reasons, oocytes from the excised ovaries are harvested from individual follicles of all sizes and stages of maturation or atresia. Initially, the methods used to

* Corresponding author.
  E-mail address: emc@colostate.edu (E.M. Carnevale).

collect oocytes from excised ovaries were developed to collect oocytes for experiments from abattoir ovaries.

Handling and transportation of ovaries

Ovaries excised from mares that have died or have been euthanized are often transported to an appropriate laboratory for the recovery and culture of oocytes. Therefore, factors associated with oocyte transportation must be considered. No study directly compares media for packaging and transportation of ovaries to the laboratory. Media that have been used for this purpose include a complete medium (tissue culture medium [TCM]-199), normal saline with antibiotics, commercial embryo flush solution, and phosphate-buffered saline [2–7]. Transportation temperature seems to play a role in subsequent oocyte quality, with temperatures of 4°C [8], 9°C to 16°C [7], 22°C to 30°C [2–4,7,9], and 30°C to 35°C [5] being reported. In a study by Pedersen and colleagues [10], ovaries were held at 20°C, 30°C, or 35°C to 37°C and cumulus morphology and granulosa cell apoptosis were evaluated. Results of the study suggest that ovaries should not be held for more than 3 hours between 20°C and 30°C to avoid granulosa cell apoptosis and that ovaries should be held less than 2 hours at 35°C to 37°C before processing to avoid morphologic changes to the cumulus. Love and coworkers [8] compared oocytes from ovaries collected immediately on arrival at the laboratory (3–9 hours) or stored overnight (15–18 hours) at room temperature or 4°C. Higher maturation rates were observed from oocytes collected immediately on arrival at the laboratory compared with oocytes from ovaries stored at room temperature or 4°C for 15 to 18 hours. Preis and colleagues [7] compared ovary storage temperatures of approximately 12° and 22°C, with no significant difference in the embryo development rates (15% at 12°C and 18% at 22°C) after transfer of in vitro matured oocytes into inseminated recipient mares. The most appropriate temperature for the storage of ovaries has not been determined. Results of studies suggest that 4°C is probably too cold for ovary storage; however, as the storage interval increases, temperature reductions are essential to maintain cell viability.

Transportation of ovaries to a laboratory requires storage time for shipping. Experimental times have varied from 1 to 24 hours, and studies have shown no effect of ovary transport times of up to 15 hours on oocyte meiotic competence [5,11]. The shortest duration of time within these studies was between 1.5 and 4 hours, however. Relatively high rates of oocyte maturation have been reported from laboratories that recover oocytes from ovaries soon after slaughter, suggesting that even a few hours of ovary storage during transportation to the laboratory could influence meiotic competence of oocytes [8,12].

The optimal temperature and method of packaging ovaries have not been determined. A possible alternative to shipping ovaries is to harvest oocytes from ovaries before shipment. The oocytes can be transported within maturation medium in a portable incubator, allowing in vitro maturation during shipment. Potentially, this method would result in oocytes that are more viable after shipment.

Collecting oocytes from excised ovaries

The materials for oocyte harvesting include media, test tubes, scalpel blades, syringes, needles, bone curettes, Petri dishes, and glass or plastic transfer pipettes. The equipment is required to be sterile and, if reused, carefully prepared to avoid substances harmful to oocytes. If oocytes are obtained at body temperature, media and equipment should be preheated in an incubator or on a dry block to minimize temperature fluctuations to the oocyte.

Media used for oocyte collections generally are simple salt solutions with added energy substrates or more complex tissue culture media, such as Ham's F-10 and TCM-199. These media are adapted from use in other species and are not specific for the horse. Media like G1/G2 [13] take into account the changing requirements of an embryo as it develops. A modification of G2, equine maturation medium (EMMI) [14], has been successfully used for holding and in vitro maturation of equine oocytes.

Equine oocytes can be removed from excised ovaries by various methods. Oocytes can be collected from follicles by aspiration [15,16], with gentle suction created by a water pump (approximately 0.1 bar) or vacuum pump (100–150 mm Hg) through an 18-gauge needle. The oocytes are aspirated into a collection vessel and identified under a stereomicroscope from the pellet at the bottom of the vessel. When collected by aspiration, most oocytes only maintained the cells immediately surrounding the oocyte, termed the *corona radiata* [17]. For ovarian slicing [18], a razor blade is used to slice the ovary into approximately 5-mm sections. The ovary is then washed in collection medium, and the fluid is pooled and searched. Scraping the inner wall of the follicle [4,5,19] seems to be more efficient than aspiration or slicing, with an oocyte collection rate of approximately 80% [5,19]. Although scraping is a slower method to process ovaries, most collected oocytes contain an intact cumulus complex [4] and most are imbedded in sheets of granulosa cells. For scraping, all visible follicles are incised with a scalpel blade. To remove the cells, the inner surfaces of follicles are scraped with bone curettes, ranging from 0.5 to 1.5 cm depending on follicular size. After all follicles visible on the surface of the ovary are scraped, the ovaries are cut into 0.5-cm sections to locate follicles within the ovarian stroma [20]. The follicular cells are washed from the bone curette into individual Petri dishes using a holding medium that maintains its pH at room temperature. Within the sheets of granulosa, cumulus oocyte complexes are located using a dissecting microscope. The cumulus oocyte complex can be dissected from granulosa cells as needed and graded as (1) compact, a sheet of tight compact cells completely surrounding the oocyte; (2) expanded, a granular or expanded cumulus layer completely surrounding the oocyte; or (3) denuded, only a partial cumulus or the corona radiata present [4].

After oocytes have been identified under the microscope, all handling procedures should be performed at a constant temperature. Groups of oocytes are pooled in Petri dishes containing a holding medium, graded according to cumulus morphology, and then transferred into an appropriate culture medium.

Cumulus oocyte complexes collected from slaughterhouse ovaries or from euthanized mares form a heterogeneous population with regard to the quality and size of the follicle from which they are collected. Irrespective of the differences in oocyte characteristics, all oocytes are generally collected and cultured in one medium. The relatively static environment in vitro is different from the environment in vivo, where supplies of nutrients change in a more dynamic manner [21]. Optimal conditions for maturation in vitro are not known. Maturation rates in vitro are generally between 50% and 70%, and the developmental capacity of in vitro matured oocytes is lower than that of in vivo matured oocytes [22].

Collection of oocytes from preovulatory follicles

For clinical procedures, oocytes are often collected after the initiation of follicle and oocyte maturation in the estrous mare. Flank and transvaginal punctures are the most common methods used to collect oocytes for clinical procedures. Flank punctures can result in good collection rates and have the advantage of minimizing equipment needs. For flank collections, a cannula is placed through the donor's flank ipsilateral to the ovary with a preovulatory follicle. The ovary is manipulated per rectum, with the large follicle firmly positioned against the end of the cannula. A needle is passed through the cannula and into the follicular antrum. The follicle can then be lavaged. This procedure is based on tactile identification and manipulation of the follicle. The procedure is limited when trying to obtain oocytes from smaller follicles, and it does not allow imaging of the needle puncture.

The method of choice for follicular aspirations in our laboratory is transvaginal follicular aspirations. Before the procedure, the donor mare is placed in a stock, her rectum is evacuated, and her perineal area is cleaned. The mare is sedated, often with a combination of xylazine and butorphanol tartrate. Rectal contractions are prevented by the administration of propantheline bromide or N-butylscopolammonium bromide. A linear or curvilinear ultrasound transducer is positioned in a plastic casing containing a needle guide. The transducer face is lubricated and placed within the anterior vagina. Care is taken to place the transducer to the side of the cervix ipsilateral to the preovulatory follicle. The ovary with the preovulatory follicle is positioned against the transducer face by manipulations per rectum. When the needle is advanced, it punctures the apex of the follicle and avoids puncturing the broad ligament and additional ovarian stroma. In our laboratory, we prefer double-lumen 12-gauge needles, allowing for the aspiration of follicular contents while the antrum is lavaged with phosphate-buffered saline (100–150 mL) or an embryo flush solution containing heparin (10 U/mL). The flush medium and all plastics are sterile and warmed to body temperature.

Oocytes are often collected approximately 20 to 36 hours after administration of human chorionic gonadotropin (hCG) or a gonadotropin releasing hormone (GnRH) analogue (deslorelin acetate). Oocytes collected 24 hours after administration of hCG are probably in metaphase I (M I) and require culture to complete maturation, whereas oocytes collected closer to 36 hours after hCG administration are probably in metaphase II (M II) and can be transferred immediately. Oocyte collection rates and embryo development rates after oocyte transfer were similar for oocytes collected 24 or 36 hours after hCG administration [23,24].

Equine oocyte

Morphologic evaluation of the cumulus oocyte complex

Morphologic evaluation of the oocyte is impaired by the presence of the surrounding cumulus cells, which impede direct imaging. Morphology of the cumulus complex can be evaluated based on the appearance and expansion of the cells, which reflect aspects of oocyte maturation and viability. The degree of cumulus expansion has been correlated with the stage of nuclear maturation of equine oocytes in several studies [9,18,25,26]. Equine oocyte maturation is associated with well-defined cytoplasmic and nuclear changes that are paralleled by increasing follicular fluid progesterone concentrations and consistently high estradiol concentrations [27,28]. The morphologic changes associated with final oocyte maturation are associated with six consecutive stages of well-defined nuclear and cytoplasmic changes: stage 1, the central spherical nucleus stage; stage 2, the presence of a spherical oocyte nucleus located at the periphery of the ooplasm; stage 3; a peripheral oocyte nucleus in stage II with a peripherally flattened nucleus; stage 4, oocyte nucleus breakdown; stage 5, M I with metaphase chromosomes peripherally located in the ooplasm; and stage 6, M II with metaphase chromosomes peripherally located and a polar body within the perivitelline space [28].

Although changes in nuclear and cytoplasmic maturation can be determined with advanced imaging procedures, the clinician relies primarily on gross morphology of the oocyte and cumulus cells to judge maturation and viability. In contrast to the embryo and on collection, the oocyte is usually surrounded by a complex of cumulus cells. Although these cells can provide valuable information regarding the oocyte's stage of maturation, they effectively prevent detailed observation of the oocyte. For such procedures as intracytoplasmic sperm injection (ICSI), cumulus cells are removed and the oocyte can be further examined. For oocyte transfer, however, the cumulus cells are left attached to the oocyte to aid in the fertilization process. Therefore, the oocyte can only be superficially examined.

Immature equine oocytes are surrounded by a nonexpanded and multilayered cumulus investment. The innermost cumulus cells have numerous projections penetrating the zona pellucida and establishing close contact with the oolemma via intermediate junctions (Fig. 1) [28]. Compact granulosa cells from the immature follicle are often in sheets with a defined edge and grainy appearance; granulosa and cumulus cells are similar in texture. The oocyte is observed within the cumulus as a gray spherically shaped area, and the clear ring of the zona pellucida may be discernible (Fig. 2). If imaged from the side, the oocyte is contained within a hillock of cumulus cells. Expanded cumulus complexes have a fuzzy or expanded appearance to the cells. Different degrees of expansion can be observed, from slight at the outer edge of cells to complete (Fig. 3). In general, oocytes with a compact cumulus yield a higher proportion of oocytes in the germinal vesicle or germinal vesicle breakdown stage than oocytes with an expanded cumulus. Therefore, the optimal maturation interval in vitro for the oocyte may differ with varying degrees of cumulus expansion. Maximum maturation rates in vitro were obtained for cumulus oocyte complexes that were expanded versus compact, respectively, at 24 and 32 hours for Hinrichs and colleagues [4] and at 24 and 30 hours for Zhang and coworkers [9].

In clinical programs, oocytes are often collected 24 to 36 hours after administration of hCG; therefore, they are usually maturing or mature at the time of collection and at the M I or M II stage of maturation. As the oocyte matures, the cumulus and granulosa cells expand. Mature granulosa cells form light sheets of cells with soft borders. As cumulus cells expand, they are intertwined in a light cellular matrix that may seem to have a yellow tint. When searching for the oocyte, granulosa cells are usually abundant and arranged in sheets of cells with a gray and grainy appearance. In contrast, the expanded cumulus is distinctly clear in appearance. Because of

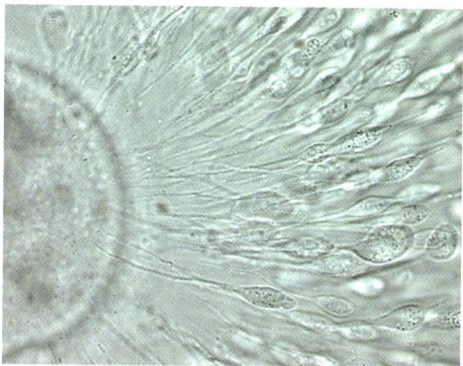

Fig. 1. Projections from the cumulus cells extend through the zona pellucida and to the oocyte.

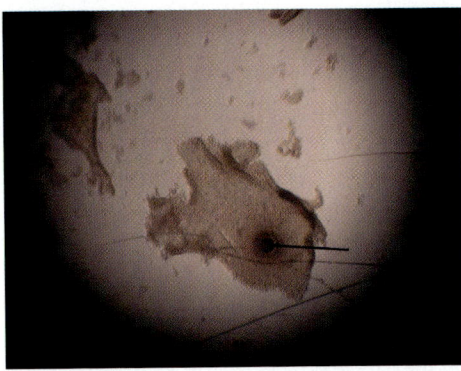

Fig. 2. An immature oocyte (*arrow*) surrounded by compact granulosa. The clear ring around the oocyte is the zona pellucida.

the expansion of cumulus cells during maturation, this complex of cells becomes large, often 3 mm or greater in diameter, and easy to identify when the bloody aspirate is spread into Petri dishes and placed over the light of a stereoscope (Fig. 4). The oocyte is small, approximately 160 μm in diameter, and sometimes difficult to image; therefore, the oocyte is often located by finding the complex of expanded cumulus cells. The dark gray oocyte can be imaged through the cumulus cells under a stereoscope. The cumulus cells directly surrounding the oocyte are called the corona radiata; these cells are often the last to expand, resulting in the appearance of a cellular ring around the oocyte (Fig. 5). As maturation is complete, cells of the corona complete their expansion, resulting in a "sunburst" appearance and easier imaging of the oocyte. The ooplasm can be different shades of gray, often with a polarized appearance caused by uneven distribution of lipid droplets and organelles (Fig. 6). Extrusion of the polar body is apparent at the M II stage of

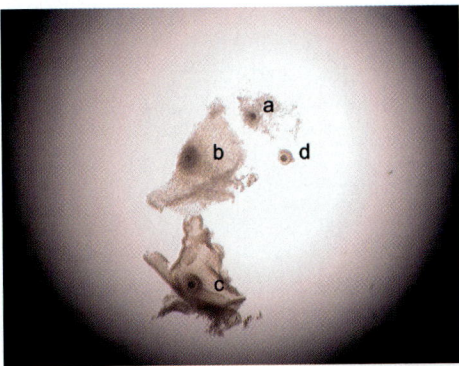

Fig. 3. Oocytes collected from excised ovaries and classified as atretic/expanded (a), expanded (b), compact (c), and mostly denuded (d).

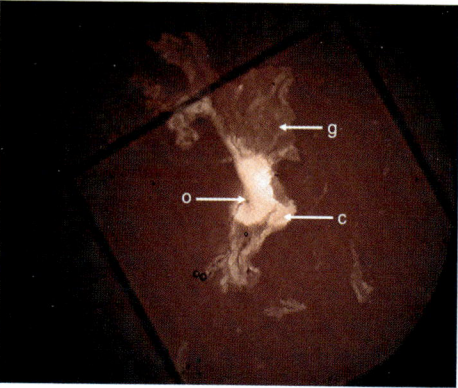

Fig. 4. An oocyte collected from a mare approximately 24 hours after induction of follicle maturation. The oocyte (o) appears as a dark circular structure within the clear cumulus cells. Granulosa cells (g) have been pulled from the follicular wall and appear as gray sheets of cells radiating from the cumulus complex (c).

maturation, signaling that the oocyte has reached the stage of nuclear maturation appropriate for fertilization (Fig. 7). The polar body is rarely imaged through the cumulus cells with a stereoscope. Occasionally, the widened perivitelline space of the mature oocyte is imaged.

With experience, identification of the oocyte becomes reliable. Some structures within the aspirate can be confused for the oocyte, however, including debris or air bubbles. Because they appear round and dark, air bubbles caught in cumulus or granulosa cells can be confused for the oocyte. Differentiation can be made by gently moving the cells for a better image. Air bubbles have a dark exterior and light interior in contrast to the oocyte, with a gray ooplasm and surrounding corona radiata (Fig. 8). Occasionally,

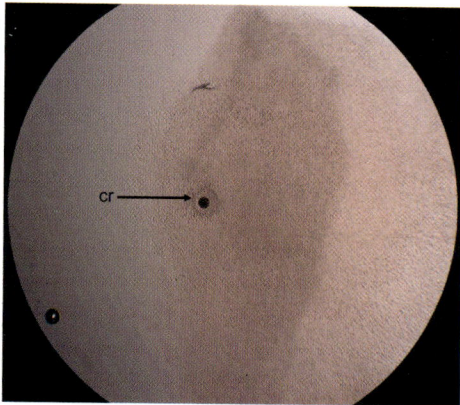

Fig. 5. A cumulus oocyte complex with an expanding corona radiata (cr).

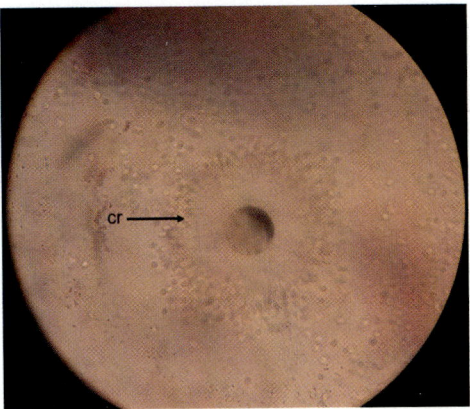

Fig. 6. An equine oocyte with the typical polarized appearance to the ooplasm and an expanding corona radiata (cr).

the oocyte fragments on collection. The ooplasm may be apparent as an elongated dark area within an oval or broken ring of cells from the corona radiata (Fig. 9).

Assisted reproductive techniques

During the past 10 years, procedures for assisted reproduction have rapidly developed for clinical use in the horse. Many of the procedures require special expertise and equipment, however, resulting in a relatively slow movement from academic to clinical settings. A clinical program in assisted reproduction was established at Colorado State University in 1998, and the basic procedures using equine oocytes and results are presented.

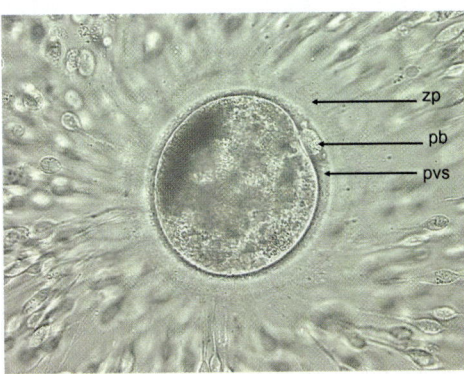

Fig. 7. The polar body (pb) is apparent in the oocyte at M II. The oolemma adjacent to the polar body is flattened, and the perivitelline space (pvs) is visible. zp, zona pellucida.

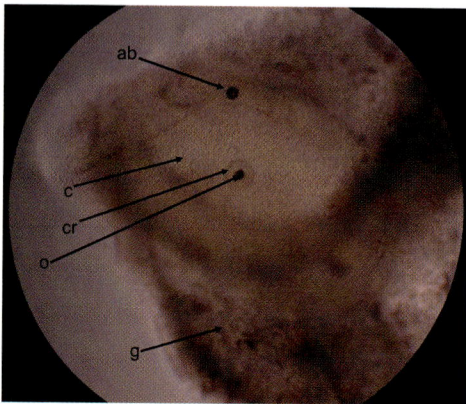

Fig. 8. An air bubble (ab) within the cumulus or granulosa cells can look similar to the oocyte (o). Note that the oocyte is gray in the center, however, with a surrounding and distinct ring of the corona radiata (cr). The central cumulus cells (c) are lighter in appearance than the surrounding layer of granulosa (g).

Oocyte transfer

Oocyte transfer involves the transfer of a donor's oocyte into the oviduct of an inseminated recipient. The primary clinical use for oocyte transfer has been to obtain offspring from mares that were not successful embryo donors or broodmares because of uterine, oviductal, or cervical problems.

At Colorado State University, approximately 150 oocyte transfers are being performed each breeding season. In our laboratory, oocytes are usually collected between 20 and 24 hours after induction of oocyte maturation. Therefore, oocytes are cultured approximately 16 hours before transfer. The procedures used for oocyte culture and transfer are based on those

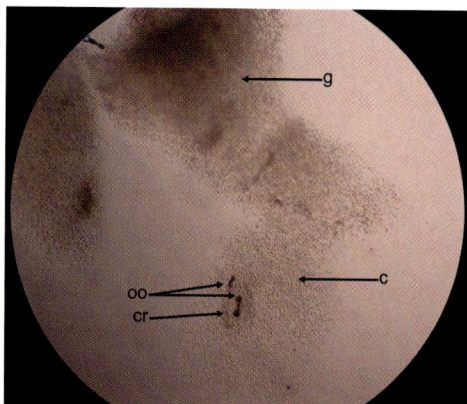

Fig. 9. The partial complex of cumulus cells (c) with attached granulosa (g) surrounds the elongated ooplasm (oo) and corona radiata (cr) of an oocyte fragmented during collection.

reported in 1995 [29], with culture in TCM-199 with additions of 10% fetal calf serum, pyruvate (0.2 mmol) and gentamicin (50 μg/mL). Oocytes are cultured at 38.5°C and in 6% carbon dioxide and air.

Cyclic and noncyclic mares have been used as recipients for oocyte transfer, with no difference in pregnancy rates [30]. If a cyclic recipient is used, the mare's oocyte is removed from the dominant follicle before transfer of a donor's oocyte. In noncyclic recipients, natural estrus is mimicked by the administration of estrogen (estradiol, 1.5–3 mg/d). Recipients are inseminated within the uterus with semen from the desired stallion approximately 12 to 16 hours before transfer and, inconsistently, approximately 2 hours after transfer. Standing flank laparotomies are performed to expose the oviductal os. A small incision is made through the skin in the flank area, muscle layers are bluntly dissected, the peritoneum is punctured, and the ovary is exposed through the incision. Oocytes are transferred using a fire-polished glass pipette and placed approximately 3 cm past the infundibular os.

Results of the oocyte transfer program at Colorado State University were recently reviewed [30]. During 4 years of the program, oocytes were collected from 86 donors, with a mean age of 19 years and histories of infertility using standard breeding methods or embryo transfer. Oocytes were collected from 77% (548 of 710) of aspirated follicles. At 16 and 50 days after transfer, pregnancy rates were 40% and 32%, respectively. One or more recipients were pregnant at 50 days for 71% of donors. Results of this program demonstrate that pregnancies can be obtained from many mares that are considered subfertile or infertile using other procedures, including embryo transfer.

Collection and transfer of oocytes from euthanized mares

The birth of a foal resulting from the culture and transfer of oocytes collected from ovaries transported across the country was first reported in 2003 [31]. Limited facilities are available to collect and transfer oocytes from euthanized mares; therefore, ovaries are often transported to a suitable facility for processing. In our laboratory, the collected oocytes are cultured in TCM-199 or EMMI [14]; media are supplemented with 10% fetal calf serum, pyruvate (0.2 mmol), gentamicin sulfate (25 μg/mL), luteinizing hormone (LH; 1 μg/mL), follicle-stimulating hormone (FSH; 15 ng/mL), estradiol (1 μg/mL), progesterone (500 ng/mL), insulin-like growth factor (IGF; 10 ng/mL), and epidermal growth factor (EGF; 100 ng/mL). Oocytes are cultured at 38.5°C in 6% carbon dioxide and air for 24 to 30 hours. One or multiple oocytes are transferred into a recipient's oviduct.

Between 2001 and 2004 in our laboratory, oocytes were transferred from the ovaries of 25 light-horse mares after the mares had died (n = 4) or were euthanized (n = 21) for medical reasons [32]. Ovaries from 6 mares were transported for less than 1 hour to our laboratory at approximately 37°C, whereas 19 mares died in distant locations. Their ovaries were transported between 8 and 26 hours, with ovarian temperatures ranging from 10°C to 23°C on arrival. On average, 11 oocytes were collected per mare. More oocytes were collected from the ovaries of younger mares (4–19 years of age, mean of 12 oocytes) than from older mares (≥ 20 years of age, mean of 5 oocytes). Approximately 5 oocytes were transferred into the oviduct of each of 46 recipients. Embryonic vesicles resulted from 15% of the transferred oocytes as detected by ultrasound 16 days after transfer. More embryos developed from the oocytes that were transported to the laboratory in less than 1 hour versus longer intervals (36% and 10% rates of embryo development, respectively). Although 30% of recipients were diagnosed as pregnant by day 16, 6 of the 14 pregnancies were lost by day 60. One or multiple foals were produced for 24% (6 of 25) of donors.

Many mares die when recipients or semen is not available. Therefore, we would ideally have methods to cryopreserve oocytes for later fertilization. Oocytes have been successfully cryopreserved, warmed, and transferred to produce foals [33]. The efficiency of the procedure is not adequate for preserving the limited oocytes collected from dead mares, however. In our laboratory as well as others, ICSI is being used to fertilize harvested oocytes in vitro. Especially during the nonbreeding season, one advantage of ICSI is that a limited amount of sperm (ie, a small section of one frozen straw) can be used. If recipients are available, the developing embryos can be transferred within a few days of fertilization into their oviducts or allowed to develop into blastocysts for a nonsurgical embryo transfer. The success of these procedures relative to oocyte transfer is yet to be determined. The vitrification of early-cleavage embryos produced after ICSI was recently reported by Campos-Chillon and colleagues [34], providing a potential method for the cryopreservation of these embryos when recipients are not available.

Intracytoplasmic sperm injection

Although in vitro fertilization has had only limited success for the horse, ICSI has provided a method to achieve fertilization in vitro for equine oocytes [35,36]. For ICSI, a single sperm is selected and injected into the ooplasm of a mature (M II) oocyte. Although fertile sperm are needed for oocyte transfer to be successful, ICSI provides a method to obtain offspring with marginal-quality or limited numbers of sperm.

Ideally, embryos resulting from ICSI could be allowed to develop in vitro until the late morula or blastocyst stage, when they would be transferred into recipient uteri, cryopreserved, or transferred back into the donor's uterus. Development of equine embryos in vitro is not yet optimal, however. Therefore, different tactics have been used for the transfer of sperm-injected oocytes. In our laboratory, we transfer injected oocytes and early-cleavage embryos into the oviducts of recipients to minimize any detrimental effect of embryo culture in vitro. In other laboratories, however, injected oocytes have been transferred into sheep oviducts for early embryo development or successfully cultured in vitro before uterine transfers [36].

Although the first foal from ICSI was reported in 1996 [35], the procedure has only recently been used consistently for commercial purposes. In recent years, commercial foals have been produced from the injection of equine oocytes from stallions with poor-quality or limited numbers of sperm collected from the epididymis of a dead stallion and from stallions with limited frozen sperm.

Summary

Rapid advances have occurred in our ability to collect and manipulate equine oocytes. Consequently, assisted reproductive procedures have been developed for the horse. Commercial applications of oocyte technologies in the horse have resulted in clinical procedures to obtain offspring from mares and stallions with poor fertility or to salvage their gametes after death.

References

[1] Hawley LR, Enders AC, Hinrichs K. Comparison of equine and bovine oocyte-cumulus morphology within the ovarian follicle. Biol Reprod Monogr 1995;1:243–52.
[2] Alm H, Torner H. In vitro maturation of horse oocytes. Theriogenology 1994;42:345–9.
[3] Lazzari G, Crotti G, Turini P, et al. Equine embryos at the compacted morula and blastocyst stage can be obtained by intracytoplasmic sperm injection (ICSI) of in vitro matured oocytes with frozen-thawed spermatozoa from semen of different fertilities. Theriogenology 2002;58: 709–12.
[4] Hinrichs K, Schmidt AL, Friedman PP, et al. In vitro maturation of horse oocytes: characterization of chromatin configuration using fluorescence microscopy. Biol Reprod 1993;48: 363–70.
[5] Del Campo MR, Donoso MX, Parrish JJ, et al. Selection of follicles, preculture oocyte evaluation, and duration of culture for in vitro maturation of equine oocytes. Theriogenology 1995;43:1141–53.
[6] Franz LC, Squires EL, Rumpf R, et al. Effects of Roscovitine in maintaining meiotic arrest in equine oocytes and subsequent maturation rates after inhibition. Theriogenology 2002;56: 679–83.
[7] Preis KA, Carnevale EM, Coutinho da Silva MA, et al. In vitro maturation and transfer of equine oocytes after transport of ovaries at 12 or 22°C. Theriogenology 2004;61:1215–23.
[8] Love LB, Choi YH, Love CC, et al. Effect of ovary storage and oocyte transport method on maturation rate of horse oocytes. Theriogenology 2003;59:765–74.
[9] Zhang JJ, Boyle MS, Allen WR, et al. Recent studies on in vivo fertilization of in vitro matured horse oocytes. Equine Vet J Suppl 1989;8:101–4.
[10] Pedersen HG, Watson ED, Telfer EE. Effect of holding temperature and time on equine granulosa cell apoptosis, oocyte chromatin configuration and cumulus morphology. Theriogenology 2004;62:468–80.
[11] Guignot F, Bezard J, Palmer E. Effect of time during transport of excised mare ovaries on oocyte recovery rate and quality after in vitro maturation. Theriogenology 1999;52:757–66.
[12] Hinrichs K, Choi YH, Love LB, et al. Chromatin configuration within the germinal vesicle of horse oocytes: changes post mortem and relationship to meiotic and developmental competence. Biol Reprod 2005;72:1142–50.

[13] Gardner DK. Mammalian embryo culture in the absence of serum or somatic cell support. Cell Biol Int 1994;18:1163–80.
[14] Maclellan LJ, Lane M, Sims MM, et al. Effect of sucrose or trehalose on vitrification of equine oocytes 12 or 24h after the onset of maturation. Theriogenology 2001;55:310.
[15] Desjardins M, King WA, Bousquet D. In vitro maturation of horse oocytes [abstract]. Theriogenology 1985;23:187.
[16] Shabpareh V, Squires EL, Seidel GE Jr, et al. Methods for collecting and maturing equine oocytes in vitro. Theriogenology 1993;40:1161–75.
[17] Hinrichs K. The relationship of follicle atresia to follicle size, oocyte recovery rate on aspiration, and oocyte morphology in the mare. Theriogenology 1991;36:157–68.
[18] Choi YH, Hochi S, Braun J, et al. In vitro maturation of equine oocytes collected by follicle aspiration and by slicing the ovaries. Theriogenology 1993;40:959–66.
[19] Okolski A, Babuski P, Tischner M, et al. Evaluation of mare oocyte collection methods and stallion sperm penetration of zona-free hamster ova. J Reprod Fertil Suppl 1987;35:191–6.
[20] Hinrichs K, Williams KA. Relationships among oocyte-cumulus morphology, follicular atresia, initial chromatin configuration, and oocyte meiotic competence in the horse. Biol Reprod 1997;57:377–84.
[21] Bavister BD. Interactions between embryos and the culture milieu. Theriogenology 2000;53:619–26.
[22] Scott TJ, Carnevale EM, Maclellan LJ, et al. Embryo development rates after transfer of oocytes matured in vivo, in vitro, or within oviducts of mares. Theriogenology 2001;55:705–15.
[23] Coutinho da Silva MA, Carnevale EM, Maclellan LJ, et al. Effect of time of oocyte collection and site of insemination on oocyte transfer in mares. J Anim Sci 2002;80:1275–9.
[24] Hinrichs K, Betschart RW, McCue P, et al. Effect of timing of follicle aspiration on pregnancy rates after oocyte transfer in mares. J Reprod Fertil Suppl 2000;56:493–8.
[25] Torner H, Alm H. Meiotic configuration of horse oocytes in relation to the morphology of the cumulus-oocyte complex. Biol Reprod Monogr 1995;1:253–9.
[26] Gable TL, Woods GL. Confocal microscopy of germinal vesicle-stage equine oocytes. Theriogenology 2001;55:1417–30.
[27] Kenny RM, Condon W, Ganjam VK, et al. Morphological and biochemical correlates of equine ovarian follicles as a function of their state of viability or atresia. J Reprod Fertil Suppl 1979;27:163–71.
[28] Grondahl C, Hyttel P, Grondahl ML, et al. Structural and endocrine aspects of equine oocyte maturation in vivo. Mol Reprod Dev 1995;42:94–105.
[29] Carnevale EM, Ginther OJ. Defective oocytes as a cause of subfertility in old mares. Biol Reprod 1995;1:209–14.
[30] Carnevale EM, Coutinho da Silva MA, Panzani D, et al. Factors affecting the success of oocyte transfer in a clinical program for subfertile mares. Theriogenology 2005;64:519–27.
[31] Carnevale EM, Maclellan LJ, Coutinho da Silva MA, et al. Pregnancies attained after collection and transfer of oocytes from ovaries of 5 euthanatized mares. J Am Vet Med Assoc 2003;222:60–2.
[32] Carnevale EM, Coutinho da Silva MA, Preis KA, et al. Establishment of pregnancies from oocytes collected from the ovaries of euthanatized mares. In: Proceedings of 50th Annual Convention of the American Association of Equine Practitioners. Denver (CO); 2004. p. 531–3.
[33] Maclellan LJ, Carnevale EM, Coutinho da Silva MA, et al. Pregnancies from vitrified equine oocytes collected from super-stimulated and non-stimulated mares. Theriogenology 2002;58:911–9.
[34] Campos-Chillon LF, Suh TK, Seidel GE Jr, et al. Use of bovine embryos to establish methods for vitrification of early equine embryos. Theriogenology 2006;66:684–5.
[35] Squires EL, Carnevale EM, McCue PM, et al. Embryo technologies in the horse. Theriogenology 2003;59:151–70.
[36] Hinrichs K. Update on equine ICSI and cloning. Theriogenology 2005;64:535–41.

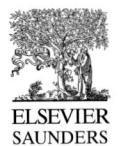

Equine Cloning
Katrin Hinrichs, DVM, PhD[a,b],*

[a]Department of Veterinary Physiology and Pharmacology, College of Veterinary Medicine and Biomedical Sciences, Texas A&M University, College Station, TX 77843–4466, USA
[b]Department of Large Animal Clinical Sciences, College of Veterinary Medicine and Biomedical Sciences, Texas A&M University, College Station, Texas, 77843–4466, USA

Cloning is applicable to equine veterinary practice as a method for saving valuable equine genetics. At the time of writing, three cloned mule foals have been produced from fetal donor cells and we are aware of 16 cloned horse foals that have been produced from adult donor cells. Thirteen of the 16 foals have developed normally; the three foals lost died from septicemia, pneumonia, and anesthetic complications. Although the first studies on cloned equine pregnancies reported poor efficiency of production of cloned foals (75%–100% of established pregnancies were lost), more recent techniques seem to be more efficient, with pregnancy rates per transferred embryo approaching those of standard embryo transfer and 50% or greater of established pregnancies going to term.

History of cloning

Cloning is defined as the process of creating an identical copy of an original. Cloning occurs commonly in nature, as seen in the production of identical twins. Cloning as a laboratory procedure has been performed for decades in nonmammalian animal species. In mammals, cloning of embryos by embryo splitting was performed soon after the development of embryo transfer techniques. Embryonic cloning by transfer of individual embryonic

---

Work performed in the authors laboratory was supported by the Link Equine Research Endowment Fund, Texas A&M University, Cryozootech SA, and the Smart Little Lena Co-managers.
  * Department of Veterinary Physiology and Pharmacology, College of Veterinary Medicine and Biomedical Sciences, Texas A&M University, College Station, Texas, 77843–4466, USA
  E-mail address: khinrichs@cvm.tamu.edu

blastomeres to enucleated oocytes was first performed in the late 1980s [1]. Cloning of mammals as it is understood generally, that is, production of a clone of an adult individual, was first reported with the publication of the birth of the sheep, Dolly, in 1997 [2]. The successful production of live offspring from a somatic cell from an adult sheep opened the doors for a remarkable amount of work in a variety of species; the list of successfully cloned species includes sheep, goats, mice, cattle, deer, cats, pigs, rhesus monkeys, dogs, and, since 2003, mules and horses.

The first equine nuclear transfer (NT) embryos produced were reported in brief communications in 2000 [3,4]. At that time, there were no established methods for equine in vitro oocyte maturation for maximum developmental competence or for equine embryo culture in vitro. Work in these areas lagged behind that for other species because in vitro fertilization was not successful in the horse. When fertilization of equine oocytes using intracytoplasmic sperm injection (ISCI) became repeatable, this was used to test the viability of in vitro matured oocytes and to provide embryos for the study of equine embryo culture requirements [5–7].

Early work in NT in the horse was frustrating because fusion rates between oocytes and donor cells were low and cleavage rates were even lower (less than 15%) [8]. In 2002, however, a collaborative group from Idaho and Utah reported pregnancies achieved by transfer of embryos produced by NT, using fibroblasts from a mule fetus as donor cells [9]. This same group reported the birth of a mule foal from this fetal cell line, the first equine clone, in 2003 [10]. The first equine clone from adult cells, a Haflinger filly, was reported by Dr. Cesare Galli's laboratory in Italy only a few months later [11]. Interestingly, this filly was carried by the same mare that was used as a cell donor; therefore, the mare was carrying its own genetic twin. The Idaho/Utah group reported that two more mule clones were born from the same cell line in 2003 [12]. No cloned equids were reported in 2004.

In 2005, the Italian laboratory produced a second viable cloned horse foal. They reported that another foal had been born but had died of septicemia within 48 hours of birth, which was apparently unrelated to its status as a clone [13]. Also, in 2005, our laboratory at Texas A&M University produced two viable cloned foals [14], bringing the number of viable cloned foals produced from adult horse donor cells to four. In 2006, our laboratory produced nine live cloned foals, of which seven survived and are developing normally, and a commercial laboratory, ViaGen, announced the birth of two healthy cloned foals.

Efficiency of equine cloning

One of the most exciting aspects of the birth of these cloned equids is that all the foals were born without assistance and the great majority have gone on to develop normally. Nevertheless, we must await the delivery of more cloned foals before we have a good idea of the proportion of cloned equine pregnancies that are viable. Although the foals that go to term seem to have good viability, there has been a high rate of embryonic and fetal loss in most reports. In the case of the mule project, 75% of established pregnancies were lost early in gestation, but all pregnancies that went past 60 days continued uneventfully to term [10]. This project used oocytes recovered after gonadotropin stimulation from the dominant preovulatory follicle of live mares, fetal donor cells, and immediate surgical transfer of recombined oocytes to the oviduct, all factors that should increase the efficiency of production of viable offspring. When this group used similar techniques with adult donor cells (cumulus cells), seven pregnancies were established from the transfer of 62 oocytes, but all pregnancies were lost before 80 days of gestation [15].

Interestingly, the efficiency reported with "standard" NT procedures (in vitro oocyte maturation, adult donor cells, and embryo culture to the blastocyst stage) in the horse has been similar to that reported for the ex vivo recovered oocytes and in vivo culture (oviduct transfer) used in the mule study. In the report of the cloned horse foal born in Italy in 2003 [11], 3% of recombined oocytes developed to blastocysts on culture in vitro. Transfer of 17 blastocysts resulted in four pregnancies, of which one was carried to term. In 2005, the same laboratory again reported a 3% blastocyst development rate after NT: transfer of 101 blastocysts resulted in nine pregnancies and the birth of one surviving foal [13].

The efficiency of equine NT may be improving as methods for recombination and activation are developed. In the study in our laboratory in 2004 that resulted in the two foals born in 2005, blastocyst development was low (4%–10% in the best treatment), but transfer of eight blastocysts from this treatment resulted in 3 pregnancies and two viable foals (25% of transferred embryos) [14]. In 2005, blastocyst development was still low (0%–13% depending on treatment). We transferred 26 cloned embryos of three different genotypes to recipient mares. Sixteen pregnancies resulted (62% pregnancy rate per transferred embryo), of which nine went to term with delivery of live foals. A commercial cloning company (ViaGen, Austin, Texas) announced in the fall of 2005 that it had more than 30 mares expecting cloned foals in 2006 from six different genotypes [16]. This company has announced the birth of two healthy cloned foals as of the time of writing (October 2006).

From these data, it seems that the rate of blastocyst development in vitro for cloned equine embryos is only 1% to 10%, which is lower than that for cloned bovine embryos and also lower than that for equine ICSI embryos (25%–35%) [7,17]. The pregnancy rate after transfer of equine cloned embryos can be quite high (from 9% to greater than 60%), however. The proportion of cloned horse pregnancies that are likely to be carried to term and produce viable offspring is not clear at this point and may vary among laboratories.

Process of cloning

When a decision has been made to clone a horse, the only role of the donor animal is to provide a tissue sample. The referring veterinarian can obtain and ship the sample; this is easily performed by preparing a small (4 cm × 4 cm) area as for surgery, making an approximately 2-cm incision, and trimming away some of the tissue exposed when the skin edges are everted. Two or three such pieces of tissue are obtained. The samples (the size of a small pea) are placed in tubes of culture media that have been cooled to refrigerator temperature and are shipped at this temperature to the laboratory. Although cell culture medium obtained from the recipient laboratory is typically used for shipping, cell samples have also been successfully transported in embryo holding media, such as ViGro (Bioniche Animal Health, Belleville, Ontario, Canada) or Emcare (ICPbio, Auckland, New Zealand). It is important to use sterile technique for acquiring and transferring the biopsy samples so as to avoid bacterial contamination. Viable biopsy samples may be obtained from animals for up to a few days after death, especially if the tissue has been refrigerated post mortem. Samples frozen without cryoprotectant have little chance of providing viable cells.

When the biopsy sample is received by the laboratory, the tissue is minced and placed in culture medium in an incubator. During the following week or so, fibroblasts (the most vigorously growing cell type in a typical skin biopsy) grow from the tissue onto the culture dish. When sufficient cells have grown, the tissue pieces are removed, the cells are suspended in the culture medium, and the suspension is used to seed additional culture dishes. Each time the cells are resuspended and additional dishes are seeded is referred to as a passage. Fibroblasts have a finite lifespan in vitro, so it is important to use or freeze the cells in early passages (typically fewer than 10).

To perform equine NT, mature horse oocytes (those in metaphase II of meiosis, the stage at which the oocyte is ready for fertilization) are required. These may be obtained from the dominant follicle of a mare just before ovulation, as was done in the study in which the cloned mules were produced [10]. Cloning is inefficient, however, and it takes a large number of mares by this method to provide enough oocytes to produce one foal. Alternatively, oocytes may be obtained from immature follicles (in vivo or from abattoir tissue) and then matured in vitro. Methods for equine in vitro oocyte maturation that allow up to 38% blastocyst development after fertilization by ISCI have been developed [7]. The genetics of the oocyte donor are not important, with the caveat that the mitochondria of the oocyte become the mitochondria of the cloned offspring.

Under a high-powered (×400) microscope, the chromosomes in the metaphase plate and polar body of the oocyte are removed using micromanipulators. This is done by placing a fine pipette into the oocyte near the chromosomes and then aspirating the cytoplasm in this area. The oocyte is checked with a DNA-specific fluorescent stain to make sure the oocyte chromatin has been removed. The enucleated oocyte is termed an *ooplast* or *cytoplast*.

Cultured cells from the donor animal are suspended in media and placed in a small drop on the dish used for micromanipulation. One somatic cell is selected from the droplet and is combined with the cytoplast. This "recombination" is typically performed by placing the donor cell under the zona pellucida and fusing the two cells by electric pulse. Alternatively, the somatic cell can be picked up and injected directly into the cytoplasm of the oocyte. For direct injection to be effective, the cell membrane of the somatic cell must be ruptured before the cell is injected.

The recombined oocyte, which now contains the nucleus of the genetic donor cell, must be activated next. Activation of an oocyte refers to the chain of events that would normally be induced by the sperm at the time an egg is fertilized, including decondensation of the chromatin and entry into the first mitotic division to form a two-cell embryo. Activation of recombined oocytes is typically achieved by causing calcium to increase within the oocyte (the action of the sperm at fertilization) and is typically further supported in vitro by inhibiting the proteins that keep the oocyte in metaphase. When the oocyte is activated, the transferred nucleus decondenses and the oocyte starts embryonic development.

The activated recombined oocyte can be transferred to the oviduct of a recipient mare by standing flank laparotomy (the technique that was used to produce the cloned mules [10]) or may be cultured in vitro for 7 to 8 days to the blastocyst stage. The advantage of in vitro culture is that the resulting blastocyst may be transferred transcervically to the uterus of a recipient mare, as for standard embryo transfer. The cloned horse foals reported were all produced using in vitro culture and transcervical transfer [11,13,14].

What can an owner expect from a cloned foal?

One of the most common questions from horse owners about cloning is "How closely is the cloned foal going to resemble the donor?" With the birth of the cloned foals this year, we can start gathering data regarding the health of the cloned foals and their similarities in behavior, conformation, and performance to the original horse and to each other. With this information, producers should be able to assess the usefulness of cloning as an aid to their breeding programs. Cloning should allow the preservation of valuable genetics, from the old mare that is the "last of her line" to endangered equids. Cloned offspring may be produced to help carry on the genetics of a filly that dies young or a stallion that is too old to reproduce. The genetics of exceptional geldings could also be saved. The availability of NT as a clinical procedure should increase the options available to veterinarians when they are faced with clinical reproductive problems that are currently insurmountable. It is certainly possible at this time to bank tissue from animals that die suddenly; this service is offered by many commercial laboratories. The decision on whether to use the cells to produce a cloned foal can be made at some time in the future.

If an owner does decide to clone a horse, it is important that he or she understands that the clone is not going to be the original horse reincarnated. There are many factors at work that may cause the phenotype and behavior of the cloned offspring to differ from those of the original genetic donor.

Epigenetic effects

Although healthy cloned offspring have been born in many species, a major problem with cloning using somatic cells in these species has been embryo loss throughout gestation and production of neonates that are nonviable or are subject to heart, lung, and other abnormalities. These problems have been best defined in cattle and sheep and are associated with abnormalities of placental formation. The cause of abnormalities in cloned fetuses is thought to be incomplete "reprogramming" of the somatic cell nucleus after it is transferred to the recipient oocyte.

The search to understand the biology behind reprogramming of transferred DNA has propelled extensive study in the field of epigenetics, that is, the regulation of gene function. A basic understanding of the role of epigenetics in cloning is important to the practitioner who wishes to advise clients effectively regarding the possible outcomes of cloning their animal. Each cell in the body contains the entire genome; this is why a skin cell can be used to produce an entire individual. A skin cell does not use every gene in the genome, however; some genes are turned on (are able to be transcribed), and others, which are not related to the function of a skin cell, are turned off. The regulation of gene transcription is controlled largely by methylation and demethylation of the DNA (methylated DNA cannot be transcribed) and by changes to the histones, the proteins around which the DNA is wrapped. The epigenetic status of genes changes throughout embryonic and fetal life as the embryo's requirements change and, of course, also changes depending on the tissue in which the cell resides.

In NT, the donor nucleus is that of a somatic cell, typically a skin cell. Before the somatic cell is transferred into the oocyte, genes important to a somatic cell are turned on and many nonessential genes are turned off. An early embryo needs a much different array of gene products than does a skin cell, however. Thus, the epigenetic markings on the DNA of the transferred somatic cell must be reprogrammed by the oocyte to turn on the genes needed by the embryo. It is this property of the oocyte (its ability to reprogram the DNA of a somatic cell) that allows cloning to be successful. The reprogramming may not be perfect in the cloned embryo, however. If the gene function in a cloned embryo is too abnormal, the embryo or fetus cannot develop and is lost. Better reprogramming may be compatible with life, but there may still be differences in gene function that cause this offspring to differ in phenotype (eg, growth rate, general health, adult size, conformation) from the original donor.

The good news is that although the cloned offspring itself may differ epigenetically from the original donor, when that offspring reproduces, the process of reprogramming for the next generation occurs normally. In all species studied so far, the progeny of cloned animals are normal. Therefore, the progeny obtained from a horse clone should be genetically and epigenetically the same as those produced by the original donor animal.

In vitro culture

In addition to epigenetic effects that are directly related to the cloning procedure, there are factors associated simply with in vitro embryo culture that have been shown in other species to affect the resultant offspring at birth and on into adulthood. In cattle and sheep, the most studied abnormality attributable to culturing of embryos in vitro is "large offspring syndrome," resulting in fetal overgrowth and delivery of large overterm calves with poor viability. In the few foals born from in vitro cultured fertilized embryos and in the cloned foals born so far, however, there has been no suggestion of a similar problem. At this time, it seems that cloned foals may be more likely than normally conceived foals to be born with some contracture in the front legs or with a large umbilical remnant that may require surgical removal. The incidence and degree of these findings should become clearer as more cloned foals are assessed.

Mitochondrial DNA

Another factor related to the NT procedure that may affect the cloned offspring is the mitochondrial DNA. Mitochondria possess their own small genome, coding for approximately 13 of the estimated 3000 proteins involved in their function. The remaining genes that control mitochondrial function are in the cell's nuclear DNA. The mitochondrial genome replicates independently from the nuclear DNA of the cell. Mitochondria are inherited along the maternal line: the mitochondria of the oocyte are the mitochondria of the resulting offspring. When NT is performed, the ooplast is the major source of mitochondria, although some mitochondria from the donor cell are also introduced. The proportion of donor cell mitochondria present in cloned offspring in other species has been reported to range from 0% to 40%. Therefore, the NT foal should have the nuclear DNA of the genetic donor but the mitochondrial DNA of the recipient oocyte or a mixture of mitochondria from the two sources. The impact of the source of mitochondria, or a mixture of mitochondria, on the traits of the progeny is currently unknown. It must be remembered that only a tiny proportion of mitochondrial genes are actually present in the mitochondrial DNA; most genes controlling mitochondrial function are still from the donor animal's nuclear DNA.

Regarding the offspring of the cloned foals, the passage of heterogeneous mitochondria differs between male and female horses. In a filly, the mitochondria are present in the oocytes, and thus are passed down to the filly's progeny. If the clone is of a stallion, however, although the heterogeneous mitochondria would be present in the cloned colt's sperm, the spermatic mitochondria are eliminated from the embryo after fertilization. Thus, a cloned colt would not pass the heterogeneous mitochondria to its progeny, and these progeny could be considered to be exactly like those that the original genetic donor would have produced.

Individual variation

Individual variation affects some aspects of a cloned foal's phenotype, most vividly the white markings. As seen in the five foals produced from one genotype in 2006, or in the few identical twin horses that have been produced by embryo splitting, white markings, such as spots, socks, and blazes, are genetically determined, but the actual size and shape of the markings differ because of migration patterns of the white cells during fetal development.

Environment

Finally, beyond changes attributable to the NT procedure itself, the cloned foal is affected by its environment during embryonic, fetal, and postnatal life. Pertinent environmental factors, such as the size and health of the uterus, difficulties at birth (eg, hypoxemia), milk production of the mare, behavior of the mare, interactions with people, nutrition and exercise programs, and training regimens, all affect the foal's health, growth, behavior, and performance. These factors affect any foal, but their influence seems to be more apparent in cloned offspring because the original donor horse or other clones of the same genotype can be used as a basis of comparison.

"Premature aging?"

Many people who have read reports in the press about Dolly, the first cloned mammal, have questions as to whether a cloned animal ages prematurely. This is because it was reported that the chromosomes in Dolly's cells had shortened telomeres in comparison to those of age-matched noncloned lambs. The telomeres are the segments of untranscribed (nonfunctional) DNA on the tips of the chromosomes that serve to protect the actual coding DNA of the chromosomes. Each time the cell replicates its DNA during cell division, the telomeres shorten. When they get too short, the last pieces of coding DNA at the ends of the chromosomes are no longer protected, the DNA is degraded, and the cell dies. The length of the telomeres is reset during gametogenesis and embryogenesis so that the next generation starts off with long telomeres again. The atypically short telomeres found in Dolly's cells led to a question of whether Dolly would age prematurely and also whether embryos produced by cloning reset their telomeres normally. Unfortunately, we were not able to find out whether Dolly would age prematurely, because at the age of 6 years, the sheep contracted a lung virus (along with many of its barnmates) and had to be euthanized. Studies in individual cattle clones found to have short telomeres showed that reproduction, milk production, and longevity of milk production were similar in these cattle to those of their noncloned herdmates [18]. Further studies in cattle showed that telomere length of cloned calves was related to the tissue used for NT: mammary gland cells (the cell type used to clone Dolly) and epithelial cells resulted in calves with shorter telomeres, whereas fibroblasts and other cell types resulted in normal telomere length [19]. Normal telomere length in offspring that were cloned from fibroblasts has been confirmed in many species [20–22]. Thus, the most typical cell used for cloning (fibroblasts) should not be associated with atypical telomere length in the resulting offspring.

Summary

In conclusion, equine cloning is now in use as a clinical technique. It is available commercially, and its efficiency seems to be increasing. The foals produced by cloning may differ in some phenotypic and behavioral traits from the original animal but should produce offspring that reflect those that the original donor animal would have produced. This is especially true in the case of male animals, where the mitochondrial DNA is not passed to the progeny. The large number of cloned foals born in 2006 should add significantly to our understanding of the factors affecting production of viable cloned foals and of the similarities and differences among cloned foals and between these foals and the donor animals.

References

[1] Willadsen SM. Cloning of sheep and cow embryos. Genome 1989;31:956–62.
[2] Wilmut I, Schnieke AE, McWhir J, et al. Viable offspring derived from fetal and adult mammalian cells. Nature 1997;385:810–3.
[3] Hinrichs K, Shin T, Love CC, et al. Comparison of bovine and equine oocytes as host cytoplasts for equine nuclear transfer. In: Proceedings of the Fifth International Symposium on Equine Embryo Transfer. Havemeyer Foundation monograph no. 3. Newmarket, UK: R&W Publications; 2000. p. 43–4.
[4] Li X, Morris LH, Allen WR. Chromatin reprogramming in enucleated horse oocytes injected with cumulus cell nuclei [abstract]. J Reprod Fertil Abstr Ser 2000;25:77.
[5] Choi YH, Love CC, Love LB, et al. Developmental competence in vivo and in vitro of in vitro-matured equine oocytes fertilized by intracytoplasmic sperm injection with fresh or frozen-thawed sperm. Reproduction 2002;123:455–65.
[6] Choi YH, Love LB, Varner DD, et al. Factors affecting developmental competence of equine oocytes after intracytoplasmic sperm injection. Reproduction 2004;127:187–94.

[7] Hinrichs K, Choi YH, Love LB, et al. Chromatin configuration within the germinal vesicle of horse oocytes: changes post mortem and relationship to meiotic and developmental competence. Biol Reprod 2005;72:1142–50.
[8] Choi YH, Shin T, Love CC, et al. Effects of initial cumulus morphology and addition of cytochalasin B on fusion, activation and cleavage of horse oocytes undergoing nuclear transfer [abstract]. Theriogenology 2001;55:261.
[9] Woods GL, White KL, Vanderwall DK, et al. Cloned mule pregnancies produced using nuclear transfer. Theriogenology 2002;58:779–82.
[10] Woods GL, White KL, Vanderwall DK, et al. A mule cloned from fetal cells by nuclear transfer. Science 2003;301(5636):1063. [Epub May 29, 2003.]
[11] Galli C, Lagutina I, Crotti G, et al. A cloned horse born to its dam twin. Nature 2003;424:635.
[12] Vanderwall DK, Woods GL, Sellon DC, et al. Present status of equine cloning and clinical characterization of embryonic, fetal, and neonatal development of three cloned mules. J Am Vet Med Assoc 2004;225:1694–9.
[13] Lagutina I, Lazzari G, Duchi R, et al. Somatic cell nuclear transfer in horses: effect of oocyte morphology, embryo reconstruction method and donor cell type. Reproduction 2005;130:559–67.
[14] Hinrichs K, Choi YH, Love CC, et al. Production of horse foals via direct injection of roscovitine-treated donor cells and activation by injection of sperm extract. Reproduction 2006;131:1063–72.
[15] Vanderwall DK, Woods GL, Aston KI, et al. Cloned horse pregnancies produced using adult cumulus cells. Reprod Fertil Dev 2004;16:675–9.
[16] Associated Press. Horse cloning hits full stride. Available at: www.msnbc.msn.com/id/10053896/. 2005. Accessed October 19, 2006.
[17] Choi YH, Love LB, Varner DD, et al. Blastocyst development in equine oocytes with low meiotic competence after suppression of meiosis with roscovitine prior to *in vitro* maturation. Zygote 2006;14:1–8.
[18] Yonai M, Kaneyama K, Miyashita N, et al. Growth, reproduction, and lactation in somatic cell cloned cows with short telomeres. J Dairy Sci 2005;88:4097–110.
[19] Miyashita N, Shiga K, Yonai M, et al. Remarkable differences in telomere lengths among cloned cattle derived from different cell types. Biol Reprod 2002;66:1649–55.
[20] Betts D, Bordignon V, Hill J, et al. Reprogramming of telomerase activity and rebuilding of telomere length in cloned cattle. Proc Natl Acad Sci USA 2001;98:1077–82.
[21] Jeon HY, Hyun SH, Lee GS, et al. The analysis of telomere length and telomerase activity in cloned pigs and cows. Mol Reprod Dev 2005;71:315–20.
[22] Tian XC, Xu J, Yang X. Normal telomere lengths found in cloned cattle. Nat Genet 2000;26:272–3.

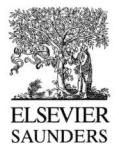

Index

Note: Page numbers of article titles are in **boldface** type.

A

Abortion, in postfixation twins in mares management, 722–723

Aging, "premature," cloning and, 864–865

Anti-inflammatory drugs, for placentitis, 769–771

Antimicrobial agents, for placentitis, 769–771

Antiprostaglandin(s), for mares at risk of preterm birth, 743

Artificial insemination, historical background of, 693

Assisted reproduction techniques
  intracytoplasmic sperm injection, 854–855
  oocytes in, **843–856**
    collection and culture of, 843–847
      from excised ovaries, 845–846
      from preovulatory follicles, 846–847
    collection of, from euthanized mares, 853–854
    culture of, 843–847
    cumulus oocyte complex, morphologic evaluation of, 847–851
    handling and transportation of ovaries in, 844–845
    transfer of, 852–853
      from euthanized mares, 853–854

B

Bacteria, in breeding-induced endometritis in mares, 708–709

Biophysical profile, in compromised equine pregnancy, 759

Birth, preterm, mares at risk for, hormone treatments for, 738–743

Bladder, measurements of, in compromised pregnancy, 757

Breeding-induced endometritis, in mares, **705–712**
  bacteria and, 708–709
  diagnosis of, 709
  pathophysiology of, 705–707
  seminal plasma and, 707–708
  treatment of, 709–710

C

Centrifugation, density gradient, 670–671

Centrifugation "cushions," 667–668

Cloning, **857–866**
  efficiency of, 858–859
  environment and, 864
  epigenetic effects of, 862–863
  history of, 857–858
  horse owners' expectations of, 861–865
  in vitro culture and, 863
  individual variation with, 864
  mitochondrial DNA and, 863–864
  "premature aging" due to, 864–865
  process of, 860–861

Colostral specific gravity, compromised equine pregnancy and, 753–754

Cortisol
  during late pregnancy, changes in, 733
  fetoplacental problems associated with, during late pregnancy, 738

Craniocervical dislocation, in postfixation twins in mares management, 717–721

Cryptorchidectomy, laparoscopic, **777–787**
  complications of, 795–796
  described, 778
  dorsally recumbent, 784–787
  presurgical preparation for, 777–778
  standing, 779–784

Cumulus oocyte complex, morphologic evaluation of, in assisted reproduction techniques, 847–851

D

Deep uterine insemination, 694–695

Density gradient centrifugation, 670–671

Deprivation theory, natural reduction and, in postfixation twins in mares management, 714–715

Diet, in postfixation twins in mares management, 715–716

Dislocation(s), craniocervical, in postfixation twins in mares management, 717–721

E

Ejaculate(s), seminal, processing of, 684–685

Electrolyte(s), mammary, compromised equine pregnancy and, 753

Embryo(s)
    collection of, 832–834
    evaluation of, 832–834
    large, small, 838–839
    small
        collection of, 834–835
        vitrification of, 838–839
    vitrification of, **831–841**
        pregnancies established from, 838–840
        procedures for, 835–837
        warming of embryos in, 837–838
    warming of, 837–838

Embryo transfer, 831

Endocrinology, in diagnosis of granulosa cell tumors of equine ovary, 802–808

Endometritis
    breeding-induced, in mares, **705–712.** See also *Breeding-induced endometritis, in mares.*
    infertility due to, in mares, 705

Environment, cloning effects of, 864

Epididymal spermatozoa, advanced insemination techniques in mares and, 697–698

Epididymal stallion sperm, collection and freezing of, **677–682**

Epididymide(s). See also *Sperm, stallion, epididymal.*
    harvesting of, 677–678
    harvesting sperm from, 678–681

Estradiol, in diagnosis of granulosa cell tumors of equine ovary, 804–805

Estrogen(s)
    compromised equine pregnancy and, 752–753
    during late pregnancy, changes in, 731–732
    fetoplacental problems associated with, during late pregnancy, 737

F

Fetal activity, compromised equine pregnancy and, 756

Fetal fluid depth, compromised equine pregnancy and, 758

Fetal heart rate, compromised equine pregnancy and, 756

Fetal presentation, compromised equine pregnancy due to, 754–756

Fetal size, compromised equine pregnancy and, 756

Fetoplacental problems, endocrine changes associated with, during late pregnancy, 734–738

Fetus(es), multiple, compromised equine pregnancy and, 758

Foal(s), cloned, horse owners expectations of, 861–865

Follicle-stimulating hormone (FSH)
    in diagnosis of granulosa cell tumors of equine ovary, 807–808
    superovulation in mares and, 821–829

FSH. See *Follicle-stimulating hormone (FSH).*

G

Glucocorticoid(s), for mares at risk of preterm birth, 740–743

Granulosa cell tumors
    described, 799–800
    of equine ovary, **799–817**
        clinical parameters of, 800–801
        complications of, 809–810
        diagnosis of, 801–808
            endocrinology in, 802–808
            estradiol in, 804–805
            FSH in, 807–808
            inhibin in, 805–807
            luteinizing hormone in, 808
            palpation in, 801–802
            progesterone in, 805
            testosterone in, 803–804
            ultrasonography in, 801–802

differential diagnosis of, 810–812
pathophysiology of, 808–809
prevalence of, 799–800
treatment of, 812

H

Heart rate, fetal, compromised equine pregnancy and, 756

Heart rhythm, fetal, compromised equine pregnancy and, 756

Hormone(s). See also specific types, e.g., *Luteinizing hormone*.
   during late pregnancy
      changes in, 728–733
      profiles and treatments with, **727–747**. See also *Late pregnancy, hormone profiles and treatments in*.
   during parturition, changes in, 728–733
   for mares at risk of preterm birth, 738–743

Hysteroscopic insemination, in mares, 695–697

I

Infertility, endometritis and, in mares, 705

Inhibin, in diagnosis of granulosa cell tumors of equine ovary, 805–807

Insemination techniques, advanced
   described, 693–694
   in mares, **693–703**
      deep uterine insemination, 694–695
      epididymal spermatozoa and, 697–698
      hysteroscopic insemination, 695–697
      intrafollicular insemination, 700
      oviductal insemination, 699
      sex-sorted spermatozoa and, 698–699

Intracytoplasmic sperm injection, in assisted reproduction techniques, 854–855

Intrafollicular insemination, 700

L

Laparoscopy, for cryptorchidectomy and ovariectomy, 773–774. See also *Cryptorchidectomy, laparoscopic; Ovariectomy, laparoscopic*.

Late pregnancy
   endocrine changes associated with fetoplacental problems in, 734–738
      cortisol, 738
      estrogens, 737
      progestagens, 734–737
      prostaglandins, 737–738
      relaxin, 738
   hormone profiles and treatments in, **727–747**
      cortisol, 733
      estrogens, 731–732
      oxytocin, 732–733
      progestagens, 728–730
      prostaglandins, 732
      relaxin, 733

Luteinizing hormone, in diagnosis of granulosa cell tumors of equine ovary, 808

M

Mammary electrolytes, compromised equine pregnancy and, 753

Manual reduction, after fixation, in postfixation twins in mares management, 715

Mare(s)
   advanced insemination techniques in, **693–703**. See also *Insemination techniques, advanced, in mares*.
   breeding-induced endometritis in, **705–712**. See also *Breeding-induced endometritis, in mares*.
   postfixation twins in, management of, **713–725**. See also *Postfixation twins, in mares, management of*.
   superovulation in, **819–830**. See also *Superovulation, in mares*.

N

Natural reduction, deprivation theory and, in postfixation twins in mares management, 714–715

O

Oocyte(s), in assisted reproduction techniques, **843–856**. See also *Assisted reproduction techniques, oocytes in*.

Ovariectomy, laparoscopic, **787–795**
   complications of, 795–796
   described, 787
   dorsally recumbent, 793–795
   laterally recumbent, 791–793

Ovariectomy (*continued*)
  presurgical preparation for, 777–778
  standing, 787–790
Ovary(ies)
  granulosa cell tumors of, **799–817**. See also *Granulosa cell tumors, of equine ovary.*
  in assisted reproduction techniques, handling and transportation of, 844–845
Oviductal insemination, 699
Oxytocin, during late pregnancy, changes in, 732–733

P

Parturition, hormone changes during, 728–733

Placentitis, **763–776**
  death due to, 763
  diagnosis of, 764–769
  pathophysiology of, 763–764
  transrectal ultrasound in, 765–767
  treatment of, 769–774
    anti-inflammatory drugs in, 769–771
    antimicrobial agents in, 769–771
    combined therapy in, 773–774
    progestins in, 771–772
    tocolytics in, 772–773
  ultrasonographic monitoring of, 764–769

Plasma, seminal, 665–666
  in breeding-induced endometritis in mares, 707–708

Postfixation twins, in mares, management of, **713–725**
  abortion in, 722–723
  craniocervical dislocation in, 717–721
  dietary manipulation in, 715–716
  manual reduction after fixation in, 715
  natural reduction in, deprivation theory and, 714–715
  surgical removal of one conceptus in, 716
  transcutaneous ultrasound-guided twin reduction in, 721–722
  transvaginal ultrasound-guided twin reduction in, 716–717

Pregnancy
  compromised
    biochemical parameters of, 752–754
    biophysical parameters and, 754–758
    biophysical profile and, 759
    bladder measurements and, 757
    colostral specific gravity, 753–754
    diagnosis of, **749–761**
    estrogens and, 752–753
    fetal activity and, 756
    fetal fluid depth and, 758
    fetal heart rate and, 756
    fetal heart rhythm and, 756
    fetal presentation and, 754–756
    fetal size and, 756
    historical parameters of, 751–752
    hormonal profiling and, 752
    identification of, risk factors for, 750–751
    mammary electrolytes and, 753
    multiple fetuses, 758
    progestagens and, 753
    stomach measurements and, 757
    ureteroplacental thickness and contrast in, 757–758
  from vitrified embryos, establishment of, 838–840
  late, hormone profiles and treatments in, **727–747**. See also *Late pregnancy, hormone profiles and treatments in.*

"Premature aging," cloning and, 864–865

Preterm birth, mares at risk of, hormone treatments for, 738–743

Progestagen(s)
  compromised equine pregnancy and, 753
  during late pregnancy, changes in, 728–730
  fetoplacental problems associated with, during late pregnancy, 734–737

Progesterone
  for mares at risk of preterm birth, 739–740
  in diagnosis of granulosa cell tumors of equine ovary, 805

Progestin(s), for placentitis, 771–772

Prostaglandin(s)
  during late pregnancy, changes in, 732
  fetoplacental problems associated with, during late pregnancy, 737–738

R

Relaxin
   during late pregnancy, changes in, 733
   fetoplacental problems associated with, during late pregnancy, 738

S

Semen
   adherence techniques, 670
   frozen, processing of, 666
   migration of, 669–670
   stallion
      collection of, 663–664
      epididymal, collection and freezing of, **677–682**
      handling and preparation of
         adherence techniques, 670
         advanced methods for, **663–676.** See also *Semen, stallion, handling and preparation of, advanced methods for.*
         centrifugation "cushions," 667–668
         density gradient centrifugation, 670–671
         frozen semen processing, 666
         processing for cooling, 664–665
         seminal plasma, 665–666
         separation techniques, 668–669
            applications of, 671–673
            sperm migration, 669–670

Seminal ejaculates, processing of, 684–685

Seminal plasma, 665–666
   in breeding-induced endometritis in mares, 707–708

Seminal preparations
   light microscopic evaluation of, 685–686
   transmission electron microscopic evaluation of, 686–687

Sex-sorted spermatozoa, advanced insemination techniques in mares and, 698–699

Specific gravity, colostral, compromised equine pregnancy and, 753–754

Sperm, stallion
   epididymal. See also *Epididymide(s).*
      collection and freezing of, **677–682**

   results of, 681
   morphology in
      indicators of common clinical aberrations, 687–690
      processing of seminal ejaculates, 684–685
   seminal preparations
      light microscopic evaluation of, 685–686
      transmission electron microscopic evaluation of, 686–687
      ultrastructure as functional and diagnostic tool, **683–692**

Spermatozoa
   epididymal, advanced insemination techniques in mares and, 697–698
   sex-sorted, advanced insemination techniques in mares and, 698–699

Stallion, semen of. See *Semen, stallion.*

Stomach, measurements of, in compromised pregnancy, 757

Superovulation, in mares, **819–830**
   equine FSH, 821–829
      day of initial treatment, 824–825
      described, 821–823
      efficacy of, factors affecting, 823–824
      problems associated with, 826–827
      protocols for, 827–829
      repetitive applications of, 825
      viability of embryos, 825–826
   historical background of, 819–821

T

Testosterone, in diagnosis of granulosa cell tumors of equine ovary, 803–804

Tocolytic(s), for placentitis, 772–773

Transabdominal ultrasound, in placentitis monitoring, 767–769

Transcutaneous ultrasound-guided twin reduction, in postfixation twins in mares management, 721–722

Transrectal ultrasound, in placentitis monitoring, 765–767

Transvaginal ultrasound-guided twin reduction, in postfixation twins in mares management, 716–717

Tumor(s), granulosa cell, of equine ovary, **799–817.** See also *Granulosa cell tumors, of equine ovary.*

Twin(s), postfixation, in mares, management of, **713–725.** See also *Postfixation twins, in mares, management of.*

U

Ultrasound
    in diagnosis of granulosa cell tumors of equine ovary, 801–802
    in placentitis monitoring, 764–769
    transabdominal, in placentitis monitoring, 767–769
    transrectal, in placentitis monitoring, 765–767

Ultrastructure, as functional and diagnostic tool, sperm morphology in stallions and, **683–692.** See also *Sperm, stallion, morphology in.*

Ureteroplacental thickness and contrast, in compromised equine pregnancy, 757–758

V

Vitrification, of equine embryos, **831–841.** See also *Embryo(s), vitrification of.*

Moving?

Make sure your subscription moves with you!

To notify us of your new address, find your **Clinics Account Number** (located on your mailing label above your name), and contact customer service at:

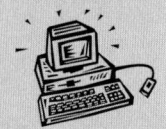

E-mail: elspcs@elsevier.com

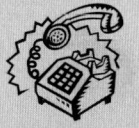

800-654-2452 (subscribers in the U.S. & Canada)
407-345-4000 (subscribers outside of the U.S. & Canada)

Fax number: 407-363-9661

Elsevier Periodicals Customer Service
6277 Sea Harbor Drive
Orlando, FL 32887-4800

*To ensure uninterrupted delivery of your subscription, please notify us at least 4 weeks in advance of move.

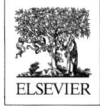